HORMONAL REGULATION OF SODIUM EXCRETION

DEVELOPMENTS IN ENDOCRINOLOGY VOLUME 10

Other volumes in this series:
Volume 1
Multiple Molecular Forms of Steroid Hormone Receptors
M.K. Agarwal Editor (1977)
Volume 2
Progress in Prolactin Physiology and Pathology
C. Robyn and M. Harter Editors (1978)
Volume 3
Hormones and Brain Development
G. Dörner and M. Kawakami Editors (1978)
Volume 4
Lipoprotein Metabolism and Endocrine Regulation
L.W. Hessel and H.M.J. Krans Editors (1979)
Volume 5
Psychoneuroendocrinology in Reproduction
L. Zichella and P. Pancheri Editors (1979)
Volume 6
Proteases and Hormones
M.K. Agarwal Editor (1979)
Volume 7
Progress in Ecdysone Research
J.A. Hoffmann Editor (1980)
Volume 8
Steroid Induced Uterine Proteins
M. Beato Editor (1980)
Volume 9
Neuroactive Drugs in Endocrinology
E.E. Müller Editor (1980)

HORMONAL REGULATION OF SODIUM EXCRETION

Proceedings of the Satellite Symposium of the 28th I.U.P.S. Congress. Regulation of Renal Sodium Excretion by Hormones held in Bratislava, Czechoslovakia, 8-12 July, 1980.

Branislav Lichardus, Robert W. Schrier and Jozef Ponec *Editors*

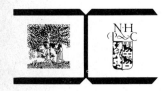

1980

ELSEVIER/NORTH-HOLLAND BIOMEDICAL PRESS
AMSTERDAM · NEW YORK · OXFORD

ISBN for this volume : 0-444-80289-4
ISBN for this series : 0-444-80009-3

Published by:
Elsevier/North-Holland Biomedical Press
335 Jan van Galenstraat, P.O. Box 211
Amsterdam, The Netherlands

Sole distributors for the USA and Canada:
Elsevier North Holland Inc.
52 Vanderbilt Avenue
New York, N.Y. 10017

Printed in The Netherlands

PREFACE

An International Satellite Symposium to the twenty-eighth International Congress of Physiological Sciences was held from July 8-12 in Bratislava, Czechoslovakia and focused on the topic of Hormonal Regulation of Sodium Excretion. It was over a decade ago when basic scientists and clinician-scientists met in a castle in Smolenice, Czechoslovakia in 1969 to discuss the same topic. The results of this second Symposium in Bratislava, Czechoslovakia which are published in these Proceedings clearly indicate that substantial progress has been made during the past decade in understanding the physiological and pathophysiological processes involved in the regulation of sodium excretion.

There now seems to be reasonable agreement in certain stress circumstances, such as the anesthetized, hemorrhaged and sodium-restricted states, that increased renal adrenergic neural activity plays an important role in renal sodium conservation. A body of evidence has also been presented over the past decade that this effect of adrenergic neural system is mediated not only by affecting renal blood flow and glomerular filtration but, in addition, by directly altering the tubular transport of sodium. A role of neuronal and non-neuronal renal dopamine may also be emerging as a factor in the control of renal sodium regulation. Extrarenal neural pathways, particularly afferent in nature, from the left atrium also seems to have been convincingly demonstrated in the dog to influence renal sodium excretion. In the Symposium, results were also presented which indicate that mixed venous PO_2 may be the best index of the elusive "effective blood volume" and that receptors in the inferior vena cava-right atrial region may sense changes in this parameter and mediate them to the central nervous system via vagal pathways. The efferent pathway(s) responsible for the natriuresis associated with left atrial distension or the sodium retention associated with a lowered mixed venous PO_2 in the vena cava-right atrial area have not been defined but may be humoral in nature.

The role of the renin-angiotensin-aldosterone system in the regulation of sodium excretion, although not dominant in some circumstances, still is evident. Results are also emerging which suggest that angiotensin II, and perhaps angiotensin III, directly enhance tubular sodium reabsorption independent of any affect on the adrenal cortex and aldosterone activity. Such an effect may be particularly evident in the setting of Goldblatt hypertension. Although unable to attend the Symposium Professors Franklyn Knox and Barry Brenner have contributed important papers to the Proceedings on the topics of the "Mechanisms of Mineralocorticoid Escape" and "Hormonal Effects on Glomerular Function" respectively. Professor Neal Bricker was invited to contribute an article to the Natriuretic Hormone section of the Proceedings because of his important contributions in this area even though he was unable to attend the Symposium.

The importance of hypothalamoneurophypophyseal hormones in the regulation of sodium and water excretion is emerging as an area of intense interest. The hypothalamus has been proposed as a potential site of production of the "Natriuretic Hormone" and hypophysectomy has been shown to enhance tubular sodium reabsorption, particularly in the collecting duct of the rat nephron. Whether a permissive role(of oxytocin and/or vasopressin in the natriuretic properties of the hypothalamoneuro hypophysis is important remains controversial. In this regard, however, evidence is emerging that the non-osmotic release of vasopressin may exert vascular, as well as antidiuretic, effects. Reversal of the antinatriuretic effects of hypophysectomy by administration of exogenous vasopressin may be at least in part due to the vascular effects of the hormone. In the Symposium in vivo evidence was presented that the vascular effect of vasopressin, as well as norepinephrine and angiotensin, is dependent on cellular calcium influx. Experimental use of blockers of calcium membrane transport also has implicated intracellular calcium in 1) sodium transport and 2) the hydroosmotic effect of vasopressin, particularly in the prostaglandin-deplete state.

The role of the prostaglandins in sodium transport was another important topic of the Symposium. There now seems little doubt that several inhibitors of prostaglandin synthesis may cause sodium retention in man, as well as other species. Mic puncture studies in the rat suggest that the prostaglandins may inhibit sodium reabsorption in the thick ascending limb and cortical collecting duct, although an effect on distal delivery rate in the juxtamedullary nephrons may also be involved. Results of in vitro studies in isolated perfused nephrons of rabbits are still controversial with respect to an effect of prostaglandins.

The role of the kallikrein-kinin system in sodium excretion is still quite controversial. While there is considerable similarity between the renin-angiotensin system and the kallikrein-kinin system, much work is necessary to demonstrate that the former renal vasoconstriction-sodium retaining system is counterbalanced by a renal vasodilator-sodium losing system, i.e. kallikrein-kinin system. Advances in techniques to measure specific renal and extrarenal kallikrein and kinin activity will provide the methodology to provide more specific answers in this potentially important area. Also, in addition to an effect on sodium reabsorption, the location of the renal kallikrein-kinin system in the distal nephron and urinary kinin measurements by radioimmunoassay in man suggest a potential role of this system in the hydro-osmotic effect of vasopressin.

The highlight of the Symposium were the various papers dealing with the Natriuretic Hormone. Over the last ten years the field has moved from asking "Is there a Natriuretic Hormone?" to "What is the chemical structure and source of the Natriuretic Hormone?" Several groups now have identified a low molecular weight substance which inhibits Na-K-ATPase in salt-loaded as well as hypertensive states. Professor Hugh de Wardener, the pioneer and perpetuator of the natriuretic hormone, has proposed that the inhibition of Na-K-ATPase in hypertension impairs cellular sodium-calcium exchange which results in increased intracellular calcium concentration. As cited above, there is now not only in vitro but also in vivo evidence that increased intracellular calcium is the primary common pathway for humorally-mediated vasoconstriction of smooth muscle. Could, therefore, "volume dependent" hypertension, such as low-renin hypertension and salt sensitive hypertension in the Dahl rat, cause hypertension by activating natriuretic hormone which inhibits

Na-K-ATPase, thus increasing intracellular calcium and thereby causing vasocon-striction of peripheral vasculature? Similarly, vasoconstriction mediated hyper-tension may also be associated with increased intracellular calcium secondary to the action of known humoral substances such as norepinephrine, angiotensin and vasopressin to enhance calcium movement across cellular membranes. In this context, de Wardener's group has preliminary demonstrated that patients with low renin hyper-tension have very elevated renal cortical G6PD levels, as measured by a new cyto-chemical assay. This is a finding quite compatible with inhibition of Na-K-ATPase and activation of the Pentose Pathway. Interestingly, normal salt-loaded subjects constitute another group which have elevated renal cortical G6PD levels. Gruber and Buckalew also reported in this Symposium that the radioimmunoassay for cardiac glycosides, known inhibitors of Na-K-ATPase, may provide a means to assay Natri-uretic Hormone.

Thus, while the chemical nature and production site for the Natriuretic Hor-mone remain to be clarified, a new assay system, namely assessment of Na-K-ATPase activity, is emerging in several laboratories. The potential biological implications of the Natriuretic Hormone also has been extended from normal sodium excretion and sodium-retaining disorders to hypertensive states.

Because of space and time, the stimulating formal and informal discussions which took place during the Symposium in Bratislava, have not been included in the Proceedings but perhaps this Preface provides some flavor of these discussions.

MUDr. B. Lichardus, DrSc.

Robert W. Schrier, M.D.

RNDr. J. Ponec, CSc.

CONTENTS

NATRIURETIC HORMONE

SYMPOSIUM ORGANIZERS

Czechoslovak Medical Society of J.E. Purkyňe
Czechoslovak Society of Endocrinology
Czechoslovak Society of Physiology
  and
Czechoslovak Society of Nephrology
  under the auspices of the
Center of Physiological Sciences of the Slovak Academy of Sciences
  and of the
Renal Commission of IUPS

This International Symposium was a Satellite Symposium to the 28th IUPS
Congress in Budapest in 1980.

Hormonal Regulation of Sodium Excretion,
B. Lichardus, R.W. Schrier and J. Ponec, eds.
© 1980 Elsevier/North-Holland Biomedical Press

NATRIURETIC HORMONES

Introductory remarks

BRANISLAV LICHARDUS

Institute of Experimental Endocrinology, Center of Physiological
Sciences, Slovak Academy of Sciences, Vlárska 3, 80936 Bratislava,
(Czechoslovakia)

THE OBJECTIVES OF THE SYMPOSIUM

The choice of the topic of the present International Satellite
Symposium of the 28th International Congress of Physiological Sciences "REGULATION OF RENAL SODIUM EXCRETION BY HORMONES" (Bratislava,
July 8-12, 1980) resulted from the evidence accumulated mainly over
the past two decades indicating that besides aldosterone other hormones may participate in the mechanism of natriuresis. The aim of
the organizers has been to review the present state of knowledge
on the as yet unidentified natriuretic hormone on the threshold of
the twentieth anniversary of the idea that such a hormone could or
perhaps should exist. At the same time the physiological aspects of
the natriuretic properties of existing hormones should be reviewed
in order to evaluate either the room left for a new natriuretic
hormone or to facilitate the establishment of the operative radius
for such a hormone once it is identified.

ALDOSTERONE AND NATRIURETIC HORMONES

Aldosterone is an antinatriuretic hormone. It had been taken
for granted for a long time that the main type of hormonally induced natriuresis resulted either from an inadeqaucy of aldosterone
production or from the impairment of its action in the kidney. Con-
trarywise, "non-aldosterone hormones" which may be involved in the
renal sodium execution are mostly of natriuretic nature and thus
natriuresis is the result of their promoting renal sodium excretion.
They differ from aldosterone also in a more rapid onset of action.
As a matter of fact there is much more evidence by now for the
existence of promptly acting natriuretic hormones than for a promp-

tly acting antinatriuretic hormone - substance "X" - which was pro-
gnosticated in 1957 by Homer W. Smith[1].

Natriuretic hormones may be divided into two groups on the basis
of whether their identity id known or unknown. To the first group
belong e.g. some prostaglandins, catecholamines, kinins, substance
P, calcitonin, parathormone and some pituitary and neuropituitary
hormones such as growth hormone, prolactin, melatonin, oxytocin and
vasopressin. It is, however, to be stressed that even if natriuretic action of the above listed hormones has been repeatedly documented, their role in the physiology or pathophysiology of renal
sodium excretion may not always be clear.

The existence of the second group consisting of natriuretic hormones of unknown identity has been so far predicted mainly on the
basis of biological evidence for a natriuretic activity in body
fluids or in various organs. When stressing the existence of an unknown natriuretic hormone, more or less convincing attempts have
been simultaneously made to exclude an obvious possibility that natriuretic activity is represented by a known hormone. For example
evidence for a blood-borne natriuretic activity was originally
claimed on the basis of results of a cross-circulation experiment
in which a signal for increasing renal sodium excretion was transferred from a donor dog with expanded extracellular fluid volume
(ECFV) with saline to a recipient dog with unexpanded ECFV and that
was achieved even if high doses of aldosterone and antidiuretic
hormone were applied to the animals[2]. However, the concomittant
hemodilution due to saline infusion was an obstacle to be overcome
for an interpretation of the results obtained less equivocally in
favour of the existence of a new hormone as hemodilution was by itself a blood-borne natriuretic signal. Therefore later a non-dilu-
ting solution for expanding ECFV of a donor dog was used such as
suspension of dog erythrocytes in isooncotic solution of bovine
albumine in saline[3,4] or homologous blood[5] or blood with which the
recipient's one had been equilibrated[6] and it was shown that also
without hemodilution a signal to raise the sodium output can be
transferred between two animals. It was, however, not decided
whether the postulated natriuretic hormone affected tubular trans-

port directly and or via affecting the renal hemodynamics. A serious analysis is also lacking why the cross-circulation experiments yielded negative results in some laboratories.

Yet another obstacle to accept more generally the idea of the existence of a natriuretic hormone was created by negative results from cross-circulation experiments in rats. Indeed those negative results were used to deny altogether the hormonal nature of natriuresis in animals with expanded ECFV[7].

Positive results in favour of the operation of a natriuretic hormone also in rats were obtained when the so-called sustained fluid volume expansion was used in which urine of the expanded donor animal was drained back into its venous system by a cannula connecting urinary bladder with a jugular vein[8,9,10]. This procedure not only sustained the fluid volume expansion but it also prevented concentration of the circulating blood[11] and presumably also a loss of a natriuretic hormone by the renal way. All those factors together could have participated in promoting natriuresis in the recipient rat. Of course, one should not underestimate the natriuretic role of urea in this type of experiments. However, it was shown by others that besides urea a more specific natriuretic factor probably also operates[12].

ATTEMPTS TO ISOLATE A NEW NATRIURETIC HORMONE

The next logical step was to clarify the basic question whether the blood borne natriuretic signal in the animals with expanded extracellular fluid volume was the result of a diminution in the concentration of an antinatriuretic substance in the blood, or of an increase of a natriuretic substance. One way to answer this question was by testing bovine deproteinized plasma, obtained from conscious cows after their intravascular volume had been expanded with 6% Dextran in physiological saline. Tests for natriuretic activity were performed on hydrated anesthetized rats. It was found that when 0.2 ml of postexpansion plasma was injected i.v. to rats their sodium and urine output increased. Such a small volume of the deproteinized plasma could evoke natriuresis neither by blood volume expansion in the test-animals, nor by any other effect which could be due to dilution of its blood. It was concluded that the natriuretic material in plasma deproteinized by trichloracetic acid was probably a small molecular substance[13,14]. This conclusion has been repeatedly confirmed and elaborated by various types of analytical methods and led to a further conclusion that natriuretic activity might be represented by a small peptide molecule (mol. weight around 1000)[15]. The advance in this direction, covered by a series of reviews[16,17,18,19,20,21,22,23,24,25,26,27,28,29] has been linked mainly with the work of Bricker and Bourgoignie, Buckalew, de Wardener and Clarkson, Gonick, Kruck and Kramer, Nizet and Godon, Pearce and Sonnenberg.

COEXISTENCE OF VARIOUS NATRIURETIC FACTORS ?

The hypothesis of the existence of an unidentified natriuretic hormone has, almost from the very beginning, been more often critizised than accepted and other explanations for the mechanism of natriuresis due to the ECFV expansion have been offered. One of the positive results of the critical approach to the new hypothesis was a modern reevaluation and elaboration of the role of renal hemodynamic and physical factors in the control of renal sodium and water excretion. Another one was a search for natriuretic properties of known hormones. It is true that formerly a tendency prevailed to stress a predominance of one of the natriuretic factors over the others. Now-it seems-that with more facts available, a more realistic tendency leads to the acceptance of a state of coexistence of various natriuretic factors. An example of such a tendency is the theory on a natriuretic hormone cascade formed by interaction of unidentified natriuretic hormone, renal nerves'activity, dopamine, kallikrein-kinin, acetylcholin, angiotensin, noradrenalin, glucagon, calcitonin and prostaglandin[30] (I.H. Mills, personal communication). Another example is a theory on the interaction of physical and hormonal factors in the mechanism of natriuresis now supported mainly by the results of experiments on acutely hypophysectomized rats [31,32] which was roughly outlined back in 1967[25]. Yet most recent example is the multifactorial theory of escape from the sodium-retaining effects of mineralocorticoids[33].

INSIDE PROBLEMS OF THE HYPOTHESIS ON NATRIURETIC HORMONE

Having more or less found a modus vivendi for various natriuretic factors, new problems are emerging from the inside of the hypothesis on the existence of a new natriuretic hormone. Evidence for a small molecular weight natriuretic hormone has been complemented by the evidence for a large molecular weight hormone not only in urine[34,35] but also in the renal tissue[20,36]. The open problems are relations between both types of suggested hormones and also between the circulating and the tissue natriuretic activity.

Furthermore the hypothalamus is the earliest suggested source of a natriuretic hormone [37,38,39]. The natriuretic substance, isolated lately from bovine hypothalamus, may be a qualitatively new and a far-reaching elaboration of the preceeding physiological studies. A problem, however, is that this substance with oubain-like properties is apparently not of a peptide nature. Thus perhaps more than one unidentified natriuretic hormone and of different chemical structures await identification. And both of them apparently equipped with oubain.like activity[40,41,42]. The aspect that a natriuretic hormone(s) posseses such an activity may open an entirely new and broad horizon for futher development and exploitation of the results which have accumulated from the search for this hormone. The still ongoing discussion of a local character as to which part of the nephron is a target for a natriuretic hormone may now be enlarged to include a general questions whether a natriuretic hormone is not an overall endogenous regulator of Na-K-ATPase activity in body cells ? If it is, then a new boom of interest in natriuretic hormone, or perhaps-more precisely - in the transport enzyme inhibitor, may be expected. And new ambitious goals besides the original one which was to understand the renal regulation of body fluid volumes may come to be set up. This is since 1969 the sixth symposium devoted to the problem of hormonal mechanism of natriuresis (1969-Smolenice near Bratislava; 1969-Stockholm-part of the 4th ISN Congress; 1972-Mexico City-part of the 5th ISN Congress; 1976--Bonn; 1978-Montreal-part of the 7th ISN Congress). May it enlarge at least in some aspects our present views on this intricate but challenging issue.

REFERENCES

1. Smith, H.W. (1957) Amer. J. Physiol., 23, 623.

2. De Wardener, H.E., Mills, I.H., Clapham, W.F., Hayter, C.J. (1961) Clin. Sci., 21, 249.

3. Lichardus, B., Pearce, J.W. (1965) Fed. Proc., 24, 404.

4. Lichardus, B., Pearce, J.W. (1966) Nature, 209, 407.

5. Lichardus, B., Nizet, A. (1972) Clin. Sci., 42, 701.

6. Bahlmann, J., McDonald, S.J., Venton, M.G., de Wardener, H.E. (1967) Clin. Sci., 32, 403.

7. Bonjour, J.P., Peters, G. (1970) Pflügers Arch. ges. Physiol., 318, 21.

8. Lichardus, B., Ponec, J. (1970) Physiol. bohemoslov., 19, 330.

9. Sonnenberg, H., Veress, A.T., Pearce, J.W. (1972) J. clin. Invest., 51, 2631.

10. Lichardus, B. (1973) Čs. Fysiol., 22, 397.

11. Ponec, J., Lichardus, B. (1970) In: Regulation of Body Fluid Volumes by the Kidney (eds. J.H. Cort, B. Lichardus), Karger, Basel, pp. 93-99.

12. Harris, R.H., Yarger, W.E. (1977) Kidney Internat., 11, 93.

13. Lichardus, B., Pliška, V., Uhrín, V., Barth, T. (1968) Lancet i, 127.

14. Lichardus, B., Pliška, V., Uhrín, V., Barth, T. (1970) In: Regulation of Body Fluid Volumes by the Kidney (eds. J.H. Cort, B. Lichardus), Karger, Basel, pp. 114-121.

15. Sedláková, E., Lichardus, B., Cort, J.H. (1969) Science, 164, 580.

16. Bourgoignie, J., Licht, A., Kaplan, M. (1978) In: Natriuretic Hormone (eds. H.J. Kramer, F. Krück), Springer, Heidelberg, pp. 122-130.

17. Buckalew, V.M. (1978) idem, pp. 131-140.

18. Gonick, H.C. (1978) idem, pp. 108-121.

19. Cort, J.H., Lichardus, B. (1968) Nephron, 5, 401.

20. Bricker, N.S. (1972) New Engl. J. Med., 286, 1093.

21. Klahr, S., Rodriguez, H.J. (1975) Nephron, 15, 387.

22. Krück, F., Kramer, H.J. (1978) Contr. Nephrol., 13, 19.

23. Lee, J., de Wardener, H.E. (1974) Kidney Internat., 6, 323.

24. Levinsky, N.G. (1974) Advances in Metab. Disord., 7, 37.

25. Lichardus, B. (1967) Endocrin. exp., 1, 181.

26. Lichardus, B. (1978) In: Hormones and Brain Development (eds. G. Dörner, M. Kawakami), Elsevier/North-Holland

Biomed. Press, Amsterdam, pp. 465-470.

27. Lichardus, B. (1978) Mechanizmy rýchlej renálnej regulácie objemu extracelulárnej tekutiny, VEDA SAV, Bratislava, pp. 1-154.

28. De Wardener, H.E. (1977) Clin. Sci. Mol. Med., 53, 1.

29. De Wardener, H.E. (1978) Amer. J. Physiol., 235(3), F 163.

30. Mills, I.H., Obika, L.F.O., Newport, P.A. (1978) Contr. Nephrol., 12, 132.

31. Lichardus, B., Ponec, J. (1976) Experientia, 32, 884.

32. Lichardus, B., Ponec, J. (1978) In: Natriuretic Hormone (eds. H.J. Kramer, F. Krück), Springer, Heidelberg, pp. 6-15.

33. Knox, F.G., Burnett, J.C., Kohan, D. E., Spielman, W.S., Strand, J.C. (1980) Kidney Internat., 17, 263.

34. Sealey, J.E., Laragh, J.H.(1971) Circulat. Res. 28/29 Suppl. II, 32.

35. Clarkson, E.M., Raw, S.M., de Wardener, H.E. (1976) Kidney Internat., 10, 381.

36. Godon, J.P. (1978) In: Natriuretic Hormones (eds. H.J. Kramer, F. Krück), Springer, Heidelberg, pp. 88-100.

37. Cort. J.H., Lichardus, B. (1963) In: Hormones and the Kidney (ed. P.C. Williams), Academic Press, London, pp. 25-39.

38. Lichardus, B., Mitro, A., Cort, J.H. (1965) Amer. J. Physiol., 208, 1075.

39. Lichardus, B., Jonec, V., Strážovcová, A. (1969) Endocr. exp., 3, 141.

40. Haupert, G.T., jr., Sancho, J.M. (1979) Proc. Natl. Acad. Sci., 76, 4658.

41. Gonick, H.C., Kramer, H.J., Paul, W., Lu, E. (1977) Clin. Sci.Mol. Med., 53, 329.

42. Cort, J.H., Lichardus, B. (1970) In: Regulation of Body Fluid Volumes by the Kidney (eds. J.H. Cort, B. Lichardus), Karger, Basel, pp. 1-10.

EFFECTS OF ADRENERGIC AND RENIN-ANGIOTENSIN-ALDOSTERONE SYSTEMS ON TUBULAR AND GLOMERULAR FUNCTION

Hormonal Regulation of Sodium Excretion,
B. Lichardus, R.W. Schrier and J. Ponec, eds.
© 1980 Elsevier/North-Holland Biomedical Press

HUMORAL REGULATION OF GLOMERULAR PERFUSION AND FILTRATION

NESTOR SCHOR AND BARRY M. BRENNER
Laboratory of Kidney and Electrolyte Physiology, Peter Bent Brigham Hospital,
721 Huntington Avenue, Boston, Massachusetts (USA)

Based on direct visual impressions in amphibia, Richards and Schmidt concluded that the renal glomerulus is a contractile structure that responds to
various stimuli by altering its pattern of intra-glomerular perfusion[1]. Following electrical stimulation or infusion of adrenalin, these workers observed
variable perfusion within individual glomeruli and proposed the concept of intermittence of glomerular urine formation based on intrinsic variation in
glomerular capillary surface area[1]. This concept soon received additional support in other studies in amphibia[2,3].

Although glomeruli are rarely visible on the surface of the mammalian kidney,
Hall[4] came to the same conclusion as Richards and Schmidt, based on studies of
the structure of the glomerulus in man, rat and dog. Recently, it has been
shown that glomeruli of several mammalian species are also capable of contraction[5-7]. Moreover, glomerular mesangial cells, specialized forms of smooth
muscle cells, are morphologically well suited to a role in regulating capillary
surface area by virtue of their rich content of intracellular myofilaments[8-10].
These filaments have been shown to contain the contractile proteins, actin and
myosin[9,10]. Furthermore, isolated mesangial cells in culture contract in
response to angiotensin II (AII) and arginine vasopressin (AVP).

With increasing recognition of the unique contractile properties of the
glomerular mesangium, it has also become evident in recent years that a variety
of vasoactive substances are capable of regulating glomerular ultrafiltration
in vivo[11-15]. In large part, these substances have been shown to modify the
glomerular capillary ultrafiltration coefficient, K_f, the product of capillary
filtering surface area and capillary wall hydraulic conductivity.

The possible pathways whereby vasoactive substances alter filtering surface
area and/or capillary hydraulic conductivity, and thus K_f, are depicted in
Figure 1.

Pathway 1 involves the direct stimulation of contraction of glomerular mesangial cells, the effect of which is to reduce glomerular capillary patency and
hence K_f. Two substances, AVP and AII, have been shown to stimulate mesangial
cell contraction in vitro[16]. In vivo, the effect of AII on K_f in the rat is

12

reversed by verapamil and manganese ion[17], known blockers of smooth muscle contraction, and by the AII antagonist, saralasin[18]. Although no antagonist of AVP action on K_f has yet been studied <u>in vivo</u>, there is evidence to suggest that K_f varies inversely with circulating AVP levels[13].

Less clear is the mechanism by which dibutyryl cAMP (DBcAMP), parathyroid hormone (PTH), prostaglandins, acetylcholine and histamine also elicit changes in K_f. Pathway 2 (Fig. 1), involving a direct effect of these substances on mesangial cell contraction seems unlikely, at least for prostaglandin E_2 and

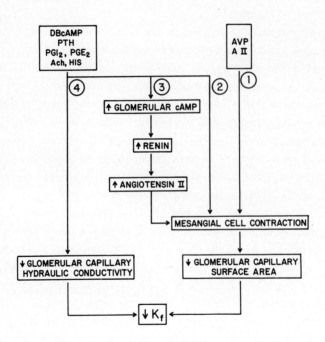

Fig. 1. Possible pathways involved in the regulation of K_f by angiotensin II (AII), arginine vasopressin (AVP), dibutyryl cAMP (DBcAMP), PTH, prostaglandins I_2 and E_2, acetylcholine (Ach), and histamine (HIS).

PTH, since Ausiello et al.[16] were unable to trigger mesangial cell contraction by these substances in vitro. Of note, however, all of the substances shown in the top left panel of Fig. 1 are known to stimulate renal renin release[19-21]. The possibility exists, therefore, as shown in pathway 3, that these vasoactive substances modulate K_f by virtue of their ability to promote local intrarenal AII formation, with the latter serving as the final mediator of mesangial cell contraction and eventual decline in K_f. Clearly, the possibility also exists that PTH, prostaglandins and the other substances shown in the top left hand panel of Fig. 1 initiate changes in K_f by some pathway independent of the mesangial cell, as in pathway 4.

It seemed to us that saralasin might be a useful agent to help distinguish which of these last three pathways is primarily involved. If this AII antagonist were to reverse the fall in K_f induced by these vasoactive drugs, pathway 2 and 4 would be unlikely and pathway 3 would be favored. Therefore, to explore these various possibilities, we employed the protocol shown in Fig. 2. Solutions containing either DBcAMP (83 µg/kg/min, n=8 rats), PTH (5 U/kg/min, n=7), Pitressin (0.6 mU/kg/min, n=7), PGI_2 (62 ng/kg/min, n=8), PGE_2 (125 ng/kg/min, n=10) or vehicle alone (tris buffer or saline, n=7), were infused into euvolemic Munich-Wistar rats. Since these vasoactive substances can stimulate prostaglandin release, a prostaglandin synthetase inhibitor (indomethacin or meclofenamate, 5 µg/kg/min) was also infused starting 45 minutes before and continued throughout the duration of each experiment. After an initial equilibration period, appropriate measurements and collections needed for the calculation of K_f were obtained in the pre-saralasin study period. Then, with continued infusion of a given vasoactive substance, a saralasin infusion (5 µg/kg/min) was begun in each rat, and after a second equilibration period, all measurements and collections were repeated.(Fig. 2).

Results obtained are summarized in Table 1.

DBcAMP vs. Control Group

Despite no significant change in systemic mean arterial pressure, $\overline{AP}$, relative to the Control Group, DBcAMP led to a small but significant increase in transglomerular hydraulic pressure difference, $\overline{\Delta P}$. Single nephron glomerular filtration rate (SNGFR) and glomerular plasma flow rate, Q_A, declined by $\sim$ 25% and $\sim$ 30%, respectively, the latter due to an impressive increase in total renal arteriolar resistance, R_{TA}. These effects are identical to those obtained previously in this laboratory[13], as was the finding also shown in Table 1 that DBcAMP infusion led to a marked decline in K_f.

These increases in $\overline{\Delta P}$ and R_{TA}, and decreases in Q_A and K_f, are typical of changes seen when AII is infused[11,17]. We therefore studied the effect of

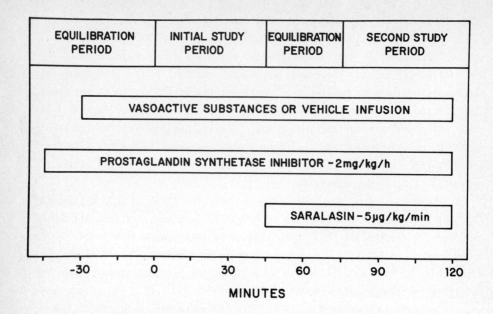

Fig. 2. Protocol employed for study of the effects of vasoactive substances (DBcAMP, PTH, ADH, PGI_2 and PGE_2) or vehicle alone, and saralasin, on the determinants of glomerular ultrafiltration.

saralasin infusion, a competitive antagonist of AII, on the actions of DBcAMP. In the presence of saralasin, the effects of DBcAMP on $\overline{\Delta P}$, SNGFR, Q_A, R_{TA} and K_f were completely reversed (Table 1). Therefore, the action of DBcAMP on the glomerular microcirculation appears to involve an intermediate action of AII. In the Control animals, however, no significant effects of prostaglandin inhibition alone or in combination with saralasin were found, suggesting that in the absence of DBcAMP infusion (or the other vasoactive substances examined in this study), endogenous AII plays little role in regulating glomerular dynamics under euvolemic conditions. An identical conclusion for the kidney as a whole has also been reported[22].

TABLE 1

SUMMARY OF SINGLE NEPHRON FUNCTION IN RATS GIVEN VARIOUS VASOACTIVE SUBSTANCES BEFORE AND DURING SARALASIN (Sar.) INFUSION

	$\overline{AP}$ mmHg	$\overline{\Delta P}$ mmHg	SNGFR nl/min	Q_A nl/min	R_{TA} 10^{10}dyn·s·cm^{-5}	K_f nl/(s·mmHg)
CONTROL (n=7)	111±4	37±1	40±2	119±6	3.9±0.1	0.081±0.010
CONTROL+Sar.	106±7	36±1	40±2	116±7	4.0±0.2	0.080±0.011
DBcAMP (n=8)	111±4	40±1^a	30±3^a	84±7^a	5.8±0.5^a	0.035±0.002^a
DBcAMP+Sar.	110±4	35±1	47±3	142±10^b	3.0±0.2^b	0.087±0.008
PTH (n=7)	113±4	40±1^a	35±2	100±7	5.1±0.4^a	0.047±0.004^a
PTH+Sar.	109±5	39±1	42±2	115±6	4.1±0.3	0.076±0.005
ADH (n=7)	122±7	42±1^a	40±3	130±12	4.0±0.3	0.046±0.006^a
ADH+Sar.	121±7	43±1^b	39±3	126±12	4.3±0.4	0.038±0.005^b
PGI$_2$ (n=8)	110±4	42±1^a	30±2^a	82±5^a	5.4±0.4^a	0.039±0.006^a
PGI$_2$+Sar.	108±4	34±1^b	50±3^b	178±9^b	2.5±0.2^b	0.088±0.006
PGE$_2$ (n=10)	108±3	41±1^a	35±3	96±7	4.7±0.2	0.032±0.003^a
PGE$_2$+Sar.	103±4	34±1	41±2	138±9	3.4±0.3^b	0.073±0.006

Values are expressed as mean±SE; ^{a}p<0.05 vs. Control and ^{b}p<0.05 vs. Control+ Sar.

PTH vs. Control Group

As also shown in Table 1, the effects of PTH infusion on $\overline{AP}$ were negligible whereas $\overline{\Delta P}$ rose slightly but significantly. Mild declines in SNGFR and Q_A were also observed, the latter due to an increase in R_{TA}. PTH also led to an impressive lowering of K_f, as noted by this laboratory previously[14]. During infusion of saralasin, these effects of PTH on SNGFR, Q_A, $\overline{\Delta P}$, R_{TA} and K_f were again largely reversed.

ADH vs. Control Group

Administration of a nonpressor dose of Pitressin, a vasoactive peptide known to exert effects on the glomerular microcirculation similar to those of the native antidiuretic hormone, AVP[13], led to a significant increase in $\overline{\Delta P}$. SNGFR, Q_A and R_{TA} did not change with Pitressin infusion. ADH also led to an impressive lowering of K_f, as noted by this laboratory previously[13]. Unlike the findings with DBcAMP and PTH, the administration of saralasin did not reverse the effects on any of the determinants of glomerular ultrafiltration induced by Pitressin. Therefore, the findings suggest that the mechanism(s) of the ADH-associated fall in K_f is independent of a pathway involving the concomitan:

action of AII, as pointed out in pathway 1 (Fig. 1).

PGI_2 vs. Control Group

The effects of PGI_2 infusion (Table 1) were qualitatively similar to those of DBcAMP and PTH in that $\overline{\Delta P}$ and R_{TA} increased whereas SNGFR, Q_A and K_f fell significantly. Once again, all of these effects were reversed by saralasin. Indeed, in the presence of saralasin, the action of PGI_2 on the glomerular microcirculation was transformed from that of a potent vasoconstrictor (low Q_A and high R_{TA}) to an equally potent vasodilator (high Q_A and low R_{TA}).

PGE_2 vs. Control Group

As shown in Table 1, during infusion of a non-hypotensive dose of PGE_2, $\overline{\Delta P}$ and R_{TA} rose. Mild declines in SNGFR and Q_A were observed, although these changes were not statistically significant. PGE_2 infusion also led to an impressive reduction in K_f. Saralasin infusion effectively antagonized the increases in $\overline{\Delta P}$ and R_{TA} and reversed the declines in K_f and Q_A induced by PGE_2 alone. Thus, saralasin also transformed the renal action of PGE_2 from vasoconstrictor to vasodilator. Therefore, as with DBcAMP and PTH, the effects of PGI_2 and PGE_2 on the glomerular microcirculation appear to involve a pathway in which AII plays a fundamental role (pathway 3, Fig. 1).

In conclusion, the evidence to date suggests the existence of two distinct pathways for the humoral regulation of K_f (Fig. 3).

One pathway involves the direct stimulation of mesangial cell contraction, and in vitro[16], AII and AVP appear to be capable of attaching to specific receptor sites on these cells to initiate contractility. The other pathway also involves a key role for AII in initiating mesangial cell contraction, but the intrarenal formation of AII in this case seems to depend on stimulation by cAMP. In support of this latter pathway, it has been shown in this laboratory that infusion of DBcAMP leads to a brisk decline in K_f[13]. This nucleotide derivative is known to mimic the action of endogenous cAMP in a number of tissues, either through a direct action or through inhibition of cAMP phosphodiesterase[23]. In addition, mammalian glomeruli are rich in adenylate cyclase[24] and isolated suspensions of glomeruli have been shown to generate cAMP in response to prostaglandins and PTH[24,25]. Moreover, since cAMP is a potent stimulus for renal renin release[19,20], the possibility is presented that these vasoactive substances modulate K_f by virtue of their ability to promote local intrarenal AII formation, with the latter serving as the final mediator of mesangial cell contraction and decline in K_f. Thus, given this evidence for parallel changes in Q_A and K_f in response to several vasoactive hormones, it seems clear that perfusion of the intimate circulation within the mammalian

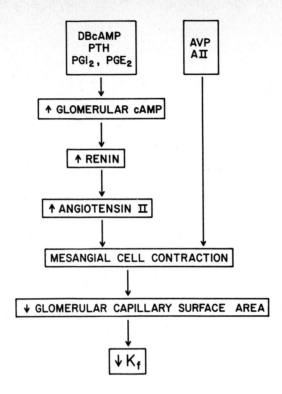

Fig. 3. Suggested pathways involved in the regulation of K_f by angiotensin II (AII), arginine vasopressin (AVP), dibutyryl cAMP (DBcAMP), PTH, and prostaglandins I_2 and E_2.

glomerulus may be more variable and intermittent than previously believed. Obviously, additional studies are required to evaluate the importance of this process of glomerular intermittence in the overall modulation of glomerular filtration in physiological and pathological states in mammals.

ACKNOWLEDGEMENTS

These studies were supported by U.S.P.H.S. Grant AM 19467 from the National Institutes of Health. Dr. Schor performed these studies during the tenure of a Postdoctoral Research Fellowship from the Fundacao de Amparo a Pesquisa do Estado de Sao Paulo, Brazil.

REFERENCES

1. Richards, A.N. and Schmidt, C.F. (1924) Am. J. Physiol., 71, 178-208.

2. Bieter, R.N. (1929-30) Am. J. Physiol. 91, 436-460.

3. Elias, H., Hossman, A., Barth, I.B. and Solmor, A. (1960) J. Urol., 83, 790-798.

4. Hall, V. (1957) Am. Heart J., 54, 1-9.

5. Bernik, M.B. (1969) Nephron, 6, 1-10.

6. Hornych, H., Beaufils, M. and Richet, G. (1972) Kidney Int., 2, 336-343.

7. Sraer, J.D., Sraer, J., Ardaillou, R. and Mimoune, D. (1974) Kidney Int., 6, 241-246.

8. Pease, D.C. (1968) J. Ultrastr. Res. 23, 304-320.

9. Becker, C.G. (1972) Am. J. Pathol., 66, 97-107.

10. Scheinman, J.I., Fish, A.J., Matas, A.J. and Michael, A.F. (1978) Am. J. Pathol., 90, 71-84.

11. Blantz, R.C., Konnen, K.S. and Tucker, B.J. (1976) J. Clin. Invest., 57, 419-434.

12. Baylis, C., Deen, W.M., Myers, B.D. and Brenner, B.M. (1976) Am. J. Physiol. 230, 1148-1158.

13. Ichikawa, I. and Brenner, B.M. (1977) Am. J. Physiol., 233, F103-F117.

14. Ichikawa, I., Humes, H.D., Dousa, T.P. and Brenner, B.M. (1978) Am. J. Physiol., 234, F393-F401.

15. Ichikawa, I, and Brenner, B.M. (1979) Circ. Res., 45, 737-745.

16. Ausiello, D.A., Kreisberg, J.I., Roy, C. and Karnovsky, M.J. (1980) J. Clin. Invest., 65, 754-760.

17. Ichikawa, I., Miele, J.F. and Brenner, B.M. (1979) Kidney Int., 16, 137-147.

18. Steiner, R.W. and Blantz, R.C. (1978) Kidney Int., 14, 703.

19. Wimer, N., Chokshi, D.S. and Walkenhorst, N.G. (1971) Circ. Res., 29, 239-248.

20. Campbell, W.B., Graham, R.M. and Jackson, E.K. (1979) J. Clin. Invest., 64, 448-456.

21. Brenner, B.M., Badr, K.F., Schor, N. and Ichikawa, I. (In Press) Mineral and Electrolyte Metabolism.

22. Mimran, A., Casellas, D., Dupont, M. and Barjon, P. (1975) Clin. Sci. Mol. Med., 48, 299S-302S.

23. Hall, D.A., Barnes, L.D. and Dousa, T.P. (1977) Am. J. Physiol., 232, F368-F376.

24. Torres, V.E., Northrup, T.E., Edwards, R.M., Shah, S.V. and Dousa, T.P. (1978) J. Clin. Invest., 62, 1334-1343.

25. Schlondorff, D., Yoo, P. and Albert, B.E. (1978) Am. J. Physiol., 235, F458-F464.

Hormonal Regulation of Sodium Excretion,
B. Lichardus, R.W. Schrier and J. Ponec, eds.
© 1980 Elsevier/North-Holland Biomedical Press

MECHANISM OF MINERALOCORTICOID ESCAPE

FRANKLYN G KNOX, M.D., Ph.D., AND JOHN C. BURNETT, JR., M.D.

Department of Physiology & Biophysics, Mayo Clinic, Rochester, Minnesota

55901 (USA)

INTRODUCTION

Ragan et al[1], in 1940, demonstrated that the chronic injection of
deoxycorticosterone acetate (DOCA) produced a syndrome of polydipsia and
polyuria in normal animals. Most importantly, they demonstrated that there
was no striking accumulation of extracellular fluid or congestive heart
failure when DOCA was administered to normal dogs; i.e., sodium retention
was only transient whereas the hypokalemia was persistent, finally leading
to paralysis and death of the animal. Clinton and Thorn, in 1941, extended
these observations by demonstrating that the chronic administration of DOCA
increased plasma volume of normal subjects by 6%[2]. In 1958, August, Nelson
and Thorn extended these observations with DOCA to the evaluation of the
response of normal subjects to aldosterone. Following an initial period of
weight gain and sodium retention, the weight gain ceased and sodium excretion returned to control levels, despite continued administration of the
hormone[3]. Relman and Schwartz, who also studied the effects of DOCA during
variations of sodium intake, concluded that the escape from the sodium-
retaining effect of DOCA was the result of regulatory mechanisms which
override the hormonal effect on the renal tubule[4]. The term "escape" was
introduced into the literature in this context. Since the term has been
widely utilized and provides a convenient description of the phenomenon, we
will use the term escape as an abbreviation in this review. Most recently,
the phenomenon of DOCA escape has been extensively reviewed by Knox, et
al[5].

NEPHRON SITES OF ALTERED SODIUM REABSORPTION

The nephron sites of enhanced sodium reabsorption subsequent to minera-locorticoid action and those responsible for escape may not be the same. Although it is certain that mineralocorticoids enhance sodium reabsorption in the cortical collecting tubule[6], a direct effect on other tubule segments remains controversial.

A proximal site of escape was suggested by Schacht et al[7] based on free-water clearance studies. Further evidence for a proximal site of mineralocorticoid escape has been presented by Wright et al[8] in which dogs given DOCA for 5 to 13 days were found to have lower (TF/P) inulin concentration ratios in the late proximal convoluted tubule than did the controls. Subsequent micropuncture studies by Knox et al[9] revealed no difference between (TF/P) inulin concentration ratios in the proximal tubules of dogs treated with DOCA and either low or high salt diets. Studies in man[10] and dogs[11] found that hypercalciuria, but not phosphaturia, occurs with escape, suggesting a decrease in sodium reabsorption at a distal, but not proximal, nephron site. Sonnenberg[12] showed no difference in proximal fluid transport between salt-loaded DOCA-treated and salt deprived rats. It appears, therefore, that an increased delivery of sodium from the proximal tubule of superifical nephrons is not responsible for escape. However, proximal tubules of deep nephrons might handle sodium differently.

Little data is available concerning sodium reabsorption by the loop of Henle during escape. Although Sonnenberg[12] observed no differences in sodium reabsorption by the loop of Henle between salt-deprived and salt-loaded DOCA escaped rats as calculated by comparison of differences between the late proximal and early distal tubule, Haas et al[13] noted greater sodium delivery in the superficial distal tubule in acutely volume expanded

DOCA escaped rats as compared with controls. Superimposed volume expansion
in the latter study may have unmasked the contribution of the loop of Henle
in escape. Thus, the loop of Henle may represent the site of altered
sodium transport in escape.

As previously mentioned, sodium transport by the isolated cortical
collecting tubule from the rabbit is markedly stimulated by mineralocorticoid pretreatment[6]. However, these same rabbits had escaped from the
sodium retaining effects of DOCA. Since sodium transport was markedly stimulated in the cortical collecting tubules, this effect was not decisive
for the final regulation of sodium excretion. Rather, the increased reabsorption in the cortical collection duct may be overcome by increased delivery of sodium to this segment.

Sodium reabsorption by the papillary collecting duct is similar in
DOCA-escaped and normal rats. In the micropuncture studies by Haas et
al[13] in which sodium reabsorption by the papillary collecting duct was not
changed by DOCA treatment; therefore, we conclude that the papillary duct
may not play an important role in escape from the salt-retaining effects of
mineralocorticoids.

THE ROLE OF HEMODYNAMIC AND PHYSICAL FACTORS

An increased glomerular filtration rate has been suggested to be
responsible for the return to sodium balance during chronic DOCA
administraton. Biglieri observed a significant increase in glomerular
filtration rate in subjects with aldosterone secreting tumors who were in
sodium balance which returned to normal values following surgical removal
of the tumors[14]. Despite the evidence implicating a role for glomerular
filtration rate in escape, other studies minimize the association.
Significant reductions in glomerular filtration rate by aortic or renal

artery constriction following acute volume expansion failed to block the natriuretic response to volume expansion[15]. In the hypophysectomized dog, Davis et al were unable to block escape despite a significant reduction in glomerular filtration rate[16]. Thus, escape may occur in the absence of an increased glomerular filtration rate.

The positive relationship between arterial blood pressure and sodium excretion may have important relevance in escape. Chronic mineralocorticoid administration and primary aldosteronism are both characterized by diastolic hypertension[3,14]. Zipser et al[17], however, have recently reported a case of primary aldosteronism associated with persistently normal blood pressure. Studies by Higgins suggest that escape is independent of alterations in arterial pressure since escape occurred in the presence of significant reduction in arterial presure by the administration of quanethidine and hydralazine[18]. An alternative explanation is that the hydralazine may have resulted in renal vasodilation, permitting an enhanced transmission of pressure to the peritubule capillaries, thus attenuating the effects of a reduced systemic arterial pressure.

Measurements during acute volume expansion clearly document a striking positive correlation between interstitial pressure and sodium excretion[19]. Perhaps, in escape, an increase in renal interstitial pressure resulting from increased renal perfusion pressure and/or expansion of the extracellular volume results in decreased sodium reabsorption either directly as a physical factor or indirectly through a humoral factor. Thus, the kidney may serve as an important volume/pressure receptor influencing intrarenal mechanisms mediating escape.

RENIN-ANGIOTENSIN SYSTEM

Recent studies have established that angiotensin II (AII) has a potent effect on sodium excretion independent of changes in aldosterone secretion. Recent studies by Hall et al[20] demonstrated that, in dogs with the renin-angiotensin system activated by sodium depletion, blockade of AII increased urinary sodium excretion fivefold without changes in circulating aldosterone concentration. Both acute and chronic infusion of AII studies[21,22] suggest that the increased absorption of sodium might be secondary to altered physical forces in which glomerular filtration is maintained in association with a decrease in renal plasma flow. A direct effect of AII, however, upon the tubule epithelium, has been suggested by others[23].

Mineralocorticoid escape may result from the suppression of AII con-centration by gradual expansion of the extracellular fluid volume occurring in response to the administration of sodium-retaining steroids. Johnston et al[24] examined the role of the importance of renin-angiotensin-aldosterone axis in escape by measuring plasma renin activity in dogs with small A.V. fistulas which escaped and in dogs with large A.V. fistulas which failed to escape from the sodium-retaining action of DOCA. Despite marked differences between dogs with small or large fistulas in response to DOCA, both groups had suppressed renin activity.

These studies suggest that the circulating renin-angiotensin system does not mediate the escape phenomenon; however, further studies remain necessary to firmly rule out a role for intrarenal AII.

RENAL ADRENERGIC SYSTEM

An effective expansion of some fluid volume compartment is widely held to be a central component of escape. This thesis leads to the question of how this volume expansion is perceived and the formulation of the concept of fluid volume receptors. Several studies have reported the importance of the sympathetic nervous system in initiating a volume reflex mechanism in controlling sodium excretion following acute volume expansion[25]. However, studies by McDonald et al[26] demonstrated a normal pattern of sodium retention followed by escape in dogs given DOCA both before and after C6 cord section, suggesting that escape is independent of input from the sympathetic nervous system.

It now seems clear, based on morphologic evidence for direct tubular innervation of the tubule[27], and on clearance and micropuncture studies[27,29] that the renal nerves can directly affect sodium reabsorption. With the establishment of the ability of the renal nerves to alter sodium excretion, the possibility that the sodium retention produced by mineralocorticoid administration leads to alterations in renal efferent nerve traffic and thereby mediates escape must be considered. Evidence supporting changes in the renal adrenergic system with chronic administration of DOCA was reported by Ljungqvist[30]. In this study, concentrations of renal adrenergic transmitter, as measured by histofluorescence, were decreased in rats treated with a high salt diet and DOCA.

Evidence against a role for the renal nerves in mediating escape was provided by Davis et al in studies where the kidney was transplanted to the neck of adrenalectomized dogs[16]. Following the administration of DOCA, usual escape occurred. The authors concluded that the mechanism cannot be neurally mediated since all nerves to the kidney were cut during transplantation. Recent studies by Katholi et al[31] support the thesis that escape is not dependent upon intact renal nerves; these studies observed escape to occur in steroid-treated rats with and without intact renal nerves. Denervated organs can exhibit a hypersensitivity to catecholamines; therefore, final judgment concerning a role for neural influences in escape await studies in which circulating catecholamines are also evaluated.

KALLIKREIN-KININ AND PROSTAGLANDINS

Kinins and prostaglandins have been considered as mediators of escape since they are so closely linked to sodium and water metabolism. The kallikrein and prostaglandin systems have been localized to the late distal and cortical collecting tubules. Thus, the strategic location of these systems provides an anatomical basis to suggest a potential interaction, not only with each other, but also with mineralocorticoids.

Initial observations by Adetuyibi and Mills demonstrated that urinary kallikrein excretion was increased in subjects during the escape from the sodium-retaining effects of mineralocorticoids[32]. At the same time, other investigators confirmed that urinary kallikrein was elevated in DOCA-salt hypertension[33]. Further, urinary kallikrein excretion was elevated in primary aldosteronism and was reduced in adrenalectomized rats. That renin was not a significant factor regulating urinary kallikrein excretion was derived from the observation that DOCA administration (low renin) and low sodium diet (high renin) were both associated with elevated kallikrein excretion. Thus, the data showed a direct relationship between mineralo-corticoids and kallikrein excretion and support the proposition by Margolius et al that mineralocorticoids are a primary factor stimulating urinary kallikrein excretion.

The contribution of renal prostaglandins to escape has been examined in several studies. Escape from the sodium-retaining effects of DOCA occurred in dogs on a high salt diet within the first day without alteration in uri-nary prostaglandin excretion[34]. By the sixth day of treatment, hypokalemia, hypernatremia, increased urinary prostaglandin E_2 and F_2

excretion increased polyuria and suppressed plasma renin activity had
developed. When potassium supplements were superimposed upon DOCA
treatment, the changes in urinary prostaglandin excretion, urine volume and
serum sodium were all attenuated. Indomethacin administration did not
affect DOCA escape or its time course in this or a previous study[35],
suggesting that prostaglandins were not a contributing factor. In a
separate study, the effect of indomethacin (2 mg/kg/day) on the increased
water turnover, characteristic of chronic DOCA treatment with a high salt
diet, was evaluated in dogs[36]. Indomethacin had no effect on the return to
sodium balance, as above, but prevented the increased water turnover. It
was concluded that prostaglandins may play a role in the increased water
turnover associated with escape and that this may be related to the concurrent hypokalemia.

In studies in humans who received either DOCA alone for 10 days or DOCA
plus indomethacin or ibuprofen for a similar duration, DOCA administration
increased urinary kallikrein excretion in the presence or absence of the
prostaglandin synthetase inhibitor[37]. Further, inhibition of urinary
prostaglandin excretion during DOCA administration appeared to facilitate
rather than to retard escape, although total weight gain and sodium retention were unaltered.

In summary, the relationship of the renal kallikrein-kinin and
prostaglandin systems to salt and water metabolism and to escape is only
partially understood. Nevertheless, the initiation of escape prior to
increased prostaglandin excretion, the reversal of this excretion with
potassium supplements, and the failure to block escape with inhibitors of
prostaglandin synthetase, all suggest that changes in prostaglandin metabolism may be secondarily induced by chronic mineralocorticoid
administration, but that prostaglandins do not mediate escape.

NATRIURETIC HORMONE

A circulating natriuretic factor has been postulated as a mediator of escape. de Wardener has recently reviewed the evidence in support of a natriuretic hormone[38]. For example, if animals are expanded with a solution which is in equilibrium with the test animal's blood, the blood of the volume-expanded animal can be used to perfuse a denervated assay kidney at constant pressure[39]. The resulting natriuresis in the assay kidney was attributed to a circulating natriuretic substance. Sonnenberg et al have performed similar experiments except that a whole animal was used as the assay preparation[40]. Again, increased sodium excretion was interpreted to indicate a change in the concentration of some substances which control urinary sodium excretion.

Additional experiments suggest the presence of a natriuretic factor rather than a decrease in an antinatriuretic factor in volume expansion. Pearce and Veress[41] evaluated the natriuretic effects of extracts from plasma obtained before and after volume expansion. The extracts from volume expanded animals were natriuretic in the assay animals. Buckalew and Lancaster evaluatd a humoral factor in plasma of dogs before and after administration of DOCA[42]. They demonstrated that escape from the salt-retaining effects of DOCA correlated with sodium transport inhibitory activity in plasma as determined in a toad bladder assay.

Despite a vigorous search for a natriuretic hormone which might mediate escape, the existence of such a natriuretic hormone remains in question. Perhaps this question will linger until the sites of origin, its affects and precise chemical nature are known. The search for a natriuretic hormone is not obligatory and yet this cannot be ruled out as one of several participating mechanisms.

28

SUMMARY OPINION

In our opinion, it is unlikely that a single factor mediates escape.
Interruption of a single system, as repeatedly demonstrated in this review,
does not prevent escape, probably due to activation of other mechanisms.
For this reason, the evidence does not firmly rule out the participation of
many of the individual mechanisms discussed in this review. Most likely,
an interplay of several compensatory mechanisms mediate escape from the
salt-retaining effect of mineralocorticoids. As stated by Smith[43], "where
multiple controls are superimposed on a function, such as sodium excretion,
it is conceived that normal regulatory mechanisms may be obscured by compensatory reactions."

The mechanisms for escape from the salt-retaining effects of mineralocorticoids is not proved. In consideration of all of the foregoing, our
current view of the mechanism for escape is as follows: Salt and water
retention leads to expansion of an effective vascular volume, stimulation
of volume receptors, and subsequent decreases in renal adrenergic activity.
This decreased renal adrenergic activity directly decreases sodium
transport as well as vasodilates the kidney, allowed increased transmission
of systemic blood pressure to the renal vasculature. These factors,
perhaps modulated by intrarenal hormones, increase sodium excretion and
thereby mediate the escape from the salt-retaining effects of
mineralocorticoids.

ACKNOWLEDGMENTS

Studies from the author's laboratory were supported by NIH grant
HL14133 and the Mayo Foundation.

REFERENCES

1. Ragan, C., Ferrebee, J.W., Phyfe, P., Atchley, D.W., Loeb, R.F. (1940)
   A syndrome of polydipsia and polyuria induced in normal animals by
   desoxycorticosterone acetate. Am. J. Physiol. 131,73-78.

2. Clinton, M., Thorn, G.W. (1943) Effect of desoxycorticosterone acetate
   administration on plasma volume and electrolyte balance of normal human
   subjects. Bull. Johns Hopkins Hosp. 72,255-264.

3. August, J.L., Nelson, D.H., Thorn, G.W. (1958) Response of normal subjects to large amounts of aldosterone. J. Clin. Invest. 37,1549-1555.

4. Relman, A.S., Schwartz, W.B. (1952) The effect of DOCA on electrolyte
   balance in normal man and its relation to sodium chloride intake. Yale
   J. Biol. Med. 24,540-558.

5. Knox, F.G., Burnett, J.C., Jr., Kohan, D.E., Spielman, W.S., Strand,
   J.C. (1980) Escape from the sodium-retaining effects of
   mineralocorticoids. Kidney Int. 17,263-276.

6. O'Neil, R.G., Helman, S.I. (1977) Transport characteristics of renal
   collecting tubules: Influences of DOCA and diet. Am. J. Physiol.
   232,F544-F558.

7. Schacht, R.G., Lowenstein, J., Baldwin, D.S. (1971) Renal mechanism for
   DOCA escape in man. Bull. NY Acad. Med. 47,1233

8. Wright, F.S., Knox, F.G., Howards, S.S., Berliner, R.W. (1969) Reduced
   sodium reabsorption by the proximal tubule of DOCA-escaped dogs. Am.
   J. Physiol. 216,869-875.

9. Knox, F.G, Schneider, E.G., Dresser, R.P., Lynch, R.E. (1970)
   Natriuretic effect of increased proximal delivery in dogs with salt
   retention. Am. J. Physiol. 219,904-910.

10. Rastegar, A., Agus, Z., Connor, T.B., Goldberg, M. (1972) Renal
    handling of calcium and phosphate during mineralocorticoid "escape" in
    man. Kidney Int. 2,279-286.

11. Knox, F.G. (1973) Role of the proximal tubule in the regulation of uri-
    nary sodium excretion. Mayo Clinic Proc. 48,565-573.

12. Sonnenberg, H. (1973) Proximal and distal tubular function in salt-
    deprived and in salt-loaded deoxycorticosterone acetate-escaped rats.
    J. Clin. Invest. 52,263-273.

13. Haas, J.A., Berndt, T., Knox, F.G. (1979) Collecting duct function in
    desoxycorticosterone-treated rats. J. Clin. Invest. 63,211-214.

14. Biglieri, E.G., Forsham, P.H. (1961) Studies on the expanded extra-
    cellular fluid and the responses to various stimuli in primary
    aldosteronism. Am. J. Med. 30,564-576.

15. Levinsky, N.G., LaLone, R.C. (1963) Mechanism of sodium diuresis after
    saline infusion in the dog. J. Clin. Invest. 42,1261-1276.

16. Davis, J.O., Holman, J.E., Carpenter, C.C.J., Urquhart, J., Higgins, J.T., Jr. (1965) Effects of saline infusion on sodium reabsorption by proximal tubule of dog. J. Clin. Invest. 4,1160-1170.

17. Zipser, R.D., Speckart, F.J. (1978) "Normolensine" primary aldosteronism. Ann. Int. Med. 88,655-656.

18. Higgins, J.T.,Jr. (1970) Escape from sodium-retaining effects of deoxy-corticosterone in hypotensive and hypertensive dogs. Proc. Soc. Exp. Biol. Med. 134,768-772.

19. Marchand, G.R. (1978) Interstitial pressure during volume expansion at reduced renal artery pressure. Am. J. Physiol. 235,F209-F212.

20. Hall, J.E., Guyton, A.C., Trippodo, N.C., Lohmeier, T.E., McCaa, R.E., Cowley, A.W.,Jr. (1977) Intrarenal control of electrolyte excretion by angiotensin II. Am. J. Physiol. 232,F538-F544.

21. Waugh, W.H. (1971) Angiotensin II: Local renal effects of physiological increments in concentration. Can. J. Physiol. Pharmacol. 50,711-716.

22. Fagard, R.H., Cowley, A.W., Jr., Navar, L.G., Langford, H.G., Guyton, A.C. (1976) Renal responses to slight elevations of renal arterial plasma angiotensin II concentration in dogs. Clin. Exptl. Pharmacol. Physiol. 3,531-538.

23. Harris, P.J., Young, H.A. (1977) Dose dependent stimulation and inhibition of proximal tubular sodium reabsorption by angiotensin II in the rat kidney. Pfluegers Arch. 367,295-297.

24. Johnston, C.I., Davis, J.O., Robb, C.A. MacKensie, J.W. (1968) Plasma renin in chronic experimental heart failure and during renal sodium escape from mineralocorticoids. Circ. Res. 22,113-125.

25. Pearce, J.W., Sonnenberg, H. (1965) Effects of spinal section and renal denervation on the renal response to blood volume expansion. Can. J. Physiol. Pharmacol. 43,211-224.

26. McDonald, K.M., Rosenthal, A., Schrier, R.W., Galicich, J., Lauler, D.P. (1970) Effect of interruption of neural pathways on renal response to volume expansion. Am. J. Physiol. 218,510-517.

27. Muller,J., Barajas, L. (1972) Electron microscopic and histochemical evidence for a tubular innervation in the renal cortex of the monkey. J. Ultrastruct. Res. 41,533-549.

28. Bencsath, P., Bonvalet, J-P., de Rouffignac, C. (1972) Tubular factors in denervation diuresis and natriuresis. IN: Recent Advances in Renal Handling of Sodium. ed. J. Wirz, F. Spinelli, Basel, Kargar. p 96.

29. Bencsath, P., Kottra, G., Szalay, L., Takach, L. (1977) Micropuncture study on the effect of chronic renal sympathectomy in the anesthetized rat. Proc. XXVII Internat. Cong. Physiol. Sciences, Paris, 13,66.

30. Ljungqvist, A. (1975) The effect of angiotensin infusion, sodium loading and sodium restriction on the renal and cardiac adrenergic nerves. Acta. Pathol. Microbiol. Scand. 83,661-668.

31. Katholi, R.E., Naftilan, A.J., Oparil, S. (1980) Importance of renal sympathetic tone in the development of DOCA-salt hypertension in the rat. Hypertension 2,266-273.

32. Adetuyibi, A., Mills, I.H. (1972) Relation between urinary kallikrein and renal function, hypertension, and excretion of sodium and water in man. The Lancet 2,203-207.

33. Margolius, H.S., Geller, R., deJong, W., Pisano, J.J., Sjoerdsma, A. (1972) Altered urinary kallikrein excretion in rats with hypertension. Circ. Res. 30,358-362.

34. Dusing, R., Gill, J.R., Jr., Bartter, F.C. (1978) The role of prostaglandins in the renal response to desoxycortisterone (DOCA) in the dog. Am. Soc. Neph. 11th Ann. Mtg., New Orleans, La., 59A.

35. Youngberg, S.P., Marchand, G.R., Romero, J.C., Knox, F.G. (1977) Mineralocorticoid escape: the role of prostaglandins. Fed. Proc. 36,627.

36. Youngberg, S.P., Marchand, G.R., Haas, J.A., Romero, J.C., Knox, F.G. (1977) The role of prostaglandins (PG) in the nephrogenic diabetes insipidus (DI)-like state following prolonged administration of minera-locorticoids (MC). Clin. Res. 25,509.

37. Zipser, R.D., Zia, P., Stone, R.A., Horton, R. (1978) The prostaglandin and kallikrein-kinin systems in mineralocorticoid escape. J. Clin. Endo. Metab. 47,996-1001.

38. deWardener, H.E. (1977) Natriuretic hormone. Clin. Sci. Mol. Med. 53,1-8.

39. Kaloyanides, G.J., Azer, M. (1971) Evidence for a humoral mechanism in volume expansion natriuresis. J. Clin. Invest. 51,1603-1612.

40. Sonnenberg, J., Verees, A.T., Pearce, J.W. (1972) A humoral component of the natriuretic mechanism in sustained blood volume expansion. J. Clin. Invest. 51,2631-2644.

41. Pearce, J.W., Veress, A.T. (1975) Concentration and bioassay of a natriuretic factor in plasma of volume expanded rats. Can. J. Physiol. Pharmacol. 53,742-747.

42. Buckalew, V.M., Jr., Lancaster, C.D., Jr. (1972) The association of a humoral sodium transport inhibitory activity with renal escape from chronic mineralocorticoid administration in the dog. Clin. Soc. 42,69-78.

43. Smith, H.W. (1957) Salt and water volume receptor. Am. J. Med. 23,623-652.

Hormonal Regulation of Sodium Excretion,
B. Lichardus, R.W. Schrier and J. Ponec, eds.
© 1980 Elsevier/North-Holland Biomedical Press

HAVE RENAL NERVES A MAJOR ROLE IN CONTROL OF SODIUM EXCRETION ?

JANUSZ SADOWSKI, JAN KURKUS and RYSZARD GELLERT
Department of Applied Physiology, Medical Research Centre
of the Polish Academy of Sciences, and Department of Medicine,
Warsaw Medical School, Warsaw /Poland/

INTRODUCTION

Despite many decades of experimental studies the phenomenon of denervation diuresis and natriuresis and the role of renal nerves in physiological control of sodium excretion remain controversial. To Homer W. Smith[1] the denervation natriuresis was nothing more than an artifact, obtained only when sympathetic tonus to the kidney is augmented and renal hemodynamics are depressed by anesthesia and surgical trauma. He argued that in conscious undisturbed animals the sympathetic input to the kidney is so slight that denervation does not lead to any increase in renal blood flow or glomerular filtration rate; hence, no denervation diuresis or natriuresis develops. Smith's criticism of experiments using anesthetized and traumatized animals did not curtail further studies which focused on elucidation of the intrarenal mechanism underlying denervation natriuresis. There was an uncertainty if it was due exclusively to higher filtration rate on the denervated side or inhibition of tubular reabsorption was also involved. This question could not be satisfactorily settled until new refined techniques were applied, including micropuncture and renal nerve stimulation. As pointed out in recent reviews[2,3,4], it was demonstrated that, at least in anesthetized animals, increased renal nerve activity enhances tubular reabsorption of sodium chloride while renal denervation results in a defect of reabsorption. Before these results are recognized as exposing an important mechanism in the overall complex control of sodium excretion, they need to be confirmed in absence of anesthesia and acute surgery. A review of such attempts shows that earlier studies with unanesthetized animals were few in number and furnished contradictory results[5]. A thorough study of effects of extracellular volume expansion and hemorrhage on the function of the innervated and denervated kidney was recently reported by Lifschitz[6]. He concluded that renal nerves do not influence kidney response to these two conditions.

During the past few years effects of renal denervation on renal function of conscious dogs were extensively studied in our laboratory. Those data from our research which bear directly on the issue of the control of sodium excretion are outlined below.

DENERVATION NATRIURESIS IN CONSCIOUS DOGS: ROLE OF GFR
AND TUBULAR REABSORPTION

In order to investigate the functional role of renal nerves in conscious undisturbed animals we performed clearance experiments

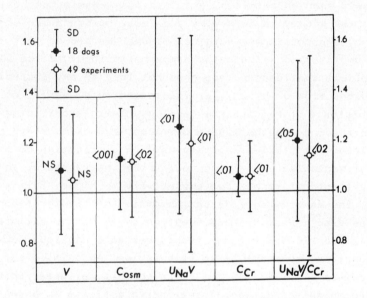

Fig. 1. Denervated-to-innervated kidney ratios for basic renal function parameters /means ± SD/. P values refer to the difference of mean ratios from 1.0 i.e. the value representing equal function of both kidneys.

in dogs with one kidney chronically denervated and the urinary bladder surgically divided. Polyethylene cannulas implanted into two hemibladders enabled separate urine collection from each kidney. To achieve complete denervation, all the visible nerve fibers entering the hilum were excised and the adventitia was stripped off the renal artery. Subsequently, the artery was thoroughly coated with 10% phenol solution in absolute ethanol and then exposed to phenol for at least 20 min. This mode of denervation resulted in a complete disappearance of renal tissue norepinephrine when tested several weeks later.

The results of preliminary studies designed to compare the function of the denervated and innervated kidney in so prepared dogs have already been published[5]. The full expanded data are presented in Fig. 1 which shows denervated-to-innervated kidney ratios / D/I / for basic renal function parameters measured in 49 experiments with 18 moderately hydrated dogs.

It is seen that for osmolar clearance $/C_{osm}/$, exogenous creatinine clearance $/C_{cr}/$ and sodium excretion expressed in absolute terms $/U_{Na}V/$ or corrected to 100 ml glomerular filtrate $/U_{Na}V/C_{cr}/$, mean D/I ratios were significantly higher than 1.0, indicating predominance of the denervated kidney. This was the case regardless of the variant of analysis applied: with each experiment treated as an individual item /n = 49/ or using means for each dog /n = 18/. However, it should be noticed that this predominance was only slight as the denervated kidney excreted but 1.15 to 1.3 times more sodium than the innervated organ. Furthermore, fairly large standard deviations surpassing the unity or equality axis indicate that in many experiments it was the innervated kidney which actually showed higher sodium excretion.

Since GFR was slightly but significantly higher on the denervated side, the data cannot answer the question whether the "denervation natriuresis" was related to a defect of reabsorption or reflected higher filtration rate of the denervated organ. An attempt to approach this question by comparing D/I ratios for GFR and $U_{Na}V$ in individual experiments is presented in Table 1.

It shows that a total of 30 experiments from quadrants /2/ and /3/ of the Table display a usual correlation: higher GFR of the denervated kidney is associated with higher $U_{Na}V$, and lower GFR with lower $U_{Na}V$. The 10 experiments of the quadrant /1/ are of more interest as here relatively higher $U_{Na}V$ of the denervated kidney was associated with its lower GFR. Accordingly, this group lends support to the view that a defect of tubular reabsorption is involved in the mechanism of natriuresis. However, the impact

TABLE 1

ANALYSIS OF INDIVIDUAL D/I RATIOS FOR $U_{Na}V$ AND GFR

Three experiments in which D/I equalled 1.0 are not included

$U_{Na}V$	Glomerular filtration rate	
	D/I < 1.0	D/I > 1.0
D/I > 1.0	/1/ 10 experiments in 9 dogs	/2/ 21 experiments in 13 dogs
D/I < 1.0	/3/ 9 experiments in 6 dogs	/4/ 6 experiments in 5 dogs

of this evidence is somewhat diminished by the six experiments of quadrant /4/ in which lower $U_{Na}V$ of the denervated kidney was associated with higher GFR. One would wish to regard such results as "aberrant" but, if so assumed, how many experiments of quadrant /1/ are also aberrant rather than indicative of tubular nature of natriuresis ? It is clear that by those favorably inclined to reabsorption defect hypothesis such results can be regarded as supporting their view while someone more skeptical would have ample basis for stressing the role of renal hemodynamics.

Irrespective of the underlying mechanism, the data show that in conscious dogs denervation natriuresis is quantitatively much less pronounced than that described in anesthetized animals subjected to surgical trauma.

A SEARCH FOR A DEFECT OF PROXIMAL REABSORPTION

Since micropuncture experiments have shown that the crucial change in the profuse denervation natriuresis of anesthetized animals is a defect of reabsorption in the proximal tubule[7,8], we made an attempt to estimate and compare proximal transport of the denervated and innervated kidney in our conscious dogs, using indirect methods that could be applied in chronic studies/J. Sadowski and J. Kurkus, Pfluegers Archiv,submitted for publication/

Experiments with water diuresis

In one series of experiments maximal water diuresis was induced by an oral water load of 35 ml/kg body wt followed by iv infusion of 3% glucose at 9 ml/min. This proved an effective means of inhibiting ADH release, for urine osmolality fell to about 70 mosm/kg H_2O and free water clearance $/C_{H_2O}/$ reached about 8 ml/100 ml glomerular filtrate per kidney. In such an experiment the absence of ADH and a reduction of renal medullary tissue hypertonicity both contribute to an inhibition of a major part of water backdiffusion in the distal and collecting tubule. Then C_{H_2O} may be used as a measure of NaCl reabsorbed from the ascending limb of Henle's loop and more distal tubule segments while sodium clearance $/C_{Na}/$ represents NaCl which escapes reabsorption. Consequently, $C_{H_2O} + C_{Na}$ is an index of sodium chloride delivery to the distal nephron.

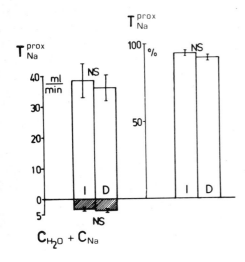

Fig. 2. Experiments with water diuresis. Distal Na delivery $/C_{H_2O} + C_{Na}$, hatched blocks/ and proximal Na transport of innervated /I/ and denervated /D/ kidney. The right diagram shows fractional proximal reabsorption of two kidneys /means±SE/.

Fig. 2 shows that in our experiments the distal delivery was quite similar for the innervated and denervated kidney and there was no significant difference between the respective proximal transport values estimated as GFR $-/C_{H_2O} + C_{Na}/$. The fractional proximal transport rates were also very close and not significantly different. An inspection of Fig. 2 shows that application of $C_{H_2O} + C_{Na}$ as a measure of distal delivery yielded an unrealistic estimate of fractional reabsorption, of about 90% of the filtered load. This was obviously due to the fact that even in absence of ADH some backdiffusion of water beyond the diluting sites does occur; hence, $C_{H_2O} + C_{Na}$ underestimates the magnitude of distal NaCl delivery and, accordingly, GFR $-/C_{H_2O} + C_{Na}/$over-estimates proximal reabsorption. However, provided that denerva-tion does not alter permeability of the distal nephron to water or hypertonicity of the renal medullary tissue, this methodologi-cal drawback might not seriously influence the validity of compa-ring the calculated reabsorption rates of the innervated and de-nervated kidney. Indeed, we found that antidiuretic responses of the two kidneys to exogenous vasopressin were quite similar, sug-gesting no change in tubule permeability or osmolality of the re-nal medullary interstitium.

Experiments with blockade of distal NaCl transport

Fifteen years ago Earley et al.[9] showed that simultaneous ad-ministration of ethacrynic acid and chlorothiazide to anestheti-zed dogs induces a virtually complete blockade of the distal tu-bular reabsorption of NaCl. The first agent apparently abolished transport in the ascending limb of Henle's loop while the other interfered with reabsorption at more distal sites. We applied such treatment in our conscious unilaterally renal-denervated dogs and, assuming total distal blockade, calculated proximal re-absorption by subtracting $U_{Na}V$ from the filtered sodium load .

Fig. 3 shows that during infusion of the two diuretics the fractional sodium reabsorption averaged 66% of the filtered load $/F_{Na}/$. This is equal to the value reported from distal blockade experiments of Earley et al.[9] and compares satisfactorily with the data from dog micropuncture studies[10]. Quite remarkably, there was no difference in the so calculated proximal sodium re-absorption between the innervated and denervated kidney. Fig. 3 shows also that water reabsorption was in these experiments inhi-bited almost equally as sodium, in spite of the presence of ADH. This was probably due to extremely high rates of tubular fluid flow along the collecting system. Again, there was no difference in "proximal" water reabsorption between the intact and denerva-ted kidney.

As a whole, both the water diuresis and distal blockade stu-dies failed to demonstrate any major inhibition of proximal

transport related to denervation of the kidney. Since clearance
studies have limited sensitivity, a small reabsorption defect
cannot be excluded. However, the data strongly suggest that under
basal conditions neural influences on renal tubular sodium reabsorption have no great importance for the control of sodium excretion.

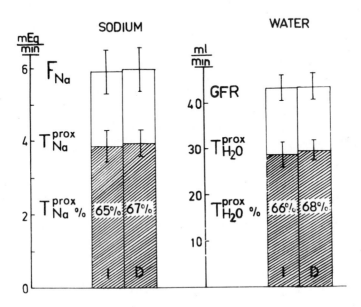

Fig. 3. Blockade of distal reabsorption with ethacrynic acid and
chlorothiazide. Filtered Na load /F_{Na}/, proximal reabsorption
/hatched area/, absolute and fractional, for innervated /I/ and
denervated /D/ kidney. On the right filtration and reabsorption
of water /means ± SE/.

RENAL NERVES IN VOLUME EXPANSION NATRIURESIS

We know from micropuncture experiments that both in the natriuresis of renal denervation observed in anesthetized animals[7,8]
and in that produced by volume expansion the crucial change is
a transport defect in the proximal tubule[11]. In the anesthetized
rat the two effects: of denervation and of volume expansion, were
reported to be additive[12]. The purpose of a part of our studies
was to assess the natriuretic response of the innervated and denervated kidney of conscious dogs to isotonic volume expansion
with saline[13].

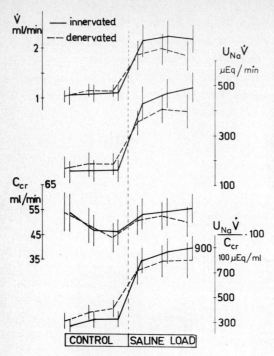

Fig. 4. Denervated and in-nervated kidney responses to saline load in six cons-cious dogs. All post-saline increments except C_{cr} chan-ge of the denervated kidney were significant /p <0.05 or less/ /means ± SE/.

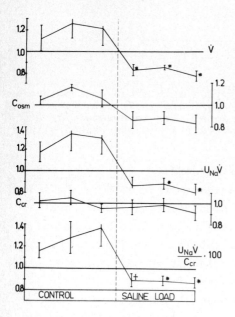

Fig. 5. Saline-induced changes in denervated-to-innervated kid-ney ratios for six conscious dogs. Asterisks and a cross indi-cate significant changes in mean D/I value compared to mean cont-rol ratio /means ± SE/.

After obtaining control data in standard clearance experiments, a load of 0.81% saline, 35 ml/kg body wt, was given iv during 15 min, followed by a maintenance saline infusion at 9 ml/min. When urine flow stabilized at a new high level, at least three clearance periods were made during sustained saline diuresis. Fig. 4 gives a comparison of intact and denervated kidney responses to saline load. In control periods $U_{Na}V/C_{cr}$ was here insignificantly higher on the denervated side. Both kidneys responded to saline with profuse natriuresis but after the load it was the intact kidney which excreted slightly more Na. The significance of this shift in relative natriuresis from the denervated to intact kidney can be best assessed through analysis of D/I ratios as illustrated in Fig. 5. It shows that after saline D/I values for urine flow and $U_{Na}V$ were significantly lower than in control periods. In additional experiments we observed an even greater fall in D/I ratios for anesthetized dogs[13].

Interpretation of the change from natriuresis of denervated kidney before saline loading to relative antinatriuresis after saline is not immediately obvious. It is known that acute volume expansion can depress renal nerve activity in rats[3,14], rabbits[15], dogs[16] and cats[17]. Possibly, in our experiments the innervated kidney responded to saline loading with a greater increment in $U_{Na}V$ because the overall response included a small but significant component relative to a fall in renal nerve activity, with an attendant increase in GFR and/or a decrease in reabsorption. The depression of renal nerves by acute volume expansion /"acute functional denervation"/ would be even more pronounced in anesthesia when control sympathetic tonus is higher; hence, a greater fall in D/I ratio after Na loading in anesthetized dogs[13].

It is seen that although, rather paradoxically, the principal finding of these experiments was greater saline diuresis of the innervated kidney, the observation is consistent with a modest but definite contribution of renal nerves to the natriuresis which follows acute massive extracellular volume expansion. It remains to be established if this effect would be important in regulation of body sodium and fluid balance with less extreme changes in extracellular volume.

ACKNOWLEDGEMENTS

The excellent technical assistance in our experiments of Mrs. Jadwiga Zwolińska is greatly appreciated.

All the studies described in the present paper were supported from the state's research problem grant No. 10.4

Sodium etacrynate /Sodium Edecrin^R/ and chlorothiazide /Diuril^R/ were generously supplied by Merck, Sharp and Dohme, West Point, Pennsylvania, U.S.A.

REFERENCES

1. Smith, H.W. /1951/ The Kidney, Oxford, New York, pp.411-460.

2. Di Bona, G.F. /1977/ Amer. J. Physiol. 233, F73-F81.

3. Colindres, R.E. and Gottschalk, C.W. /1978/ Fed. Proc. 37, 1218-1221.

4. Takacs, L. et al. /1978/ Proc. 7th Internat. Congr. Nephrol. Karger, Basel, pp. 553-558.

5. Sadowski, J. et al. /1979/ Arch. Internat. Physiol. Bioch. 87, 663-672.

6. Lifschitz, M.D. /1978/ Clin. Sci. Mol. Med. 54, 567-572.

7. Bencsath, P. et al. /1972/ Recent Advances in Renal Physiology /ed. Wirz, H., Spinelli, F./ Karger, Basel, pp. 96-106.

8. Bello-Reuss, E. et al. /1975/ J. Clin. Invest. 56, 208-217.

9. Earley, L.E. et al. /1966/ J. Clin. Invest. 45, 1668-1684.

10. Bennet, C.M. et al. /1967/ Amer. J. Physiol. 213, 1254-1262.

11. Dirks, J.H. et al. /1965/ J. Clin. Invest. 44, 1160-1170.

12. Bello-Reuss, E. et al. /1977/ Amer. J. Physiol. 232, F26-F32.

13. Sadowski, J. et al. /1979/ Amer. J. Physiol. 237, F262-F267.

14. Kottra, G. et al. /1978/ Acta Physiol. Acad. Sci. Hungar. 51, 142.

15. Clement, D.L. /1972/ Circ. Res. 31, 824-830.

16. Judy, W.V. et al. /1971/ Physiologist 14, 169.

17. Schad, H. and Seller, H. /1976/ Pfluegers Arch. 363, 155-159.

Hormonal Regulation of Sodium Excretion,
B. Lichardus, R.W. Schrier and J. Ponec, eds.
© 1980 Elsevier/North-Holland Biomedical Press

CATECHOLAMINES AND SODIUM EXCRETION

Andrew Baines and Nikolas Morgunov
Department of Clinical Biochemistry, University of Toronto,
100 College St., Toronto, Ontario, Canada, M5G 1L5.

INTRODUCTION

There is now no doubt that renal nerves and the sympathetic nervous system (SNS) influence sodium excretion.[20] This influence is evident in sodium retaining disease states. For example renal denervation, ganglionic blockade and intrarenal α-adrenergic blockade all increase sodium excretion from animals with low-output circulatory failure.[17] Furthermore, β-blockade reduces the sodium retention produced by chronic bile duct ligation.[44]

Guyton's portrait of the kidney as ultimate regulator of blood pressure has made us aware that the balance between sodium excretion and arterial pressure must be reset in hypertensive individuals.[21] Evidence of the significant role played by catecholamines (CATS) and renal nerves in this process is found in animal models of hypertension as well as in the fact that human hypertension responds to sympatholytic therapy. Norepinephrine (N) infused chronically into the renal artery produces hypertension and resets the pressure-natriuresis curve.[13] The same dose of N given intravenously does not exert a pressor effect. A specific role for renal nerves is evident from the observation that renal denervation slows the onset of hypertension in rats with spontaneous[28] or DOCA-salt hypertension.[26] These observations and others, to be discussed, indicate an intimate connection between CATS in the kidney and glomerulotubular Na balance.

To thoroughly review CATS and Na excretion would require discussion of systemic volume and baroreceptors and the integrative brain centres with their modulation of SNS activity.

Space limits us to an examination of interactions between Na^+ excretion and the three renal CAT inputs: renal nerves, circulating CATS and arteriovenous anastomoses between adrenal and kidney. It should be remembered that CATS are outnumbered considerably by other neurotransmitters including amino acids, peptides and nucleotides. Some effects associated with neural stimulation or denervation may be produced by non-CAT neuro-transmitters.

Renal Nerves. Chronic denervation (DNX) of a rat kidney reduced norepinephrine (N) and dopamine (D) delivery to renal venous plasma and urine.[42] Reduced urinary CAT excretion was evident in both hydropenic (HY) and volume-expanded (VE) states (10% bodyweight with 0.15M saline) but the difference between innervated (INX) and DNX was reduced in the latter case. Epine-phrine (E) excretion from both INN and DNX kidneys was the same.

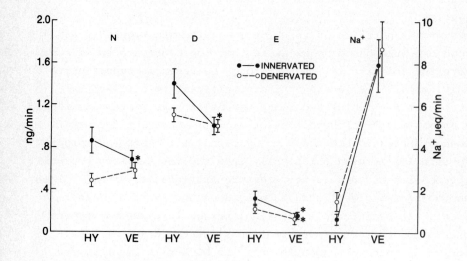

Fig.1. CAT & Na excretion by INN & DNX kidneys. *$p < 0.05$.

Response to neurally released CATS depends upon their con-centrations at receptor sites within and outside the neural cleft; therefore, it is important to know what these concentra-tions are.

Neurotransmitters in a neural cleft may be transported back into the nerve or enter the target tissue or diffuse laterally into the surrounding tissue. Lateral diffusion is proportional to cleft width.[9] Neural clefts are wide in the adventitia of large arteries and veins, similar to those found in the cortico-medullary area. Here CAT concentrations rise inside and outside the cleft to the same level (10^{-7}M) during strong electrical stimulation.[9] Neural junctions with renal arterioles and tubules are narrow (1000-6000 Å)[6]; concentrations outside 1000 Å clefts may be only 6 x 10^{-9}M when concentrations within are 10^{-5}M.[9]

In the kidney CATS diffuse from neural clefts into vascular lumens, lymphatics or peritubular fluid. From peritubular fluid they are secreted probably into the proximal tubule.[5] After entering the tubular fluid by secretion or glomerular filtration, CATS are unlikely to re-enter the general circulation.[5]

The fate of CATS which diffuse into the peritubular cortical space can be followed by microinjecting radioactive CATS beneath the capsule of one kidney and collecting urine from both kidneys. With this approach we showed that N and D secretion is inhibited by raising the concentration of circulating D (fig 2).

From the quantity of radioactivity entering the ipsilateral urine corrected for recirculation, we estimated fractional secretion rates for endogenous CATS in anesthetized diuretic rats: 20±4% for N, 66±4% for D and 47±1% for E. Tubular secretion of labelled CAT was not altered by chronic DNX. Earlier studies, in which radioactive CATS were microinjected into peritubular capillaries, yielded lower secretion rates.[5] The relative orders of magnitude for N and E excretion agree with those derived from labelled CAT clearance by isolated perfused rat kidneys.[40] During the secretion process CATS were methylated and to a lesser extent deaminated.[5,40] The methylated metabolites were also secreted.[5]

Although we know the amounts of N and D escaping from renal neural clefts we do not know what fraction this constitutes of the total released. We can measure the rate of escape in 3 ways.

Neural CAT escape was estimated from the difference in urinary CAT excretion (UCAT) by INN and DNX kidneys. |Neural escape = UCAT (INN-DNX) ÷ fractional secretion of labelled CAT|. According to this method renal nerves of VE rats release N

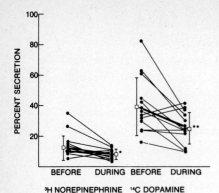

PERCENT SECRETION

BEFORE   DURING   BEFORE   DURING

³H NOREPINEPHRINE   ¹⁴C DOPAMINE

Fig.2. Tubular secretion of ³H-N and ¹⁴C-D before and during intravenous infusion of non-labelled D at 0.1-0.3uM/min. *p<0.05 ** <0.01

at 0.9±0.2 and D at 0.4±0.1 ng/min. N and D escape from renal nerves is increased 25% and 50% respectively by baroreflex stimulation (carotid artery ligation).[33] Another estimate of neural CAT escape was obtained from endogenous UCAT and renal venous plasma CAT in INN and chronically DNX kidneys. |Neural escape = (renal plasma flow (RPF) x venous CAT + UCAT) - (RPF x arterial CAT)|. According to this equation non-diuretic kidneys release N at 0.8±0.3 and D at 0.4±0.1 ng/min. In the absence of renal nerves no N is released by the kidney. However, the DNX kidney continues to release D at 0.7±0.1 ng/min. Therefore 50% or more of urinary D is produced by non-neuronal sources in the kidney.

N escape calculated by both methods agrees well with N turnover of 1.2±0.1 ng/min in kidneys of conscious rats after inhibition of N synthesis with α-methyl-p-tyrosine. (M. Sole, pers. com.). These release rates can be compared with those found in the densely innervated saphenous vein which contains 30 times more N/g than renal tissue. Strips of vein stimulated electrically (9 volts,5Hz,2msec) release 6 ng N/g tissue/minute. This is only 6 times the race of release in kidneys. Thus it appears that renal nerves are among the more active nerves of the body; this probably ensures high CAT concentrations not only within neural clefts but also in the area around the cleft.

A constant high CAT turnover may explain neural D production in the kidney, since noradrenergic terminals become partially dopaminergic when nerve impulse flow is markedly increased.[41] The response of conscious rats to a high salt diet is consistent with this explanation for neural D production. Such a diet produced an increase in both N and D excretion. (Table 1)

TABLE 1

DAILY CATECHOLAMINE EXCRETION/KIDNEY

Rats fed a low salt diet with distilled water (LS) or 0.15M
saline (HS) or 5% glucose (GL) or 0.15M $NaHCO_3$ (BI) for 7-9 days.

Diet	N ng/min	D ng/min	Na uEq/min	H_2O ul/min	pH
LS	0.16±.01	0.80±.06	0.10±.03	5±1	6.67±.13
HS	0.22±.01*	1.21±.06*	2.33±.87*	10±5*	6.26±.17*
GL	0.36±.16*	1.39±.20*	0.04±.01	26±6*	6.30±.70
BI	0.22±.03	0.98±.16*	3.46±.75	20±7	8.20±.20*

*$p < 0.05$ t-test comparing LS-HS, LS-GL, HS-BI.

These results and others in the literature suggest that
urine flow, urine pH[38] and carbohydrate[15] as well as salt intake
modify CAT excretion.

Intrarenal CAT concentration. Lower bounds for intrarenal
concentrations can be obtained from renal lymph and venous
plasma. Under basal conditions in Inactin-anesthetized rats
renal venous and lymph concentrations of N and D in INN kidneys
were similar to arterial concentrations (fig 3). Vagotomy
stimulated renal nerves and increased N but not D or E concentrations.

Canine renal venous N + E concentration was slightly lower
than the arterial level in the basal anesthetized state but
rose to 7×10^{-8}M when electrical nerve stimulation was associated with a 90% decrease in RPF.[12] The same escape rate
into a kidney with normal RPF would produce 1/10th this venous
concentration. From this we conclude that in kidneys with
normal RPF CAT concentrations are high only in the immediate
vicinity of neural clefts.

An estimate of cortical CAT concentration under stress was
obtained by measuring the fluid exuded from the decapsulated
surface of dog kidneys. Atrial fibrillation raised N and E
concentration in this fluid from arterial levels to 8×10^{-9}M.
This concentration is below the threshold for effects on isolated proximal tubules,[7] vide infra.

Renal venous and lymph concentrations are consistent with

a vascular site for D release. D concentration in venous plasma from INN kidneys was slightly higher than in arterial plasma. Denervation lowers venous D concentration considerably. D concentration in lymph from INN kidneys was less than or equal to arterial concentrations even when renal nerves were stimulated. In contrast, N concentrations during stimulation were higher in lymph than in plasma which may indicate a peritubular site of release (fig 3).

Of course a number of other factors influence CAT concentrations in venous plasma and lymph. Among these factors are: higher protein concentrations in plasma than in lymph and therefore more bound catecholamine in plasma[37]; higher tubular secretion rates for D than for N and therefore more effective clearance of D from peritubular fluid; different drainage patterns for lymph and venous plasma.

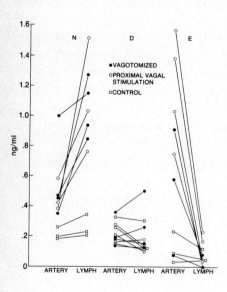

Fig.3. CAT concentrations in femoral artery and renal lymph[22] of HY rats. Lymph protein 1.0±.1 g%.

Another important influence on intrarenal D concentration is production by non-neuronal tissue. Acid labile conjugates of D[20] or free L-DOPA[4] or both may be the source of urinary and renal venous D produced by non-neuronal tissue in the kidney. Circulating free endogenous DOPA could provide 30% or more of total urinary D[4]. We find that acute adrenalectomy does not reduce urinary D excretion, therefore the adrenal is not a major source of urinary D under basal conditions.[21,41] Nonetheless there is, with circulating DOPA and conjugated D, a plethora of sources for non-neuronal D production.

It is evident to the naked eye that there are anastomoses between adrenal gland and kidney.[16,27] Flow in these vessels may go in either direction and may be regulated to vary the interchange of hormones.[16,27] So far the only direct evidence for the physiological significance of these anastomoses comes from finding high E concentration in subcapsular fluid following intense SNS stimulation.[27] The anastomoses could also provide a route for renal D to enter the adrenal. Perhaps it is via this pathway that D travels to inhibit angiotensin stimulated aldosterone secretion.[10]

We found no evidence of E entering rat kidneys directly from the adrenal gland. Our rats were prepared for micropuncture by removing the adrenal from its renal attachments; the opposite kidney was left untouched. There was no difference in E excretion from the two kidneys under basal conditions but we have not tested the effect of SNS stimuli.

<u>Circulating Catecholamines</u>.

Threshold concentrations for vascular reactivity to catecholamines in vitro are in the order of $10^{-8}M$[9] and those for tubular reabsorption are $10^{-7}M$ in isolated perfused tubules[7] and $10^{-8}M$ or less in isolated perfused rat kidneys.[8] Circulating concentrations of N and E are normally one to two orders of magnitude less than this although with extreme stress concentrations may rise to $10^{-8}M$. Nonetheless N infused in vivo at rates which raise plasma concentrations by only $2.5 \times 10^{-9}M$ produces changes in vascular resistance.[23]

N infused into rats at 1-4 µg/kg/min raised systemic pressure by 20 mmHg and increased renovascular resistance in rats.[4,35] The resulting pressure natriuresis was converted to an antinatriuresis when perfusion pressure was kept constant with an adjustable clamp about the abdominal aorta.[4] High concentrations of circulating N did not increase fractional reabsorption and may even have reduced absolute reabsorption rate from the proximal tubule and Henle's loop (fig 4). Despite this lack of effect there was a significant decrease in fractional sodium excretion.[4] Undetectable decreases in GFR may have reduced sodium excretion but it is also possible that N stimulated salt reabsorption distal to Henle's loop. No matter which explanation is true it is evident that proximal tubular reabsorption was not sensitive to large increases in circulating N. This result is to be expected if N receptors on the proximal tubule are located primarily within and adjacent to neural clefts, and are therefore exposed continuously to concentrations in excess of 10^{-8}M.

The rise in vascular resistance shows that renovascular N receptors are sensitive to physiological changes in circulating CATS.

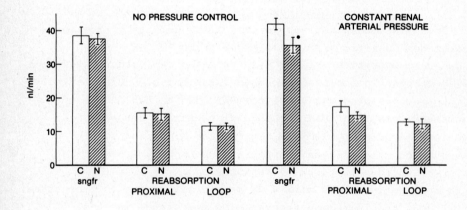

Fig.4. Single nephron glomerular filtration rate and tubular fluid reabsorption rates before (C) and during infusion of N at 1-4 µg/kg/min.

Adrenergic Influence on Na Excretion. N stimulates fluid reabsorption in isolated proximal convoluted rabbit tubules via a β adrenergic mechanism.[7] Sodium reabsorption is stimulated via a β mechanism in isolated perfused rat kidneys but in this tissue the stimulus appears to act on a segment of the distal nephron since free water formation is increased.[8] Chloride transport in the isolated rabbit cortical collecting tubule is also stimulated via a β receptor.[25] These in vitro observations may explain the natriuretic effect of β antago-

nists administered acutely to anesthetized rats.[11] Propra-
nolol's natriuretic effect in water diuretic rats is associated with decreased free water clearance[11] which is consistent
with B mediated Na transport in the distal nephron.

The natriuretic effect of β antagonists suggests that renal
nerves exert a tonic stimulatory action on sodium reabsorption.
In conscious dogs, with unilaterally DNX kidneys, the neural
antinatriuretic effect may be produced by small reductions in
GFR but in anesthetized dogs the effect is clearly tubular as
well as glomerular.[39] Clearance studies on dogs point to α
receptors as the predominant regulators of CAT effects.[17]

Further evidence for an association between neural N release
and renal sodium reabsorption appears when renal nerves are
acutely severed. The resulting natriuresis is accompanied by
a significant decrease in N excretion and a transient increase
in D excretion.[33] Interestingly the contralateral antinatriuretic response which is probably mediated by a reno-renal
neural reflex, is associated with an increase in N excretion
as sodium excretion decreases.[33]

It is clear that renal nerves alone do not play an important
role in the response to large changes in salt or fluid intake.
The response of INN and DNX to volume expansion is almost identical (fig 1). However, the inability of patients with autonomic insufficiency to conserve sodium reveals a role for the
SNS in sodium homeostasis.[43] A similar deficiency in sodium
homeostasis is produced by ganglion blockade[17] but not by α
blockade.[24] Salt depleted patients with autonomic insufficiency could not maintain sodium balance even when they received supplemental mineralocorticoid; they lost sodium at
night. In this context it is interesting to note that β
blockade increases nocturnal sodium excretion.[19]

If the SNS is so important in regulating sodium balance why
do we not find a more pronounced defect in DNX kidneys? The
answer probably can be found in the hypersensitivity to circulating CAT which develops in DNX kidney.[29]

VE reduces traffic in renal nerves and should diminish the
response to denervation, but acute DNX reduces proximal reabsorption to the same extent in VE and HY rats.[20] This surpri-

sing result indicates that the physiological role of renal nerves is far from being understood. Some of the mystery may result from interactions between N and D.

Recent investigations suggest the following roles for D: vasodilator,[2] presynaptic inhibitor of renal nerves,[32] inhibitor of aldosterone formation,[10] stimulator of aldosterone's action on distal Na and K transport,[1] stimulator of renin release. Most of these more or less tentative suggestions assign a natriuretic role to D.

A physiologically significant natriuretic role for D has been deduced from the direct relationship between urinary D and Na excretion in humans.[2] Abnormal D formation has been implicated in the pathogenesis of hypertension[14] and idiopathic edema.[36] However, baroreceptor mediated D release in the rat doesn't produce a natriuresis. Furthermore we find that in the rat D excretion is related to urine flow and pH more than to Na excretion (Table 1).

SUMMARY

Renal nerves release both N and D. N reacts with α or β receptors in proximal and distal parts of the nephron to stimulate Na and Cl reabsorption. Tubular stimulation requires high CAT concentrations and therefore renal nerves probably have only a localized effect on reabsorption. Circulating CATS do not influence proximal reabsorption but they may alter distal reabsorption. Circulating and neurally released CATS alter renal vascular tone probably through α and β stimulation. Under stressful conditions E enters the kidney directly from the adrenal via vascular anastomoses. More than half the D produced in the kidney comes from non-neuronal tissue, but the physiological significance of both neural and non-neural D is unknown.

ACKNOWLEDGEMENTS

This work was supported by the Medical Research Council of Canada and the Kidney Foundation of Canada.

REFERENCES

1. Adam, W.R. and Goland, G. (1979) Clin. Exp. Pharm. Physiol., 6, 631-638.

2. Alexander, R.W., Gill, J.R. Jr., Yamabe, H., Lovenberg, W. and Keiser, H.R. (1974) J. Clin. Invest., 54, 194-200.

3. Baines, A.D. (1978) Kidney Int., 14, 255-262.

4. Baines, A.D. and Chan, W. (1980) Life Sc., 26, 253-259.

5. Baines, A.D., Craan, A., Chan, W. and Morgunov, N. (1979) J. Pharmacol. Exp. Ther., 208, 144-147.

6. Barajas, L. (1978) Fed. Proc., 37, 1192-1201.

7. Bello-Reuss, E. (1980) Amer. J. Physiol. 238, F347-F352.

8. Besarab, A., Silva, P., Landsberg, L. and Epstein, F.M. (1977) Amer. J. Physiol., 233, F39-F45.

9. Bevan, J.A. (1979) Circ. Res., 45, 161-171.

10. Carey, R.M., Thorner, O. and Ortt, E.M. (1979) J. Clin. Invest., 63, 727-735.

11. Carrara, M.C. and Baines, A.D. (1976) Can. J. Physiol. Pharm., 54, 683-691.

12. Carriere, S. (1978) Kidney Int., 14, 692.

13. Cowley, A.W. and Lohmeier, T.E. (1979) Hypertension, 1, 549-558.

14. Cuche, J.L., Kuchel, O., Barbeau, A., Langlois, Y., Boucher, R. and Genest, J. (1974) Circ. Res., 35, 281-289.

15. DeHaven, J., Sherwin, R., Hendler, R. and Felig, P. (1980) New Eng. J. Med., 302, 477-482.

16. Dempster, W.J. (1978) Jap. Heart J., 19, 426-433.

17. DiBona, G.F. (1977) Amer. J. Physiol., 233, F73-F81.

18. Dinerstein, R.J., Vannice, J., Henderson, R.C., Roth, L.J., Goldberg, L.I. and Hoffman, P.C. (1979) Science, 205, 497-499.

19. Epstein, S.E. and Braunwald, E. (1966) Ann. Int. Med., 65, 20-27.

20. Gottschalk, C.W. (1979) Ann. Rev. Physiol., 41, 229-240.

21. Guyton, A.C., Coleman, T.G., Young, D.B., Lohmeier, T.E. and DeClue, J.W. (1980) Ann. Rev. Med., 31, 15-35.

22. Hargens, A.R., Tucker, B.J. and Blantz, R.C. (1977) Amer. J. Physiol., 233, F269-F273.

23. Hjemdahl, P., Belfrage, E. and Daleskog, M. (1979) J. Clin. Invest., 64, 1221-1228.

24. Hollenberg, N.K., Adams, D.F., Rashid, A., Epstein, M., Abrams, H.L. and Merrill, J.P. (1971) Circ., 43, 845-851.

25. Iiono, Y. and Brenner, B.M. (1979) Kidney Int., 16, 821.

54

26. Katholi, R.E., Naftilan, A.J. and Oparil, S. (1980) Hypertension, 2, 266-273.

27. Katholi, R.E., Oparil, S., Urthaler, F. and James, T.N. (1979) J. Clin. Invest., 64, 17-31.

28. Kline, R.L., Ciriello, J. and Mercer, P.F. (1980) Fed. Proc., 39, 962.

29. Kline, R.L. and Mercer, P.F. (1980) Amer. J. Physiol., 238, R353-R358.

30. Kuchel, O., Buu, N.T., Hamet, P., Nowaczynski, W. and Genest, J. (1979) Hypertension, 1, 267-273.

31. Kvetnansky, R., Weise, V.K., Thoa, N.B. and Kopin, I.J. (1979) J. Pharmacol. Exp. Ther., 209, 287-291.

32. Lokhandwala, M.F. and Jandhyala, B.S. (1979) J. Pharmacol. Exp. Ther., 210, 120-127.

33. Morgunov, N. and Baines, A.D. (1979) The Physiol., 22, 90.

34. Muldoon, S.M., Tyce, G.M., Moyer, T.P. and Rorie, D.K., (1979) Amer. J. Physiol., 236, H263-H267.

35. Meyers, B.D., Deen, W.M. and Brenner, B.M. (1975) Circ. Res. 37, 101-110.

36. Norbiato, G., Bevilacqua, M., Raggi, U., Micossi, P., Nitti, F., Lanfredinin, M. and Barbieri, S. (1979) J. Clin. Endo. Metab., 48, 37-42.

37. Powis, G. (1974) J. Pharm. Pharmacol., 26, 344-347.

38. Reynolds, G.P., Ceasar, P.M., Ruthven, C.R.J. and Sandler, M. (1978) Clin. Chim. Acta, 84, 225-231.

39. Sadowski, J., Kurkus, J. and Gellert, R. (1977) Amer. J. Physiol., 237, F262-F267.

40. Silva, P., Landsberg, L. and Besarab, A. (1979) J. Clin. Invest., 64, 850-861.

41. Snider, S.R., Miller, C., Prasad, A.L.N., Jackson, V. and Fahn, S. (1977) Nauyn-Schm. Arch. Pharm., 297, 17-22.

42. Stephenson, R.K., Sole, M.J. and Baines, A.D. (1980) Clin. Res., 28, 462A.

43. Wilcox, C.S. (1977) Clin. Sc. Mol. Med., 53, 321-328.

44. Winaver, J., Chaimovitz, C. and Better, O.S. (1978) Clin. Sc. Mol. Med., 54, 603-607.

Hormonal Regulation of Sodium Excretion,
B. Lichardus, R.W. Schrier and J. Ponec, eds.
© 1980 Elsevier/North-Holland Biomedical Press

NOREPINEPHRINE EFFECT ON Na^+ EXTRUSION IN CELLS FROM GUINEA-PIG KIDNEY CORTEX
SLICES.

G.I. YARIS and F. PROVERBIO

Centro de Biofísica y Bioquímica. Instituto Venezolano de Investigaciones Cien-
tíficas (IVIC), Apartado 1827, Caracas 1010A, Venezuela.

INTRODUCTION

During the last years experimental evidence has been accumulated which suggests that adrenergic innervation of tubular cells plays a direct role in the
regulation of renal tubular sodium reabsorption. By electron microscopy and
fluorescence histochemical studies it has been demonstrated that a direct adren
ergic innervation of the proximal and distal convoluted tubules exist[1-3]. In
the dog it was found that stimulation or inhibition of the efferent renal sympa
thetic nerve activity can produce stimulation or inhibition of renal tubular
sodium reabsorption with no changes in renal hemodynamics[4-8]. Even more, acute
renal denervation produces diuresis and natriuresis on the rat[9]. Finally, addition of norepinephrine (NE) to renal artery infusate of the dog[10] or to isolated rat kidney[11] resulted in increase of sodium reabsorption and excretion of a
dilute urine. Unfortunately, the fact that catecholamines display secondary effects on kidney function[12,13,14], makes it very difficult to ascertain a direct
effect of these molecules on Na^+ movements. Among the several possible mechanisms which have been suggested, three of them seems to be particulary interesting to explain these effects: one, accelaration of the reabsorption of sodium
in proximal tubule[9,15], two, increment of the reabsorption of sodium in the dis
tal tubule[11] and three, permeability changes of tubular membranes to sodium[16].
Searching for an understanding of kidney regulation, two modes of net Na^+ extrusion from guinea-pig kidney cortex slices, rich in proximal tubules, have
been previously described: One, is the cardiac glycoside-sensitive mechanism,
which exchanges intracellular Na^+ for extracellular K^+, obtaining its energy
from the hydrolysis of ATP[17-24]. The other is the ethacrynic acid-sensitive,
ouabain-insensitive mechanism, which extrudes Na^+ from the cell, accompanied
with Cl^- and water, obtaining also its energy from the hydrolysis of ATP[25-28].
In the present work it was studied the effect of norepinephrine on the two
mechanisms of Na^+ extrusion present in guinea-pig kidney cortex slices. It was
found that norepinephrine acts enhancing the extrusion of Na^+ accompanied by
Cl^- and water, while the mechanism which extrudes Na^+ interchanged by K^+, is
slightly inhibited by the treatment.

MATERIAL AND METHODS

In general, the experimental and analytical procedures were those previously described[19]. Outermost slices of thickness 0.2-0.3 mm. were obtained from kidneys of guinea-pig (*Cavia porcellus*). The slices were immersed in a medium with no K^+ at 0.6°C for 90 minutes, in order to induce a gain of Na^+ and Cl^- and a loss of K^+. After this treatment, a group of slices was removed for analysis. The other pieces of tissue were reimmersed at 25°C in different bath media, in the presence or not of 1×10^{-6} M norepinephrine (Sigma Chemical Company, St. Louis, Mo., U.S.A.). At the end of the experiment, these slices were separated for analysis.

In some experiments, 1 mM ouabain (Sigma Chemical Company) or 2 mM ethacrynic acid (Merck, Sharp and Dohme, Rahway, N.J., U.S.A.), was added to the incubation medium.

The chemical composition of all media was the following: Na acetate, 9 mM; $NaHCO_3$, 15 mM; NaH_2PO_4, 2.4 mM; $MgSO_4$, 1.2 mM; Na_2SO_4, 0.6 mM; Ca gluconate, 1 mM; glucose, 5 mM. To this basic medium, the required amount of NaCl and KCl were added to obtain media with the following Na^+, K^+ and Cl^- concentrations: OK^+ medium: 0 mM K^+, 150 mM Na^+ and 120 mM Cl^-; $16K^+$ medium: 16 mM K^+, 134 mM Na^+ and 120 mM Cl^-. The osmolalities were 295 ± 2 mOsm/Kg. As usual, a mixture of 95% O_2 and 5% CO_2 was passed through the solutions during the experimental periods. The pH was maintained between 7.2 and 7.6. Tissue water was calculated from the weight loss on drying. Ions were extracted in 1 N HNO_3. Na^+ and K^+ were determined by flame photometry, and Cl^- by potentiometric titrations. The extracellular space, e, was taken as 0.26 [19].

RESULTS

Table 1 shows the cell water and ion content of the kidney slices after 90 minutes of cooling period in the OK^+ medium and after rewarming at 25°C for time periods of 2, 4 and 6 minutes, in the $16K^+$ medium in the presence or absence of 1×10^{-6} M norepinephrine (NE). The net movements of water and ions, induced by the rewarming process, can be calculated by subtraction from the zero time in each case. It may be seen that even if the extrusion of Na^+ from the cells is about the same in the presence of NE, this is not the case for K^+, Cl^- and water, which movements show a transient variation in the presence of the hormone. In fact, for the first 2 minutes, the presence of NE induces a lower gain of K^+ (61 ± 4 control, 42 ± 4 experimental) and an enhanced extrusion of Cl^- (-38 ± 6 control, -68 ± 6 experimental) and water (-0.36 ± 0.04 control, -0.53 ± 0.04 experimental). In all cases, $P<0.01$.

TABLE 1

CELL WATER AND ION CONTENT OF KIDNEY SLICES REWARMED IN THE PRESENCE OR ABSENCE OF NOREPINEPHRINE (NE) IN THE MEDIUM $16K^+$.

Groups of slices were analyzed at the end of the cooling period (row a): the others were rewarmed at 25°C in the medium $16K^+$ in the presence (c) or not (b) of 1×10^{-6} M norepinephrine for 2, 4 and 6 minutes, and then analyzed.

Condition		Cell ion and water content*			
		W $\frac{g \text{ water}}{g \text{ solids}}$	Na^+ µmoles/g solids	K^+	Cl^-
a 0.6°C, OK^+		2.83 ± 0.03	440 ± 8	103 ± 2	209 ± 5
	2 min.	2.47 ± 0.02	350 ±10	164 ± 4	171 ± 3
b 25.0°C, $16K^+$	4 min.	2.19 ± 0.04	265 ± 8	209 ±10	143 ± 5
	6 min.	2.01 ± 0.04	238 ± 8	234 ± 6	120 ± 4
c 25.0°C, $16K^+$	2 min.	2.30 ± 0.02	336 ± 7	137 ± 4	141 ± 4
+ NE	4 min.	2.05 ± 0.03	269 ± 4	198 ± 6	116 ± 7
	6 min.	1.96 ± 0.03	240 ± 2	215 ± 8	106 ± 3

* Values are mean ± standard error of the mean. n = 8.

The stimulation of the NaCl extrusion induced by NE was also seen when the slices were rewarmed in the absence of K^+, as we can see in Table 2: during the 2 min. incubation at 25°C in the absence of K^+, the slices rewarmed in the presence of NE significantly extruded more Na^+, Cl^- and water, than the control slices.

TABLE 2

EFFECT OF NOREPINEPHRINE (NE) ON CELL WATER AND ION CONTENT OF KIDNEY CORTEX SLICES REWARMED IN THE MEDIUM OK^+.

Slices preincubated in the cold and then rewarmed at 25°C for 2 min. in the medium OK^+ with or without 1×10^{-6} M, NE.

Condition	Cell ion and water content*			
	W $\frac{g \text{ water}}{g \text{ solids}}$	Na^+ µmoles/g solids	K^+	Cl^-
a 0.6°C, OK^+	2.76 ± 0.03	422 ± 4	109 ± 2	200 ± 4
b 25.0°C, OK^+	2.48 ± 0.02**	391 ± 6**	100 ± 3	171 ± 3**
c 25.0°C, OK^+ + NE	2.31 ± 0.04**	365 ± 2**	106 ± 4	137 ± 6**

*Values are mean ± S.E. of the mean. (n = 8). **P<0.001.

The effect of ethacrynic acid (EA), which it is known to inhibits the NaCl extrusion in this tissue, was also studied. The results are shown in Figure 1. The presence of EA in the medium, produced only 16% inhibition on the extrusion of Na^+ interchanged by K^+, while it inhibited 54% the extrusion of NaCl in the control slices. In the presence of norepinephrine, EA, inhibited the Na^+-K^+ interchange by 10% and the extrusion of NaCl by 63%; indicating that the NE stimulation effect was abolished by EA. As shown before (Tables 1 and 2) water always followed the movement of Cl^- (data not shown).

The effect of ouabain, inhibitor of the Na^+-K^+ interchange, but not of the NaCl extrusion, is shown in Table 3: ouabain, as expected, inhibited the Na^+-K^+ interchange and did not affect the extrusion of NaCl, which, again, was enhanced by norepinephrine.

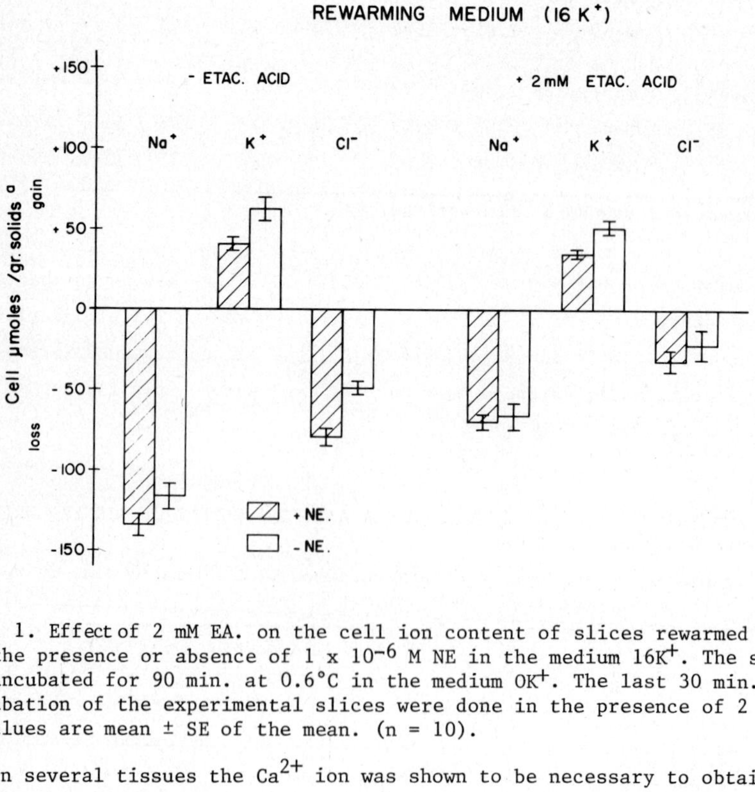

Fig. 1. Effect of 2 mM EA. on the cell ion content of slices rewarmed for 2 min. in the presence or absence of 1×10^{-6} M NE in the medium $16K^+$. The slices were preincubated for 90 min. at 0.6°C in the medium OK^+. The last 30 min. of preincubation of the experimental slices were done in the presence of 2 mM EA. * Values are mean ± SE of the mean. (n = 10).

In several tissues the Ca^{2+} ion was shown to be necessary to obtain the catecholamine effects mediated by alpha-adrenergic receptors. Even more, these effects have been explained involving the Ca^{2+} ion as a second messenger[29-32].

To investigate the possibility of a Ca^{2+} mediated mechanism in our system, the following experiment was performed. In order to deplete the cells, the slices were preincubated for 90 min. at 0.6°C in the medium OK^+ with no Ca^{2+}, and then rewarmed for 2 min. at 25°C in the medium $16K^+$ with 0, 1 or 5 mM Ca^{2+}, in the presence or absence of norepinephrine. The results are shown in Figure 2.

TABLE 3

EFFECT OF NOREPINEPHRINE (NE) ON CELL WATER AND ION CONTENT OF KIDNEY CORTEX SLICES REWARMED IN $16K^+$ MEDIUM IN THE PRESENCE OF 1 mM OUABAIN (ouab).

Slices preincubated in the cold and then rewarmed at 25°C for 2 min. in the medium $16K^+$ with 1 mM ouabain, with or without 1×10^{-6} M NE.

Condition	Cell ion and water content*			
	W g water g solids	Na^+	K^+ µmoles/g solids	Cl^-
a 0.6°C, OK^+ + ouab.	2.80 ± 0.04	427 ± 3	90 ± 3	203 ± 4
b 25.0°C, $16K^+$ + ouab.	2.43 ± 0.02**	397 ± 4**	80 ± 6	167 ± 3**
c 25.0°C, $16K^+$ + ouab.+ NE	2.28 ± 0.02**	373 ± 4**	74 ± 5	140 ± 4**

*Values are mean ± SE of the mean. (n = 10). **P<0.001.

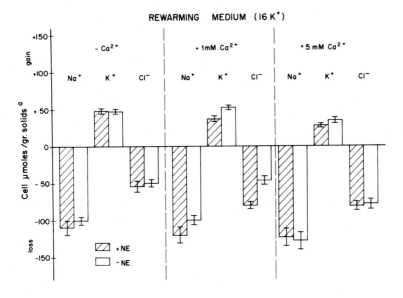

Figure 2. Effect of different concentrations of Ca^{2+} on cell ion content of kidney cortex slices rewarmed for 2 min. in the presence or absence of 1×10^{-6} M NE in the medium $16K^+$. The slices were preincubated for 90 min. at 0.6°C in the medium OK^+ with no Ca^{2+}.
*Values are mean ± SE of the mean (n = 7).

On rewarming the cells in Ca^{2+} free medium, the two proposed Na^+ extrusion mechanisms were observed to be equally insensitive to the presence of NE. As expected, the hormone effect appears if the incubation medium contains 1 mM Ca^{2+}, this is shown in Figure 2. However, independent of the presence of NE, partial inhibition of the Na^+-K^+ exchange and enhancement of the Na-Cl extrusion can be also obtained if the cells are incubated in medium containing 5 mM Ca^{2+}.

DISCUSSION

The data presented in this paper indicate that 1×10^{-6} M norepinephrine has the effect to stimulate one of the two described mechanisms of Na^+ extrusion in guinea-pig kidney cortex slices[19]. In fact, norepinephrine increases the Na^+ extrusion accompanied by Cl^- and water, while the Na^+ extrusion interchanged by K^+ was inhibited to some extent (Table 1). The enhanced NaCl extrusion induced by NE, is also apparent when the slices are rewarmed in a K^+ free medium (Table 2) or with 16 mM K^+, in the presence of 1 mM ouabain (Table 3). These results suggest that the norepinephrine stimulating effect is not associated with the running of the Na^+-K^+ pump, which is inhibited under the above mention ed conditions: $0K^+$ or $16K^+$ + 1 mM ouabain. In addition, the norepinephrine enhancing effect is not observed when 2 mM ethacrynic acid (preferential inhibitor of this mode of Na^+ extrusion[19]), is added to the rewarming medium (Figure 1).

The fact that the norepinephrine effect is not observed in the absence of external Ca^{2+} and that it can be paralelled by an increased Ca^{2+} concentration (5 mM) in the rewarming medium (Figure 2) may be taken as an indication that the observed phenomenon is produced by an enhanced Ca^{2+} influx to the cells, mediated, either by the presence of norepinephrine or by the Ca^{2+} concentration gradient.

An increased intracellular Ca^{2+} concentration may produce drastic changes in the cellular properties. In fact, in liver[33], nervous cells[34] and red cells[35], the increase of the intracellular Ca^{2+} concentration produces an increment on the membrane permeability to K^+ ions. This effect could explain the apparent inhibition observed in the K^+ gain. K^+ would be gained, but also lost immediate ly because of its increased membrane permeability.

The enhanced Ca^{2+} influx could produce, by counter-transport, an enhanced Na^+ extrusion. The Ca^{2+}, then would be actively pumped out of the cell accompanied by Cl^-, and the net result would be an enhanced extrusion of NaCl. Since the extrusion of Na^+ accompanied by Cl^- is seen also in the absence of external Ca^{2+} (Figure 2), it must be considered that only the enhanced extrusion of NaCl is driven by this mechanism. If this was the case, the source of energy responsible for the final effect, which is the enhancement of NaCl extrusion, would be a Ca^{2+}-stimulated ATPase. Since this enhancement is inhibited by ethacrynic acid (Figure 1), the involved Ca^{2+}-stimulated ATPase should also be inhibited by this agent. In relation to that, unpublished results from our laboratory (del Castillo and Proverbio, manuscript in preparation) have shown that the Ca^{2+}-stimulated ATPase, present in basal-lateral plasma membranes of this tissue, is only 35% inhibited by 2 mM ethacrynic acid. This fact suggests that the mechanism proposed above doesn't seem to be enough to explain the ion movement that are taking place.

At the present further investigations are being realized in our laboratory in the hope to learn about the possible physiological role of the observations reported in this paper.

ACKNOWLEDGEMENTS

Thanks are due to Dr. Leonardo Mateu and Reinaldo Marin for the reading and criticism of this paper. We also acknowledge the assistance of Mrs. Teresa Proverbio, the secretarial help of Mrs. Ana Maria Kübelböck and the drawings of Mr. Tommy Salgrero. This work was supported in part with grant for project N? D.F. S1-749 from CONICIT.

REFERENCES

1. Muller, J. and Barajas, L. (1972) J. Ultrastruct. Res., 41, 533-549.
2. Barajas, L. and Muller, J. (1973) J. Ultrastruct. Res., 43, 107-132.
3. DiBona, G.F. (1977) Am. J. Physiol., 233, F73-F81.
4. Zambrasky, E.J. and DiBona, G.F. (1976) Am. J. Physiol., 231, 1105-1110.
5. Zambrasky, E.J., DiBona, G.F. and Kaloyanides, G.J. (1976) Proc. Soc. Exptl. Biol. Med., 151, 543-546.
6. Zambrasky, E.J., DiBona, G.F. and Kaloyanides, G.J. (1976) J. Pharmacol. Exptl. Therap., 198, 464-472.
7. DiBona, G.F., Zambrasky, E.J., Agilera, A.J. and Kaloyanides, G.J. (1977) Circulation Res., 40, Suppl. I, I-127-I-130.
8. Prosnitz, E.H. and DiBona, G.F. (1978) Am. J. Physiol., 235 (6), F557-563.
9. Bello-Reuss, E., Colindres, R.E., Pastoriza-Muñoz, E., Mueller, R.A. and Gottschalk, C.W. (1975) J. Clin. Invest., 56, 208-217.
10. Gill, J.R.Jr. and Casper, A.G.T. (1972) Am. J. Physiol., 223 (5), 1201-1205.
11. Besarab, A., Silva, P., Landsberg, L. and Epstein, F.H. (1977) Am. J. Physiol., 233 (1), F39-F45.
12. Assaykeen, T.A. and Ganong, W.F. (1971) Frontiers in Neuroendocrinology, L. Martini and W.F. Ganong, New York, Oxford, pp. 67-102.

13. Schrier, R.W. and Berl, T. (1973) J. Clin. Invest., 52, 502-511.

14. Schrier, R.W., Lieberman, R. and Ufferman, R.C. (1976) Archiv. Internal Med., 136, 25-29.

15. Bello-Reuss, E., Trevino, D.L. and Gottschalk, C.W. (1976) J. Clin. Invest., 57, 1104-1107.

16. Aurbach, G.D. (1976) Hormone receptors in the kidney membranes and diseases. L. Bolis, J.F. Hoffman and A. Leaf, Raven Press, New York.

17. Whittam, R. and Willis, J.S. (1963) J. Physiol. Lond., 168, 158-177.

18. Kleinzeller, A. and Knotkova, A. (1964) J. Physiol., 175, 172-191.

19. Whittembury, G. and Proverbio, F. (1970) Pflügers Arch. 316, 1-25.

20. Macknight, A.D.C. (1968) Biochim. Biophys. Acta, 150, 263-270.

21. Willis, J.S. (1966) Biochim. Biophys. Acta, 163, 506-515.

22. Wheeler, K.P. and Whittam, R. (1964) Biochem. J., 93, 349-363.

23. Charnock, J.S. and Post, R.L. (1963) Australian J. Exp. Biol. Med. Sci., 41, 547-560.

24. Proverbio, F., Robinson, J.W.L. and Whittembury, G. (1970) Biochim. Biophys. Acta, 211, 327-336.

25. Munday, K.A., Parsons, B.J. and Poat, J.A. (1971) J. Physiol., 215, 269-282.

26. Whittembury, G. and Fishman, J. (1966) Pflügers Arch., 307, 138-153.

27. Torretti, J., Hendler, E., Weinstein, E., Longnecker, R.E. and Epstein, F.H. (1972) Am. J. Physiol., 222, 1398-1405.

28. Proverbio, F., Condrescu-Guidi, M. and Whittembury, G. (1975) Biochim. Biophys. Acta, 394, 281-292.

29. Bencsath, P., Bozena, A., Szalay, L. and Takacs, L. (1979) Am. J. Physiol., 236 (6), F513-F518.

30. Francoise, D., Assimacopoulos, J., Blackmore, P.F. and Eaton, J.H. (1977) J. Biol. Chem., 252 N° 6, 2662-2669.

31. Selinger, Z., Eimerl, S. and Schramm, M. (1974) Proc. Nat. Acad. Sci. USA., 71 (1), 128-131.

32. Selinger, Z., Batzri, S., Eitmerl, S. and Schramm, M. (1973) J. Biol. Chem., 248 (1), 369-372.

33. Van Rossum, G.D.V. (1970) Nature, 225, 638-639.

34. Carpenter, D.O., Suorer, S.W. and Barker, J.L. (1971) Proc. XXV Cong. Physiol. Sci. Vol. IX, 101.

35. Lew, V.L. (1970) J. Physiol. London, 206, 35P.

Hormonal Regulation of Sodium Excretion,
B. Lichardus, R.W. Schrier and J. Ponec, eds.
© 1980 Elsevier/North-Holland Biomedical Press

THE POSSIBLE MECHANISM OF ATRIAL NATRIURESIS - EXPERIMENTS ON CHRONICALLY INSTRUMENTED DOGS -

HANS-WOLFGANG REINHARDT, GABRIELE KACZMARCZYK, RAINER MOHNHAUPT, BRUNO SIMGEN
Arbeitsgruppe Experimentelle Anästhesie, Klinikum Charlottenburg, Freie
Universität Berlin, 1000 Berlin 19, Spandauer Damm 130, Germany

INTRODUCTION

In the present time our understanding of volume- and osmocontrol in mammalian organisms is based on 3 major concepts:

1. Osmocontrol by osmoreceptors located in the brain
   (Verney 1948 (19))

2. Volumecontrol by receptors located in the left atrium
   (Gauer und Henry 1956 (5))

3. Control of sodium and volume by change of the arterial pressure
   (Guyton 1976 (7))

But obviously these theories are not linked, so that many questions are unanswered. Therefore it could be useful to discuss some new results concerning the short-term control of sodium balance again.

This paper will especially focus on the function of intrathoracic receptors and their possible (physiological ?) importance for the adjustment of sodium balance. This new approach was possible because a special method was applied.

MATERIALS AND METHODS

Chronically instrumented dogs: The procedures of instrumentation and maintenance of the dogs were described extensively in several publications (9,10,12,13,14,15,17), but they should be summarized briefly: All studies were performed on female beagle dogs (body-weight 9-12 kg). Before the dogs were kept in metabolic cages, positioned in an air-conditioned room, they were dewormed and vaccinated. A daily protocol including control of body temperature and weight served to test the health of the dogs. When the dogs were not used for experiments, they had to performe daily exercises on a treadmill.

The food consisted of rice, horsemeat and water. The amount was as high as it was necessary to maintain a constant body weight (bw). The dogs received 0.5 mmol Na/kg bw/day with the food. This was a low sodium intake (LSI). If the dogs were kept on a high sodium intake (HSI), 14.0 mmol Na/kg bw were added to the food. The water, always given together with the food, was

91 ml/kg bw/day. The dogs were fed at 9.00 a.m., on the experimental days between noon and 2.00 p.m..If the food-intake was not complete 3 hours after the dogs had received their meal, the leftover was given by a gastric tube connected with a special force-feeding-machine.

The surgical procedures were performed under sterile conditions: Standard instrumentation was: 1. carotid loop, 2. thoracotomy with purse string around the left atrium some millimeters above the mitral valve and an implanted catheter in the left atrium to record the pressure (LAP). Pulling of the string was followed by mild mitral stenosis and a rather exactly adjustable increase in LAP (eLAP↑) (14). In a 3. step, one of the following instrumentations were performed: Electromagnetic flowprobe around the left renal artery together with a pneumatic cuff for measurements of renal blood flow (9). A pneumatic cuff above the renal arteries and a catheter below the renal arteries to control the renal perfusion pressure by means of an external device (13, 17). Adrenalectomy to open the feed-back loop on the level of the adrenals (15). Cardiac denervation, to exclude the influence of cardiac receptors (this procedure was carried out together with the thoracotomy)(3). Renal denervation, to exclude the influence of the renal nerves (18).

The first experiment was performed 3 weeks after the last major surgery, the time, necessary for the whole preparation procedure was sometimes more than 8 weeks. If after this time everything was operating the dogs could be used mostly for more than 3 months.

The daily protocol of the experiments was as followed:
3 periods for 60 min each: 1. control period (CP), beginning by about 9.00 a.m. with 3 urine collection periods for 20 min each, and measurement of other parameters. 2. Elevation of left atrial pressure (eLAP↑, or distension period, DP). 3. After distension period (ADP). Sometimes this protocol was performed twice.

RESULTS AND DISCUSSION

One of the first results was, that even under LSI-conditions during eLAP↑ a diuresis and a pronounced natriuresis occurred (14). This finding was confirmed under HSI-conditions (16) (fig. 1). The increase in the excretion of sodium (UNaV) seemed to be due to eLAP↑.When we described this finding, the literature was controversial (reviewed in (14)), and it was not a common result that eLAP↑ was followed by a natriuresis. Fig. 2 contains an example that contributes to the explanation of this controversy:

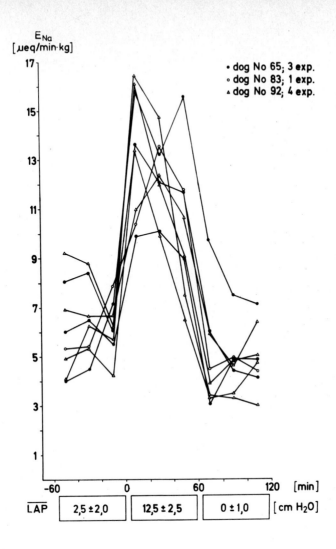

Fig. 1. Sodium excretion (ENa) after elevation of left atrial pressure
(eLAP ⬈) in chronically instrumented dogs, kept on a high Na intake (HSI).
The natriuretic response after eLAP ⬈ is the "atrial natriuresis".

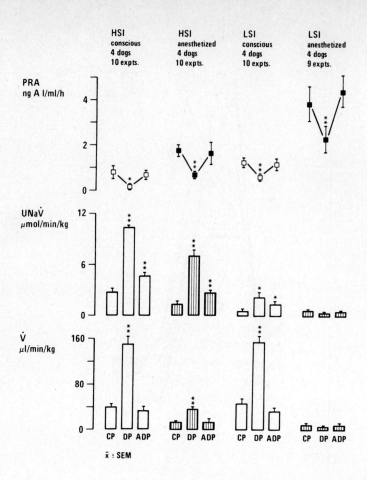

Fig. 2. The effect of an experimental increase in left atrial pressure (eLAP ↗) on plasma renin activity (PRA), sodium excretion (UNaV̇), and urine volume (V̇) in chronically instrumented dogs, kept on a low or a high Na-intake (LSI, HSI). PRA was elevated by anesthesia more in LSI-dogs than in HSI-dogs. After eLAP ↗ under both conditions a decrease in PRA could be demonstrated, but the natriuretic response of eLAP ↗ was diminished in HSI-dogs and abolished in LSI-dogs.

Dependent on the sodium intake a halothane-anesthesia without surgical stress,
reduces or abolishes the natriuretic eLAP↗ response, probably by stimulation
of the renin-angiotensin-system (RAS).

Maybe that among others these controversial results led K.Goetz in his
review (1975!) to the final conclusion that cardiac receptors are of minor
importance for the control of kidney function (6).

Another important question was now, to find out how these atrial receptors
produce the "atrial natriuresis" (AN) ? If the same experiments, as described
above, were performed in HSI-dogs, it became evident, that the eLAP↗ induced
natriuresis lasted longer in LSI-pretreated dogs. The reason was not clear.
The plasma renin activity (PRA) was measured and a marked depression of PRA
was observed during eLAP↗ . Therefore it was supposed that the renin-angiotensin-system (RAS) was involved in AN. Furthermore the different time course
of the eLAP↗ induced natriuresis made it likely that different natriuretic
effects were operating depending on the preceding diet. We believed that
the slower acting natriuretic process was due to changes in mineralocorticoid
activity.

We tested this hypothesis in adrenalectomized dogs, kept in good
conditions by gluco- and mineralocorticoid injections. If we applied the
same protocol of eLAP↗ as it was decribed above, it was found that AN was
undiminished compared with intact dogs. Furthermore, the injection of
high amounts of DOCA into intact dogs did not prevent AN either, this means
that the opening of the feed back loop on the level of mineralocorticoid
secretion did not modify AN, and we had to look for other possible mechanisms
Studies with measurements of renal blood flow during eLAP↗ failed to detect
changes (9).

Unfortunately the reversible mitral stenosis was accompanied with an
increase in heart rate and mean arterial blood pressure (Part.). The
increase in Part was in the range of 10 to 20 mmHg (14). Therefore the
increase in Part was as high that it could be responsible for the increase
in UNaV. We therefore performed studies in which the arterial perfusion pressure
of the kidneys(Pren) was kept constant over DP. This was achieved by computerized
calculating of a time, during which a motordriven pump inflated or deflated
an implanted pneumatic cuff above the renal arteries. Though this control
procedure was accompanied with a severe reduction in pulse pressure.
AN was absolutely undiminished compared to the controls.
These results were very reliable, since "controls" and "experimentals"
were performed in the same dogs (13, 17). This means, that neither changes

in mineralocorticoid secretion, renal blood flow, nor an increase in Pren was responsible for AN.

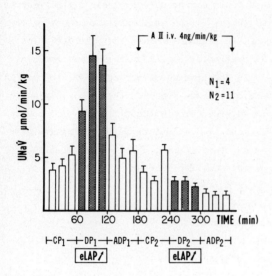

Fig. 3. Sodium excretion (UNaV) after elevation of left atrial pressure (eLAP ⬈) with and without infusion of angiotensin II (AII).

N_1 number of dogs

N_2 number of experiments

But another component of the renin-angiotensin-aldosterone-axis could be involved: Since Johnson and Malvin (8), Fagard et al. (4), and Lohmeier et al. (11) it is supposed that AII has a direct effect on renal sodium reabsorption. The question is open whether renal sodium reabsorption is primarily due to hemodynamic changes or to changes in tubular reabsorption. But nevertheless, we opened the loop by infusion of angiotensin II in very small amounts. This dosage (4 ng/min/kg) did not influence Part as long as no sodium was given (1). This finding was confirmed in these experiments, but the natriuretic effect of eLAP⬈ was completely suppressed (Fig. 3). In these experiments the first eLAP ⬈ was followed by a second one. In a lot of control experiments the diuretic effect of the second eLAP ⬈ was always by about 80 % of the first one. In the "angiotensin" study the diuresis was much more reduced, this means, that angiotensin II has influenced the diuretic response to eLAP↗ also. The mechanism is unknown. These results support the hypothesis that AN is due to a suppression of PRA. But the RAS acts on sodium retention in a twofold manner: by aldosterone and angiotensin II, the latter is the faster acting one. But this conclusion can be misleading: It cannot be excluded that the antinatriuretic activities of AII and aldosterone override natriuretic processes of other origin. This could be for example the "natriuretic hormone" (2) which could be liberated by eLAP↗.

There is one set of experiments which supports the existance of natriuretic activities other than the suppression of AII and aldosterone secretion. After chronic HSI-treatment the dogs begin soon after the food intake with a very rapid sodium excretion. We tested eLAP↗ at the peak of the post-prandial sodium excretion (Fig. 4). eLAP↗ was followed by a further in-crease in UNaV̇ up to a range, never reached in other comparable postprandial experiments.

The question arises, if under these conditions a further suppression of the renin secretion by the kidneys is possible and if this is possible the supposed reduction can be responsible for the additional increase in UNaV̇ ?

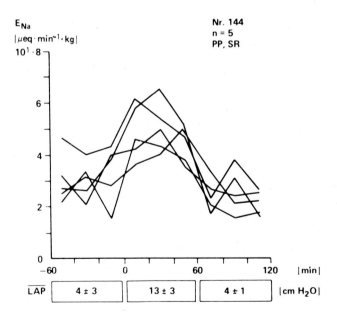

Fig. 4. Sodium excretion (ENa) after elevation of left atrial pressure (eLAP↗) during the peak of postprandial Na-excretion (HSI). Please note the different scale for ENa, compared to Fig. 1,2,3.

After blockade of the converting enzyme with SQ 14 225* some experiments
showed an undiminished AN, which is incompatible with the hypothesis that
All should be responsible for AN.

On the other hand, and this seems to be very important, AN can be completely
abolished by cardiac denervation (3), this means, that the effects of the
simulation of an increased intrathoracic blood volume, by means of the
reversible mitral stenosis are completely generated by receptors located
in the left atrium (or right ventricle), but not in the vascular bed of
the lungs. The natriuretic information is conducted via nerves to the
central nervous system. But the efferent pathway of the "natriuretic"
information, or the mechanism of PRA-suppression remains unexplained, because renal denervation failed to influence the eLAP↑ induced natriuresis.
If we summarize our knowledge concerning the control of sodium balance
by cardiac receptors, we can give the following statements:

The experimental elevation of the left atrial pressure is mostly followed
by an increase in sodium excretion. If the total body sodium is reduced,
eLAP↑ fails to increase sodium excretion (20). It is rather shure, that
eLAP↗ suppresses plasma renin secretion. This finding is more pronounced
in LSI-dogs, since PRA is primarily higher during the controls. A quantitative relationship between AN and PRA did not exist, but this may be due
to the fact, that plasma renin activity did not reflect the real intrarenal activity of the system.

'Atrial natriuresis' was not prevented by removal of the adrenals,
but the infusion of angiotensin II in very small amounts, not modifying
the arterial pressure, abolished AN completely. Since an increase of
arterial pressure was not responsible for AN it is very likely that All
is the fast acting antinatriuretic component of the renin-angiotensin-
aldosterone-system and at least partly involved in the mechanism of
'atrial natriuresis'.

It remains unexplained whether this potent natriuretic reflex acts solely
by suppression of the RAS or by activation of other natriuretic processes.
Quantitatively the reflex could be able to control a big part of the
isotonic expanded extracellular fluid by removal of sodium and water, but
the physiological importance is still unknown, since other potent mechanisms,
influencing the adjustment of sodium balance are operating (19).
Therefore it is rather clear, that the cardiac receptors are not unique
in the control of extracellular volume or osmolality.

---

*Gratitude is expressed to the SQUIBB-Institute

REFERENCES

1. DeClue, J.W., Guyton, A.C., Cowley, A.W., Coleman, G., Norman, R.A., McCaa, R.E. (1978) Subpressor angiotensin infusion, renal sodium handling, and salt-induced hypertension in the dog, Circ.Res., 43, 504-512.

2. De Wardener, H.E. (1977) Natriuretic hormone, Clin.Sci.Mol.Med., 53, 1-8.

3. Drake, A.J., Eisele, R., Kaczmarczyk, G., Mohnhaupt, R., Noble, M.I.M., Reinhardt, H.W., Simgen, B., Stubbs, J. (1980) The role of cardiac afferent nerves in the regulation of sodium balance in conscious dogs, Proc.Physiol.Soc., 135 P.

4. Fagard, R.H., Cowley, A.W., Navar, L.G., Langford, H.G., Guyton, A.C. (1976) Renal responses to slight elevations of renal arterial plasma angiotensin II concentration in dogs, Clin.Exp.Pharmacol.Physiol., 3, 531-538.

5. Gauer, O.H., Henry, J.P. (1956) Beitrag zur Homöostase des extra-arteriellen Kreislaufs, Klin.Wochenschr. 34, 356-366.

6. Goetz, K.L., Bond, G.C., Bloxham, D.D. (1975) Atrial receptors and renal function, Physiol.Rev. 55, 157-205.

7. Guyton, A.C. (1976) Physics of blood, blood flow, and pressure: hemodynamics, Textbook of medical physiology (A.C.Guyton, ed.), (Philadelphia-London-Toronto: W.B.Saunders Comp.) 235.

8. Johnson, M.D., Malvin, R.L. (1977) Stimulation of renal sodium reab-sorption by angiotensin II, Am.J.Physiol., 232, F298-F306.

9. Kaczmarczyk, G., Eigenheer, F., Gatzka, M., Kuhl, U., Reinhardt, H.W. (1978) No relation between atrial natriuresis and renal blood flow in conscious dogs, Pflügers Arch. 373, 49-58.

10. Kaczmarczyk, G., Schimmrich, B., Mohnhaupt, R., Reinhardt, H.W. (1979) Atrial pressure and postprandial volume regulation in conscious dogs, Pflügers Arch. 381, 143-150.

11. Lohmeier, T.E., Cowley, A.W., Trippodo, N.C., Hall, J.E., Guyton, A.C. (1977) Effects of endogenous angiotensin II on renal sodium excretion and renal hemodynamics, Am.J.Physiol. 233, F388-F395.

12. Lydtin, H., Hamilton, W.F. (1964) Effect of acute changes in left atrial pressure on urine flow in unanesthetized dogs, Am.J.Physiol. 207, 530-536.

13. Mohnhaupt, R., Eisele, R., Kaczmarczyk, G., Reinhardt, H.W. (1979) Sodium and water excretion during acute experimental elevation of left atrial pressure (eLAP $\nearrow$) with constant renal perfusion pressure (Pren), Pflügers Arch.Suppl. 379, R 15.

14. Reinhardt, H.W., Kaczmarczyk, G., Eisele, R., Arnold, B., Eigenheer, F., Kuhl, U. (1977) Left atrial pressure and sodium balance in conscious dogs on a low sodium intake, Pflügers Arch. 370, 59-66.

15. Reinhardt, H.W., Eisele, R., Kaczmarczyk, G., Mohnhaupt, R., Oelkers, W., Schimmrich, B. (1980) The control of sodium excretion by reflexes from the low pressure system independent of adrenal activity. Pflügers Arch. 384, 171-176.

16. Reinhardt, H.W., Eisele, R., Kaczmarczyk, G., Mohnhaupt, R., Schimmrich, B., Wegener, S. (1980) Zur extrarenalen Regulation des Natriumbestandes, Zentral-vegetative Regulationen und Syndrome (R.Schifter, ed.), Springer, Berlin-Heidelberg-New York.

17. Reinhardt, H.W., Kaczmarczyk, G., Mohnhaupt, R., Simgen, B. (1980) Atrial natriuresis under the condition of a constant renal perfusion pressure - Experiments on conscious dogs - Pflügers Arch., accepted.

18. Simgen, B., Kaczmarczyk, G., Mohnhaupt, R., Schulze, Reinhardt, H.W. (1979) The contribution of the renal nerves to adjustments of the sodium balance, Pflügers Arch.Suppl. $\underline{382}$, R 17.

19. Verney, E.B. (1948) The antidiuretic hormone and the factors which determine its release, Proc.Royal Soc. 135, 26-105.

20. Wegener, S., Kaczmarczyk, G., Schimmrich, B., Mohnhaupt, R., Reinhardt, H.W. (1978) Suppression of atrial natriuresis after acute and chronic reduction of total body sodium (TBS).- Experiments on conscious dogs on a high or a low sodium intake, Pflügers Arch.Suppl. 377, R 15.

Hormonal Regulation of Sodium Excretion,
B. Lichardus, R.W. Schrier and J. Ponec, eds.
© 1980 Elsevier/North-Holland Biomedical Press

INFLUENCE OF THE RENIN-ANGIOTENSIN SYSTEM ON SODIUM EXCRETION IN NORMAL AND GOLDBLATT HYPERTENSIVE RATS.

L. GABRIEL NAVAR, WANN-CHU HUANG, AND DAVID W. PLOTH

Nephrology Research and Training Center, Department of Physiology and Biophysics, and Veterans Administration Medical Center. University of Alabama in Birmingham, Birmingham, Alabama, U.S.A.

In recent years, there has been an increased interest regarding the specific role exerted by the renin-angiotensin system in the regulation of renal hemodynamics and sodium execretion[1-4]. In this review, emphasis will be placed on the contribution of the renin-angiotensin system to the control of sodium excretion. The influence of angiotensin on renal hemodynamics[3,4] will be discussed only as it is germane to the present topic. In addition, the indirect influence of angiotensin on sodium excretion mediated through aldosterone release will not be addressed although it is certainly of major significance[5].

It is now generally accepted that the juxtaglomerular cells of the renal arterioles are the site of renin formation[5-7]. Renin acts on circulating angiotensinogen to form the decapeptide, angiotensin I, which is then converted to octapeptide, angiotensin II, by the action of converting enzyme. There is also a pathway by which a heptapeptide, angiotensin III,[8] is formed, but the quantitative role of angiotensin III remains uncertain. Because of the unique anatomical arrangements of the juxtaglomerular complex, it has been suggested that angiotensin could be formed directly within the kidney and exert its action as a local hormone[1,2,7,9,10]. Since converting enzyme is present on the endothelium of the renal vasculature[7,11], there could be local formation of angiotensin II within the vascular system or in the surrounding interstitium. Alternatively, the presence of large quantities of converting enzyme in the endothelium of the lung capillaries[12,13] has suggested that much of the angiotensin I may be converted into angiotensin II within the lung and subsequently act as a systemic hormone. This latter possibility is of interest with regard to control of sodium excretion since it provides one means by which an interaction could exist between the two kidneys[14]. These are not mutually exclusive possibilities and presumably both effects may coexist under certain conditions. Studies of this problem have involved evaluation of the direct effects of administration of angiotensin[1,14-19] and of the effects caused by administration of various pharmacological blockers or inhibitors of the renin-angiotensin system[3,4,9,10,20-24]. Most studies attempting to assess the potential local effects of angiotensin have utilized inhibitors or antagonists which block the local formation or action of angiotensin II and thus unmask any pre-existing physiological influence being exerted by angiotensin.

EFFECT OF ANGIOTENSIN ON SODIUM EXCRETION

The effects of renin and angiotensin administration on renal excretory function have been confusing because both natriuretic and antinatriuretic responses have been demonstrated[1,14-19]. Most studies indicate that the antinatriuretic and antidiuretic effects of angiotensin occur when low doses (20 ng/kg/min) are administered[16-19] while infusions of larger concentrations usually lead to a duiresis and marked natriuresis[15,16,19]. Since there are usually associated reductions in RBF and GFR, the antidiuretic effects of angiotensin could simply be the consequence of primary hemodynamic effects. However, several recent studies have suggested that this explanation does not fully account for the effects of angiotensin on sodium excretion. Johnson and Malvin[17] reported that low doses of angiotensin II reduced urine flow and sodium excretion significantly. Although there were associated hemodynamic responses, the changes in GFR, renal plasma flow and filtration fraction did not correlate with the observed excretory responses. Harris and Young[19] provided evidence indicating that angiotensin may exert direct effects on tubular reabsorption. Using stationary microperfusion techniques, the authors demonstrated that low concentrations (1-100 pg/ml) increased sodium reabsorption by the proximal tubule while higher concentrations (.3-3 µg/ml) decreased proximal sodium reabsorption back toward or below control levels. These studies support the concept that local administration of low doses of angiotensin to the peritubular surface leads to augumented tubular fluid absorption.

EFFECTS OF ANGIOTENSIN BLOCKERS ON ANTAGONISTS ON SODIUM EXCRETION

Although the systemic administration of angiotensin allows an assessment of actions exerted by circulating angiotensin, an alternative approach for evaluating the potential local actions of angiotensin involves the application of inhibitors or competitive antagonists of the renin-angiotensin system[20]. Studies utilizing these agents are compromised by the relatively modest sodium excretion responses in normal animals and the rather dramatic hypotensive effects observed in animals having high plasma renin activity (PRA) levels. However, several studies have now reported that blockade of the renin-angiotensin system results in increased renal sodium excretion when the associated decreases in arterial pressure are not severe[9,10,20-22,24].

In recent experiments by Ploth et al.[22,25], the effects of angiotensin blockers on tubular function were evaluated in normal rats. Micropuncture techniques were used to delineate the changes in tubular fluid flow and segmental reabsorption in the proximal and distal nephron segments. These experiments were accomplished with two different agents that have been demonstrated to block the renin-angiotensin system, the converting enzyme inhibitor (CEI, SQ 20881) or the end-plate antagonist, Saralasin (P-113). Administration of both of these agents resulted in increases in renal blood flow and GFR of about 30% above control hydropenic levels. An impressive diuresis and nearly 10 fold increase in sodium excretion were observed during infusion of these agents. The increase in GFR was much less that the increase in sodium excretion and fractional sodium excretion increased significantly. Potassium excretion rates also increased indicating that inhibition of aldosterone activity was not the source of the increased sodium excretion. Microvascular hydrostatic presures were not changed from control values during blockade and whole kidney filtration fraction did not change; thus, there was no evidence to support the possibility that changes in peritubular physcial factors were responsible for the altered tubular absorptive function.

The characteristics of sgemental absorptive function were determined from proximal and distal tubular fluid collections and are summarized in Table I.

TABLE I

SEGMENTAL ABSORPTIVE EFFECTS OF CONVERTING ENZYME BLOCKADE

	CONTROL	CONVERTING ENZYME INHIBITOR
	Volume Delivery (nl/min)	Volume Delivery (nl/min)
Filtered Load	26.8 ± 1.8 nl	28.9 ± 1.2*
Late Proximal Tubule	18.2 ± 1.4	20.7 ± 1.8
Early Distal Tubule	5.7 ± .6	7.9 ± 1.0*
Urine	4.8 ± .9 µl/min	7.4 ± 1 µl/min

* denote significant change from control

Nephron GFR, measured at distal tubule sites, was significantly increased during angiotensin blockade. There was no significant alteration in absorptive function in the accessible portion of the proximal tubule; however, significant increases in delivery of fluid to the early distal tubule were observed. The data suggested reduced fractional and absolute absorption by the segments interposed between early distal and late proximal tubule micropuncture sites. Fractional and absolute volume delivery to the early distal tubule were increased and fractional absorption of the cumulative upstream segments was significantly reduced from 81% to 73%. During angiotensin blockade with Saralasin, chloride excretion increased in parallel with sodium excretion from 166 ± 87 µEq/min to 1442 ± 545 µEq/min. Absolute Cl^- delivery to the early distal tubule was increased from 323 ± 35 to 367 ± 38 nEq/min. These observations indicate that acute inhibition of the renin-angiotensin system results in increased renal sodium excretion that appears to be, in part, the result of decreased absorptive function of nephron segments between late proximal and early distal micropuncture sites. In addition, reduced absorption by segments downstream from the early distal puncture is suggested by the relatively greater changes in the urinary excretion patterns observed.

EFFECTS OF ANGIOTENSIN BLOCKADE ON BILATERAL RENAL FUNCTION RESPONSES IN ONE CLIP TWO KIDNEY GOLDBLATT HYPERTENSIVE RATS

The experiments on normal rats support the hypothesis that angiotensin exerts an influence on tubular reabsorptive processes. However, it has not been possible to determine if these effects are due to the influence of angiotensin II formed outside the kidneys and acting as a systemic hormone or to the local actions of angiotensin II formed within the kidney and acting as an endogenous hormone. As one means of evaluating this problem further, experiments were conducted using the two kidney one clip renal hypertensive rat model. This model exhibits the unique and physiologically interesting circumstance of having one kidney that is "renin depleted" existing in an overall environment of elevated plasma renin and angiotensin concentrations caused by the imposition of the renal clip on the other kidney[25]. Thus, the clipped kidney has a reduced renal perfusion pressure and elevated or high normal tissue renin content while the contralateral non-clipped kidney has reduced tissue renin content and is exposed to an elevated renal perfusion pressure. To the extent that the renal tissue renin content is a reflection of endogenous angiotensin activity it would be expected that the responses to angiotensin blockade would be greater in the kidneys with the higher tissue renin content.

Alternatively, the responses observed from the non-clipped kidney could be considered to reflect the inhibited influences of circulating angiotensin II. Since these studies involved examination of a renin depleted kidney that might be particularly susceptible to the agonist activity of end-plate receptor blockers, these experiments were conducted using the converting enzyme inhibitor, SQ 20881. For comparison, studies were also performed in normal control rats.

Goldblatt hypertensive rats (GHR) were prepared by placing a silver clip (.25 mm I.D.) around one renal artery. Hypertension was allowed to develop for 3 to 4 weeks. In one group of rats (7 GHR and 6 normal), plasma samples were collected for the measurement of plasma renin activity and the kidneys were harvested for measurement of tissue renin content. In another series (13 GHR and 12 normal), rats were prepared to allow separate urine collections and clearance measurements from both kidneys. GFR, urine flow and sodium excretion were measured for at least two control periods and for up to $3\frac{1}{2}$ hours during infusion of CEI. The SQ 20881 was administered as an initial bolus of 1 mg and followed by a constant infusion of .3 mg/100 g of body weight per hour. Since converting enzyme blockade resulted in profound decreases in arterial blood pressure in the GHR, a third group of GHR were examined to assess the direct effects of arterial pressure decreases similar to those observed during infusion of CEI. These experiments were conducted by placing an adjustable constrictor clip around the aorta above the origin of the two renal arteries.

Tissue renin content was clearly different in the two kidneys of the GHR[26]. In normal rats, kidney renin activity averaged 239 ± 54 ng AI/mg/hr. The clipped kidneys had only slightly higher values of 293 ± 40 ng AI/mg/hr. In contrast, the nonclipped contralateral kidneys of GHR demonstrated a marked reduction in kidney renin content to 14 ± 5 ng AI/mg/hr. In accord with previous results, PRA levels were higher in the GHR (24 ± 2.7 ng AI/ml/hr) than in the normal rats (12.8 ± 3.4 ng AI/ml/hr).

Infusion of CEI resulted in decreases in arterial pressure of the GHR from the control values of 153 ± 6.9 mmHg to 137 ± 7.3 mmHg after 30 minutes and 126 ± 4 mmHg by the end of the infusion. The normal rats exhibited a much smaller decrease in arterial pressure. Control arterial pressure averaged 119 ± 3 mmHg and decreased to 111 ± 3 mmHg. The decrease of 27 ± 4 mmHg was substantially greater than that observed in normal rats (8.4 ± 3.4 mmHg). Considering the decrease in arterial pressure, the clearance and excretory responses from the contralateral kidney of the GHR were surprising. Specifically, there was a marked increase in GFR that reached a maximum of 72% above control levels. Urine flow reached a maximum of 104% above control levels compared to 45% in normal rats. The sodium excretion responses were even greater reaching a maximum of 870% as compared to 480% for control rats. The average values obtained by the end of CEI infusion are shown in Table II.

TABLE II

RENAL RESPONSES TO CEI INFUSION IN NONCLIPPED AND CLIPPED

KIDNEYS OF GHR AND IN NORMAL RATS

	Nonclipped (n=13)		Clipped (n=13)		Normal (n=12)	
	Control	CEI	Control	CEI	Control	CEI
GFR ml/min	1.5 ± .06	2.1 ± .32	1.2 ± .14	.82 ± .07	1.5 ± .13	1.8 ± .24
Urine Flow µl/min	4.8 ± .7	7.4 ± 1.4	3.4 ± .4	1.8 ± .34	3.9 .26	5.5 ± .82
Sodium Excretion µl/min	.10 ± .02	.97 ± .28	.09 ± .01	.05 ± .02	.08 ± .02	.47 ± .14
Fractional Sodium Excretion	.05 ± .02	.37 ± .10	.07 ± .01	.04 ± .01	.03 ± .004	.16 ± .04

The increases in GFR, urine flow, sodium excretion and fractional sodium excretion occurring in the nonclipped kidney of the GH rats were all significantly greater than those exhibited by the corresponding kidneys from normal rats. In particular, the increase of sodium excretion was approximately twice as great in the nonclipped kidneys of GH rats than in normal rat kidneys. In contrast, the clipped kidney uniformly exhibited decreases in GFR, urine flow and sodium excretion. Fractional sodium excretion by the clipped kidney was slightly reduced.

In order to determine the extent to which observed responses were modified as a consequence of the associated decrease in arterial pressure, another group of GHR was evaluated before and during reduction of arterial pressure by aortic clamping to the same values seen during the CEI infusion. The sodium excretion responses are shown in Figure 1. For comparison, the data obtained during CEI administration are also plotted as a function of arterial pressure.

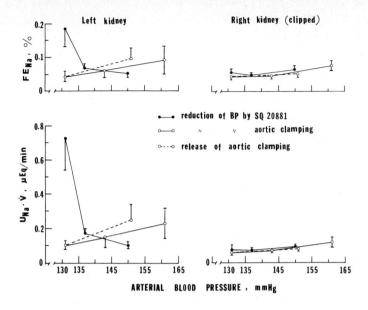

Figure 1. Relationships between arterial pressure and sodium excretion during aortic constriction and CEI infusion.

In the clipped kidneys, the decreases in GFR, urine flow and sodium excretion that occurred with clamp induced decreases in arterial pressure were similar to those observed during CEI infusion. Thus, the reductions in arterial pressure can adequately explain the alterations in function that were observed in the clipped kidney during CEI infusion. In the non-clipped kidneys, the marked GFR and urine excretory responses occurred in spite of the large arterial pressure reductions which, in the absence of converting enzyme inhibition, resulted in changes in renal function opposite to those observed during CEI infusion.

These experiments indicate that the non-clipped kidneys of GHR, characterized by decreased tissue renin content, are highly responsive to blockade of the renin-angiotensin system. To the extent that the reduced renal renin content reflects the endogenous activity of the renin-angiotensin system, these studies suggest that the influence of the renin-angiotensin system on the contralateral kidney is effected thorough systemic delivery of angiotensin. The observation that fractional sodium excretion from the non-clipped kidney increased markedly during CEI infusion is consistent with findings described in earlier sections and suggests a direct influence of angiotensin on tubular reabsorption. However, concomitant GFR responses would also be expected to contribute to the increased sodium excretion. Thus, the vascular and tubular effects of angiotensin could be operating synergistically to regulate sodium excretion rate.

ACKNOWLEDGEMENTS

This study was supported by grant #HL18426 from the NHLBI, by the Alabama Heart Association, and by the Veterans Administration. The authors thank Dr. Horowitz and the Squibb Company, Princeton, N.J., for providing us with the SQ 20881. Special thanks to Ms. Becky Smith and Mona Wright for their expert secretarial assistance.

REFERENCES

1.   Leyssac, P.P. (1976) The renin angiotensin system and kidney function: a review of contributions to a new theory. Acta. Physiol. Scand. Supp 442.

2.   Thurau, K. (1974) Intrarenal action of angiotensin. In: Angiotensin (Handbook of Experimental Pharmacology Vol. 37), edited by by I.H. Page and F.M. Bumpus. New York: Springer-Verlag, p. 475-489.

3.   Ploth, D.W., and L.G. Navar. (1979) Intrarenal effects of the renin-angiotensin system Fed. Proc. 38:2280-2285.

4.   Baer, P.G., and J.C. McGiff. (1980) Hormonal Systems and Renal Hemodynamics. Ann. Rev. Physiol. 42:589-601.

5.   Davis, J.O. (1974) The renin-angiotensin system and the control of aldosterone secretion, In: Angiotension (Handbook of Experimental Pharmacology, Vol. 37), edited by I.H. Page and F.M. Bumpus. New York: Springer-Verlag. pp. 322-336.

6.   Cook, W.F. (1967) The detection of renin in juxtaglomerular cells. J. Physiol. (London) 194:73p-74p.

7.   Thurau, K. and J. Mason. (1974) The intrarenal function of the juxtaglomerular apparatus. In: MPT Int. Rev. Sci. Physio., Ser. 1, 6:367-368.

8.   Freeman, R.H., J.O. Davis, T.E. Lohemier and W.S. Spielman. (1977) Desp-Asp[1] Angiotensin II: Mediator of the renin angiotensin system? Fed. Proc. 36:1766-1770.

9.   Hall, J.E., A.C. Guyton, N.C. Trippodo, T.E. Lohmeier, R.E. McCaa, and Cowley, A.W. (1977) Intrarenal control of electrolyte excretion by angiotensin II. Am. J. Physiol. 232:F538-F544.

10. Kimbrough, H.M. Jr., E.D. Vaughn, R.M. Carey, and C.R. Ayers. (1977) Effects of intrarenal angiotensin II blockade on renal function in conscious dog Circ. Res. 40:174-178.

11. Caldwell, P.R.B., B.C. Seegal and K.C. Hsu. (1976) Angiotension-converting enzyme: Vascular endothelial localization. Science 191:1050-1051.

12. Erdos, E.G. (1977) The angiotensin I converting enzyme. Fed. Proc. 36:1760-1765.

13. Ryan, J.W., and U.S. Ryan. (1978) Humoral control of arterial blood pressure: A role for lung. Cardiovas. Med. 3:531-550.

14. Fourcade, J.C., L.G. Navar, and A.C. Guyton. (1971) Possibility that angiotensin resulting from unilateral disease affects contralateral renal function. Nephron 8:11-16.

15. Navar, L.G., and H.G. Langford. (1974) Effects of angiotensin on the renal circulation. In: Angiotensin (Handbook of Experimental Pharmacology Vol. 37), edited by I.H. Page, and F.M. Bumpus. New York: Springer-Verlag, p. 455-474.

16. Barraclough, M.A., N.F. Jones and C.D. Marsden. (1967) Effect of angiotensin on renal function in the rat. Am. J. Physiol. 212:1153-1157.

17. Johnson M.D., and R.L. Malvin. (1977) Stimulation of renal sodium and reabsorption by angiotensin II. Am. J. Physiol. 232:F298-F306.

18. Malvin, R.L., and A.J. Vander. (1967) Effects of angiotensin infusion on renal function in the unanesthetized rat. Am. J. Physiol. 213:1205-1208.

19. Harris, P.J., and J.A. Young. (1977) Dose-dependent stimulation and inhibition of proximal tubular sodium reabsorption by angiotensin II in the rat kidney. Pfluegers Arch. 367:295-297.

20. Hollenberg, N.K. (1979) Pharmacologic interruption of the renin-angiotensin system. Ann. Rev. Pharmacol. Toxicol. 19:559-582.

21. Navar, L.G., R.A. LaGrange, P.D. Bell, C.E. Thomas, and D.W. Ploth. (1979) Glomerular and renal hemodynamics during converting enzyme inhibition in the dog. Hypertension 1:371-377.

22. Ploth, D.W., J. Rudulph, R. LaGrange, and L.G. Navar. (1979) Tubuloglomerular feedback and single nephron function after converting enzyme inhibition in the rat. J. Clin. Invest. 64:1325-1335.

23. Freeman, R.H. and J.O. Davis (1979) Physiological actions of angiotensin II on the kidney. Fed. Proc. 38:2276-2279.

24. Steiner, R.W., B.J. Tucker, and R.C. Blantz. (1979) Glomerular hemodynamics in rats with chronic sodium depletion. J. Clin. Invest. 69:503-512.

25. Ploth, D.W., R. Roy, and L.G. Navar. (1979) Renal hemodynamic and tubuloglomerular feedback responses following angiotensin blockade with Saralasin (P-113) in the rat. Clin. Res. 27:427A.

26. Brunner, H., P.A. Desaulles, D. Regoli and F. Gross. (1962) Renin content and excretory function of the kidneys in rats with experimental hypertension. Am. J. Physiol. 202:795-799.

Hormonal Regulation of Sodium Excretion,
B. Lichardus, R.W. Schrier and J. Ponec, eds.
© 1980 Elsevier/North-Holland Biomedical Press

THE ACTION OF ANGIOTENSIN III ([DES-ASP']-ANGIOTENSIN II) ON PROXIMAL TUBULAR
SODIUM REABSORPTION IN THE RAT KIDNEY

P.J. HARRIS

Department of Physiology, University Medical School, Teviot Place, Edinburgh,
U.K.

INTRODUCTION

The question of whether angiotensin has a direct action on renal tubular
sodium and water reabsorption has been the subject of much investigation and
debate. Until the application of micropuncture techniques the results of
studies using whole kidney methods such as renal clearance[1,2] remained
equivocal because of difficulties in separating the hemodynamic effects of the
peptide from possible actions on transport. Results obtained using a variety
of isolated epithelial preparations[3] although establishing the dose-dependent
nature of the response to angiotensin failed to clarify the question in relation
to the kidney.

There is now more convincing evidence from micropuncture experiments that at
least in the rat kidney angiotensin II has a direct effect on proximal tubular
sodium and water reabsorption[4,5,6]. Harris and Young[5] showed that angiotensin
II perfused into the peritubular capillaries has a direct, dose-dependent
action on proximal tubular sodium reabsorption. At 10^{-11}M, there was a
significant increase in steady-state sodium concentration gradient ($\Delta_{C_{Na}}$)
while at 3×10^{-6}M an inhibitory effect was observed.

It seemed reasonable to propose that this action might be involved in the
biphasic effect on sodium and water excretion observed following infusion of
different doses of angiotensin[1]. Here also was evidence to substantiate the
hypothesis that angiotensin II might be involved in the control of tubulo-
glomerular feedback possibly by mediating changes in proximal tubular sodium
reabsorption as a primary variable having a secondary effect on glomerular
filtration rate[7].

However, immunological studies[8] have shown that of the circulating plasma
immunoreactive angiotensin only 33% was angiotensin II while 58% was the
heptapeptide (des-asp')-angiotensin II (angiotensin III) and the remaining 9%
a mixture of the hexa-and penta-peptides. In order to relate the proximal
tubular transport actions of angiotensin II to either systemic or peritubular
plasma concentrations it therefore becomes necessary to compare the actions of

the two predominant analogues (the hepta-and octa-peptides).

METHODS

Two series of micropuncture experiments were performed using Inactin anaesthetised male Wistar rats in the weight range 250-300 g.

1. Stationary microperfusion technique. Stationary microperfusion between oil droplets was combined with simultaneous perfusion of the peritubular capillaries[9]. The intratubular perfusion fluid contained Na^+ (120 mm kg^{-1}), Ca^{2+} (1.5 mm kg^{-1}), Cl^- (105 mm kg^{-1}), HCO_3^- (8 mmol kg^{-1}) and acetate (10 mmol kg^{-1}) and was made isotonic by addition of raffinose (59 mmol kg^{-1}). The peritubular perfusion fluid had approximately plasma-like electrolyte composition and contained acetate[9]. Different concentrations of (des-asp')-angiotensin II (Calbiochem) were added as required. All glassware was siliconised to minimise adsoprtion of the peptide. In each experiment four control and four test samples (with angiotensin III included in the peritubular perfusate) were taken after 20 seconds contact time. Sodium concentrations in the recollected droplets were measured by picomole flame photometry[9] and enabled calculation of the steady-state sodium concentration gradient ($\Delta_{c_{Na}}$) across the proximal tubular epithelium. These experiments were thus carried out using an identical protocol to that described previously by Harris and Young[5] in the previous study on angiotensin II to allow direct comparison of the results.

2. Shrinking split oil-droplet technique. The method described by Gertz[10] and modified by Györy"[11] was used with simultaneous perfusion of the peritubular capillaries. The intratubular and peritubular perfusion fluids used had the same composition as those described above for the stationary droplet experiments except that raffinose was omitted from the intratubular fluid. Droplets were photographed using a 16 mm cine camera (Vinten) triggered to expose one frame per second. The shrinking droplet sequences were analysed by projection using a single-frame motion analysis projector. Measurement of the radii and distance between menisci was then made using a vernier caliper. Reabsorptive half-times ($t\frac{1}{2}$) were calculated as described by Györy"[11] and since comparisons were to be made between tubules within each rat and also between different rats the rate of reabsorption expressed as flux per unit area ($Jv_{(a)}$). At least four droplets were photographed during peritubular perfusion with the control solution (no angiotensin) and then at least four test droplets during perfusion with angio-tensin. This order of control and experimental perfusions was alternated in successive animals.

RESULTS

The results obtained using the stationary microperfusion technique are shown in Table 1.

TABLE 1

Ang. III conc^n. (mol. kg^{-1})	No. of animals	Mean ΔC_{Na} (mmol. kg^{-1}) Control	Test	P(paired 't' test)
10^{-12}	4	16.62 ± 1.22[a]	13.27 ± 0.85	< 0.02
10^{-11}	6	19.65 ± 1.02	14.41 ± 1.13	< 0.02
10^{-9}	6	15.91 ± 0.72	16.88 ± 1.52	> 0.4

[a] Results are shown as mean $\pm$ S.E.M.

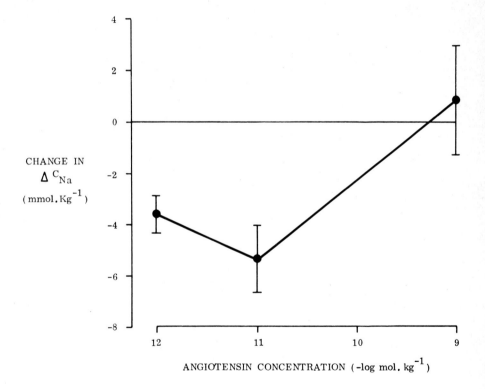

CHANGE IN
ΔC_{Na}
(mmol.Kg^{-1})

ANGIOTENSIN CONCENTRATION (-log mol. kg^{-1})

Fig. 1. Effect of angiotensin III on steady-state sodium concentration gradient (ΔC_{Na}). Differences between control and test data shown in Table 1 expressed as mean $\pm$ S.E.M.

The data summarised in Table 1 and Figure 1 show that angiotensin III at both 10^{-11} and 10^{-12}M caused a significant decrease in $\Delta_{C_{Na}}$ when compared with control perfusions in the same animal. The maximum effect was observed with 10^{-11}M angiotensin.

TABLE 2

Ang. III concn. (mol. kg^{-1})	No. of animals	Mean $J_{v(a)}$ ($\times 10^{-4}$.mm^3.mm^{-2}.sec^{-1})		P (paired 't')
		Control	Test	
10^{-13}	5	3.17 ± 0.18^{a}	2.85 ± 0.19	> 0.1
10^{-12}	5	2.54 ± 0.29	2.11 ± 0.15	> 0.1
10^{-11}	5	3.00 ± 0.34	1.31 ± 0.51	< 0.005
10^{-10}	5	2.55 ± 0.21	1.91 ± 0.22	< 0.05
10^{-8}	4	2.53 ± 0.07	2.64 ± 0.50	> 0.4

[a] Results are shown as mean $\pm$ S.E.M.

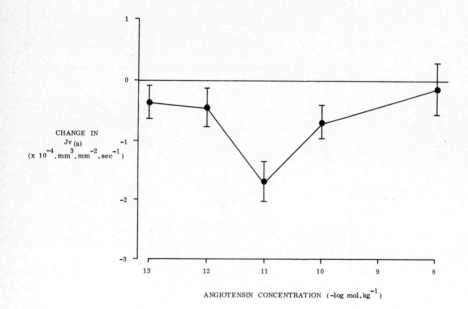

CHANGE IN $J_{v(a)}$ ($\times 10^{-4}$.mm^3.mm^{-2}.sec^{-1})

ANGIOTENSIN CONCENTRATION ($-\log$ mol.kg^{-1})

Fig. 2. Effect of angiotensin III on proximal tubular fluid reabsorption ($J_{v(a)}$). Differences between control and test data shown in Table 2 expressed as mean $\pm$ S.E.M.

The data presented in Table 2 and Figure 2 show that peritubular perfusion with 10^{-10} and 10^{-11} M angiotensin III caused a significant reduction in transepithelial fluid reabsorption when compared with control perfusions using fluids containing no angiotensin. Maximum reduction was observed at 10^{-11} M but no significant effect was seen either at higher (10^{-8} M) or at lower (10^{-12}, 10^{-13} M) concentrations.

DISCUSSION

These two series of experiments have shown that angiotensin III caused a significant decrease in both $J_{v_{(a)}}$ and $\Delta_{C_{Na}}$ with a maximum effect at 10^{-11} M. The interpretation of results obtained using these techniques has been the subject of considerable study. A decrease in $J_{v_{(a)}}$ could be the result of either lowered water permeability or a reduction in sodium reabsorption rate, although the latter effect is more likely. Changes in $\Delta_{C_{Na}}$ have been interpreted as alterations in the rate of active sodium reabsorption provided that there are no associated changes in either transepithelial potential difference or in sodium permeability. In the experiments described here no attempt was made to evaluate either of these factors. However, the observation that angiotensin III reduced both $J_{v_{(a)}}$ and $\Delta_{C_{Na}}$ suggests an action on active sodium reabsorption.

Previous studies on the relative potencies of angiotensin II and angiotensin III have been reviewed by Peach[12]. A variety of tissues and assay preparations have been used and in all cases the heptapeptide has shown a qualitatively similar action to the octapeptide although the effects have often been quantitatively different. It is now generally accepted that angiotensin III has only 25-50% of the pressor activity of angiotensin II but that it is at least equipotent if not more potent as a stimulus for aldosterone biosynthesis. This observation has formed the basis for a number of studies showing that the pressor and adrenal receptors for angiotensin are different[13-16]. However while there is considerable evidence that des-asp' angiotensin II may be the mediator of the adrenal steroid response[17] and act on specific angiotensin III receptors[18] there has been little support for a similar mechanism either in the kidney[19] or in epithelial preparations such as toad skin[20].

Figure 3 shows the data from Figure 1 compared with data obtained in a previous similar study[5]. While both analogues have maximum effects at the same concentration (10^{-11} M) their actions are clearly opposite. This observation is rather surprising in view of the evidence that these analogues have qualitatively similar effects in other tissues. The rate of proximal tubular

88

sodium and water reabsorption would thus appear to depend on the ratio between the heptapeptide and octapeptide concentrations. If the relative proportions of angiotensins reported by Semple and Morton[8] for arterial plasma in the rat are any indication of the peritubular concentrations then both angiotensins II and III would be important in regulating the rate of tubular transport. The relation between arterial and peritubular plasma angiotensin concentrations is difficult to predict since it would depend on both the pathway and rate of production of the heptapeptide and on the relative breakdown rates of the two peptides. These factors are known to be species dependent and could account for the unusually high proportion of angiotensin III found in rat plasma compared with other species. It would follow that any physiological significance of angiotensin III found in the rat may also be peculiar to this species.

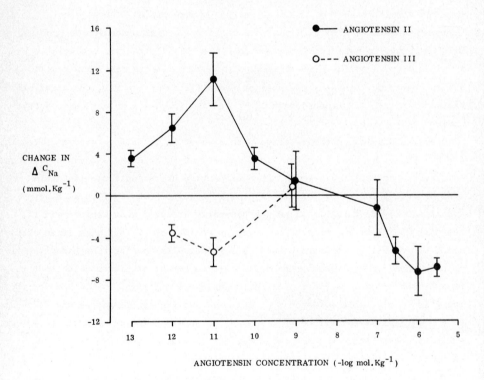

Fig. 3. Effects of angiotensins II and III on steady-state sodium concentration gradients ($\Delta_{C_{Na}}$). Results are shown as mean $\pm$ S.E.M.

The results summarised in Figure 3 are open to several interpretations and lead to some intriguing questions. It may be proposed that associated with the proximal tubule there is one population of angiotensin receptors with different affinities for angiotensins II and III. The complete dose-response curve for angiotensin III would therefore be a similar shape to that for angiotensin II but shifted to the left. This would imply that a stimulatory effect of angiotensin III would be predicted at about 10^{-16}M, a rather low concentration for this effect to have any physiological significance.

There is however another possible hypothesis that the biphasic response to angiotensin II is due to dose-dependent activation of two different angiotensin receptors, a transport receptor and a vascular receptor. At low concentrations of angiotensin II (10^{-12}-10^{-10}M) a stimulatory effect is observed perhaps associated with activation of a transport receptor. This may be related to the stimulatory effect of 10^{-11}M angiotensin II observed on sodium transport in cultured MDCK cell monolayers[21].

When the peritubular capillaries are perfused with angiotensin II at concentrations of 2×10^{-8}, Jensen and Steven[22] showed that the capillaries contract and peritubular hydrostatic pressure increases. It is likely that this increase in pressure would inhibit fluid reabsorption from the proximal tubule ($J_{v_{(a)}}$) and might also affect the attainment of equilibrium in the steady-state microperfusion experiments. This vascular effect may be proposed to account for the disappearance of the stimulatory action of angiotensin II at about 10^{-9}M and the development of an inhibitory response at higher concentrations. The shape of angiotensin II dose-response curve would thus represent the sum of responses associated with the two types of receptor. Using this model the action of angiotensin III over the range tested would be predominantly on the vascular receptor. Further studies with antagonist analogues of both octapeptide and heptapeptide that have previously been used to examine the adrenal and peripheral vascular receptors would be useful to test this hypothesis.

Several other factors may also be involved in the hormonal control of proximal tubular sodium reabsorption. In particular the contribution of the effects of angiotensin on the adrenergic and dopaminergic nerve terminals known to be closely associated with the tubular epithelium have received little investigation. The potentiation of adrenergic stimuli by angiotensin II and their interactions with prostaglandins have been clearly demonstrated but little understood, particularly in the kidney[23]. The possibility of interactions between angiotensin and adrenergic nerve terminals is especially interesting in the light of evidence that stimulation by angiotensin II of intestinal fluid transport in the rat is possibly mediated by noradrenaline[24].

CONCLUSIONS

(i) Angiotensin III perfused into the peritubular capillaries surrounding rat proximal tubules caused significant inhibition of both transepithelial volume flux ($J_{v(a)}$) and steady-state sodium concentration gradient (Δc_{Na}). A maximum effect was observed at 10^{-11} M.

(ii) When the angiotensin III results were compared with previous data obtained using angiotensin II it was evident that in the physiological range these two peptides had opposite effects.

(iii) It is proposed that in the rat a direct tubular action of angiotensin III may be of some physiological significance in the hormonal control of sodium excretion.

ACKNOWLEDGEMENTS

The work described in this paper was carried out with the aid of grants from the National Health and Medical Research Council of Australia and the Medical Research Council. The expert technical assistance of Miss J. Munro is gratefully acknowledged.

REFERENCES

1. Barraclough, M.A., Jones, N.F. and Marsden, C.D. (1967) Am. J. Physiol., 212, 1153-1157.

2. Johnson, M.D. and Malvin, R.L. (1977) Am. J. Physiol., 232, F298-F306.

3. Navar, L.G. and Langford, H.G. (1974) Angiotensin. Handbuch der exp. pharmakol Bd. 37. Springer, Berlin-Heidelberg-New York, pp. 455-474.

4. Steven, K. (1974) Kidney International, 6, 73-80.

5. Harris, P.J. and Young, J.A. (1977) Pflügers Arch., 367, 295-297.

6. Spinelli, F. (1977) Proc. I.U.P.S., 13, 711.

7. Leyssac, P.P. (1976) Acta physiol. scand. suppl. 442, pp. 5-52.

8. Semple, P.F. and Morton, J.J. (1976) Circ. Res., 38, 122-126.

9. Gyory, A.Z., Lingard, J.M. and Young, J.A. (1974) Pflügers Arch., 348, 205-210.

10. Gertz, K.H. (1962) Pflügers Arch., 276, 336-356.

11. Gyory, A.Z. (1971) Pflügers Arch., 324, 328-343.

12. Peach, M.J. (1977) Physiol. Reviews, 57, 313-370.

13. Bravo, E.L., Khosla, M.C. and Bumpus, F.M. (1975) J. Clin. Endocrinol. Metab., 40, 530-533.

14. Freeman, R.H., Davis, J.O., Lohmeier, T.E. and Spielman, W.S. (1977) Fed. Proc., 36, 1766-1770.

15. Blumberg, A.L., Nishikawa, K., Denny, S.E., Marshall, G.R. and Needleman, P. (1977) Circ. Res., 41, 154-158.

16. Caldicott, W.J.H. and Hollenberg, N.K. (1979) Life Sciences, 24, 503-512.

17. Goodfriend, T.L. and Peach, M.J. (1975) Circ. Res., 36, Suppl. 1., 38-48.

18. Devynck, M-A., Koreve, V., Matthews, P.G., Meyer, P. and Pernollet, M-G. (1977) Adv. Nephrol., 7, 121-135.

19. Hall, J.E., Coleman, T.G., Guyton, A.C., Balfe, J.W. and Salgado, H.C. (1979) Am. J. Physiol., 236, F252-F259.

20. Coviello, A., Raisman, R., Elso, G. and Orce, G. (1978) Biochem. Pharmacol., Pharmacol., 27, 611-612.

21. Simmons, N.L. (1978) J. Physiol., 276, 28P-29P.

22. Jensen, P.K. and Steven, K. (1977) Pflügers Arch., 371, 245-250.

23. Zambraski, E.J. and Dibona, G.F. (1979) Proc. Soc. exp. Biol. Med., 162, 105-111.

24. Levens, N.R., Munday, K.A., Parsons, B.J., Poat, J.A. and Stewart, C.P. (1979) J. Physiol., 286, 351-360.

Hormonal Regulation of Sodium Excretion,
B. Lichardus, R.W. Schrier and J. Ponec, eds.
© 1980 Elsevier/North-Holland Biomedical Press

KIDNEY FUNCTION DURING CAROTID CHEMORECEPTOR STIMULATION -
INFLUENCE OF UNILATERAL RENAL NERVE SECTION

ARNOLD HONIG and MANFRED SCHMIDT
Institute of Physiology, Ernst-Moritz-Arndt-University,
DDR - 2200 Greifswald, German Democratic Republic

INTRODUCTION

Young and healthy humans and mammals under resting conditions
acutely exposed to moderate arterial hypoxia show an increase of
renal sodium and water excretion, a decrease of the plasma volume
and a rise of the hemoglobin and protein concentration in the
blood[1,2,3,4]. Since hypoxic hypoxia is accompanied by a stimulation of the arterial chemoreceptors we supposed that there might
exist a reflex influence of these receptors on renal sodium excretion[4,5,6]. Indeed in previous studies we could show that stimulation of the vascularly isolated carotid chemoreceptors increases renal sodium excretion. This response resulted from an
inhibition of renal tubular sodium reabsorption and proved to be
independent of the reactions of breathing and systemic arterial
blood pressure, the behaviour of renal blood flow and glomerular
filtrations rate, and the integrity of the vagal nerves[4,5,6]. Section of the carotid sinus nerves prevented the natriuresis due to
carotid chemoreceptor stimulation. Thus the arterial chemoreceptors were supposed to have a reflex influence upon renal sodium
excretion[4,5,6]. The experiments presented here investigated into
the possible efferent pathways of this natriuretic reflex.

MATERIALS AND METHODS

We studied the influence of unilateral renal nerve section
upon the kidney effects of a prolonged hypoxic- hypercapnic perfusion of the vascularly isolated carotid bodies in chloralosed,
spontaneously breathing, nonvagotomized cats, undergoing saline
diuresis (0.3 ml/min/kg). The left kidney was exposed by a flank
incision and all visible nerves in the vicinity of the main renal
vessels were cut after infiltration of this area with procaine.
The urine from both kidneys was sampled separately. The methods

ror perfusing the carotid bifurcations and for stuying renal
functions are described in detail elsewhere[4,5]. The carotid
bodies were perfused successively with the animals' own arterial
blood, with their own venous blood and again with arterial blood
(Figs 1 and2). The perfusion pressure at the carotid sinuses was
always held about 1.3 kPa above the systemic arterial pressure.

RESULTS AND DISCUSSION

During the last clearance-period before beginning the hypoxic
perfusion of the carotid bodies (base-lines in Figs. 1 and 2)
there were no significant differences between the innervated and
denervated kidneys with respect to the effective renal plasma
flow (C_{PAH}), the glomerular filtration rate (C_{IN}), filtration
fraction, and renal vascular resistance. During the same time,
however, the denervated kidneys show significantly higher fractional excretions for urine (ca.+80%), sodium (ca.+90%), potassium (ca.+30%), and the fractional osmolar clearance (ca.+60%).
Urine osmolality was lower at the denervated side.

The hypoxic perfusion of the carotid bodies was accompanied by
an enforcement of breathing and a transient increase (+0.8 kPa)
of the mean systemic arterial blood pressure (MBP). The behaviour
of renal hemodynamics (Fig. 1) was characterized by an increase
of the vascular resistance (ca.+28%) at the innervated side. The
reaction of the vascular resistance in the denervated kidneys was
only one fifth of that of the innervated vascular bed. These results support the hypothesis that the renal vasoconstriction due
to arterial chemoreceptor stimulation is mainly mediated by the
renal nerves.

As it is shown in Fig. 2 there was no clear reaction of the
fractional urine excretion and the fractional osmolar clearance
in the innervated kidneys during chemoreceptor stimulation,
whereas the fractional potassium excretion increased. This behaviour of the potassium excretion probably depends on the
breathing reaction and the accompanying respiratory alcalosis[6].
The significant decrease of the fractional sodium excretion of
the innervated kidneys may be explained by the fall of glomerular
filtration rate and renal blood flow (Fig. 1). In contrast to
these (anti-natriuretically effective) reactions of the renal

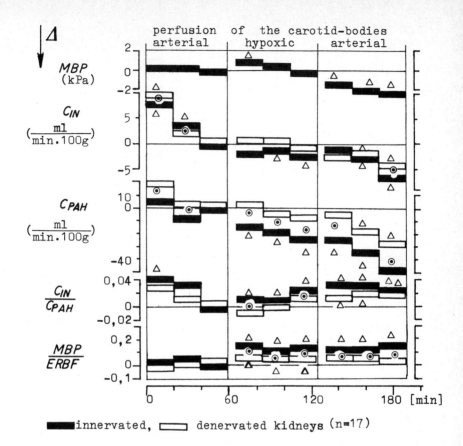

Fig. 1. Changes of the mean systemic arterial blood pressure, glomerular filtration rate, effective renal plasma flow, filtration fraction, and renal vascular resistance (MBP/ERBF) during stimulation of the carotid chemoreceptors; average values (n=17), ⊙ = differences between the reactions of the denervated and innervated kidneys significant (p < 0.05), △ = deviation from base-line significant (p < 0.05).

Hemodynamics in the innervated kidneys, the stimulation of the carotid chemoreceptors was not accompanied by such changes of GFR and RBF in the denervated kidneys and here we found significant increases of the fractional excretion presented in Fig. 2. From these results we conclude that acute renal nerve section fails to prevent the inhibition of tubular sodium reabsorption due to stimulation of the carotid chemoreceptors in spontaneously breathing nonvagotomized cats. Thus the mechanism of this response remains

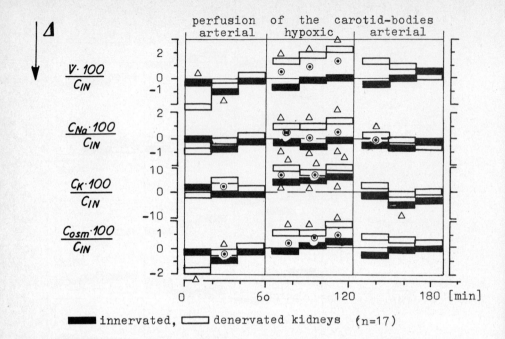

Fig. 2. Changes of the fractional urine volume, the fractional sodium excretion, the fractional potassium excretion, and the fractional osmolar clearance during stimulation of the carotid chemoreceptors. - All other data as in Fig. 1.

to be investigated. In this respect it is of interest that following adrenalectomy the increase in potassium excretion upon exposure to highaltitude hypoxia continues to occur, but the striking increases in sodium and chloride excretion are no longer observed[7,8]. Some questions related to this problem and to the involvement of the arterial chemoreceptors in the control of body fluid volumes and renal function in acute hypoxic hypoxia are discussed elsewhere[4].

Our results suggest that the natriuresis due to acute high-altitude exposure and the accompanying decrease of the plasma volume might be the result of the stimulation of the arterial chemoreceptors. These reactions could possibly explain, why humans who live at high altitudes have both lower blood pressure and a lower incidence of hypertension than individuals of similar age living at sea levels[9,10,11,12], and why simulated high-alti-

tude hypoxia protects rats against the development of renal
hypertension[13].

But on the other hand the question arises whether function and
reflex effects of the arterial chemoreceptors are altered in
hypertension? This seems to be an important problem, because due
to their influence on the sodium metabolism a changed activity
of the arterial chemoreceptors would in turn affect the development of systemic hypertension. So far in post-mortem studies an
enlargement and striking catecholamine concentrations of the carotid bodies have been described in hypertensive individuals[14,
15,16]. In both human hypertensives and spontaneously hypertensive
rats (Okamoto-strain/SHR) altered hemodynamic and breathing
responses due to exposure to hyperoxia or hypoxia have been observed[17,18,19,20,21], suggesting changed reflex effects of the
arterial chemoreceptors in hypertension. In own experiments (unpublished data) we found the carotid bodies of spontaneously
hypertensive rats (SHR, 30-40 wks) to be significantly greater
(ca +70%) than those of age-matched, normotensive Wistar rats
(random-bred strain), and we could also confirm the finding[19]
that SHR exhibit alveolar hyperventilation as compared with
normotensive animals.

The finding that systemic hypertension is accompanied by chronic stimulation of the arterial chemoreceptors would explain, why
both hypertensive humans and animals show many symptoms that are
very similar to those of normal mammals living at high alti-
tude. For instance, the behaviour of renal hemodynamics (Fig.1.)
of the innervated kidneys during chemoreceptor stimulation (particularly the increase of the vascular resistance and the higher
filtration fraction) resembles the picture of renal hemodynamics
in patients with hypertension[22], in spontaneously hypertensive
rats (SHR)[23,24], and in normal individuals living at high alti-
tude[25,26].

REFERENCES

1. Assmussen, E. et al. (1945) Acta physiol. scand., 9, 75
2. Berger, E.Y. et al. (1949) J. Clin. Invest., 28, 648
3. Bursaux, E. et al. (1976) Pfluegers Archiv, 365, 213
4. Honig, A. (1979) Acta physiol. pol. suppl., 18, 93
5. Honig, A. et al. (1975) Acta biol. med. germ., 34, 907

98

6. Flemming, B. et al. (1976) Ergebn. Exp. Med., 23, 251
7. Langley, L.L. et al. (1942) Yale J. Biol. Med., 14, 529
8. Lewis, R.A. et al. (1942) J. Clin. Invest., 21, 33
9. Makela, M. (1978) J.Chron. Dis., Ⅱ 31, 587
10. Meerson, F.Z. et al. (1975) Dokl. Akad. Nauk. USSR 220/3,749
11. Moret, P.R. et al. (1978) Coeur et Med. Int. XVII,(suppl),75
12. Ruiz, L. et al. (1977) Mayo Clin. Proc., 52, 442
13. Fregly, M.J. (1970) Proc. Soc. Exp. Biol. Med., 134, 78
14. Edwards. C. et al. (1971) J. Pathol., 104. 1
15. Lange, F. (1962) Dtsch. Med. Wschr., 87, 13
16. Steele, R.H. et al. (1972) J. Lab. Clin. Med., 80, 63
17. Full, H. et al. (1923) Klin. Wschr., 2, 69
18. Kirchhoff, H.W. (1964) Truppenpraxis-Wehrmed. Mittlg., 2, 23
19. Przybylski, J. (1978) IRCS Med. Sci., 6, 315
20. Przybylski, J. et al. (1980) Acta physiol. pol., (in press)
21. Walsh, G.M. et al. (1978) Amer. J. Physiol., 234, H 275
22. Reubi, F.C. et al. (1978) Amer. J. Med., 64, 556
23. Beierwaltes, W.H. et al. (1978) Circul. Res., 42, 721
24. DiBona, G.F. et al. (1978) Amer. J. Physiol., 235, F 409
25. Becker, E.L. (1957) J. Appl. Physiol., 10, 79
26. Monge, C.C. et al. (1969) Fed. Proc., 28, 1199

Hormonal Regulation of Sodium Excretion,
B. Lichardus, R.W. Schrier and J. Ponec, eds.
© 1980 Elsevier/North-Holland Biomedical Press

THE INFLUENCE OF MIXED VENOUS pO_2 VARIATIONS ON SODIUM HANDLING
- INVESTIGATIONS ON THE AFFERENT PATHWAY

DIETER ROLOFF, BERT FLEMMING, JOSE A. MENENDEZ
Institute of Physiology, Humboldt University, Hessische Str.3/4
1040 Berlin, GDR

INTRODUCTION

Many authors have suggested that the cardiac output may regulate water and sodium excretion by the kidney. Confirmatory
evidence has been obtained during inferior vena cava constriction, low output heart failure and during blood volume expansion. Contradictory evidence has been found in exercise and in
chronic conditions like anemia, arteriovenous fistula and high
output heart failure. The common factor in all the above conditions appeared to us to be an alteration of the mixed venous
pO_2 ($pO_{2\bar{v}}$). We had previously demonstrated that an isolated
change of $pO_{2\bar{v}}$ influences the renal sodium excretion. The present study is an attempt to determine the localisation of such
pO_2 sensitive structures in the central venous circulatory
region and to explore possible afferent pathways.

MATERIALS AND METHOD

Experiments were performed on chloralose anesthetized cats.
The trachea was cannulated for spontaneous breathing with room
air. The animals received a continuous infusion into the left
femoral vein to induce an osmotic basic diuresis (176 mmol/l
Mannit, 178 mmol/l Glucose, PAH, Inulin and Heparin; 0.1 ml per
min and kg body wt).

Blood from the other proximal and distal femoral veins
flowed by gravity into a rolling oxygenator from which it was
pumped into the cat's jugular vein; the catheter top was placed
2 cm below the right atrium into the inferior vena cava or in

the other mode 2 cm above the right atrium into the superior vena cava.

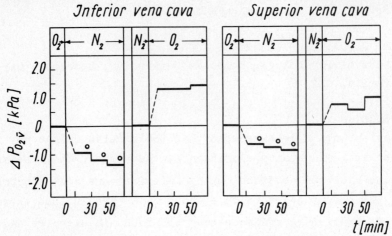

Fig. 1. Change in absolute mixed venous pO_2 ($pO_{2\bar{v}}$) measured in the right ventricle after alteration of oxygenator's gas mixture from oxygen to nitrogen (O_2-N_2) and from nitrogen to oxygen (N_2-O_2). (o) - differences between both changes are significant (2p < 0.05).

The infused blood was pumped through a heat exchanger and a blood filter near the jugular vein. The extracorporal volume was kept constant.

The gas mixture in the oxygenator was changed every hour and contained 95 % O_2 and 5 % CO_2 or 95 % N_2 and 5 % CO_2.

In a few investigations the animals were cervical vagotomized before beginning the experimental procedure.

The blood pressure was measured in the brachial artery. Blood samples were obtained from the right ventricle and the femoral artery.

The results are expressed as the mean. Dates for significance were tested by the WILCOXON-test. Values of 2 p < 0.05 were considered significant (o).

TABLE 1

THE ABSOLUTE BASIC VALUES

These levels are the mean basic values to which the others are related after changing the $pO_{2\bar{v}}$

Parameter	i.v.c.[a]		s.v.c.[b]	
	O_2-N_2[c]	N_2-O_2[d]	O_2-N_2[c]	N_2-O_2[d]
$pO_{2\bar{v}}$ (kPa)	5.7	4.4	7.1	6.9
BPm (kPa)	16.0	14.8	15.5	14.9
c_{In} (ml/min)	7.7	5.9	9.6	8.6
c_{PAH} (ml/min)	34.2	28.3	32.6	33.4
R_{ren} ($\frac{MPa.s}{l}$)	26.6	31.9	19.6	21.2
$\dot{V}_U$ (ml/min)	0.42	0.35	0.41	0.42
$U_{Na}\dot{V}$ (μmol/min)	5.08	4.90	5.74	4.19
$U_K\dot{V}$ (μmol/min)	11.21	6.00	10.65	11.47

[a] inferior vena cava infusion
[b] superior vena cava infusion
[c] change from oxygen to nitrogen gas phase in the oxygenator
[d] change from nitrogen to oxygen gas phase in the oxygenator

RESULTS

The absolute values before changing the gas mixture in the oxygenator are shown in Table 1.

The mixed venous pO_2 ($pO_{2\bar{v}}$) measured in the right ventricle was altered with assistance of the oxygenator nearly about 1.4 kPa during inferior vena cava infusion and nearly about 0.8 kPa during superior vena cava infusion (Fig. 1). The arterial pO_2 and the acid base status, however, did not demonstrate any dependence on the composition of gas in the oxygenator.

A decrease of $pO_{2\bar{v}}$ during inferior vena cava infusion was followed by a reduced mean arterial pressure (BPm), glomerular

102

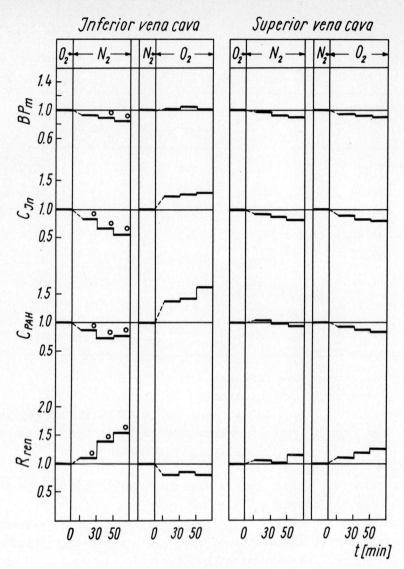

Fig. 2. Mean relatively changes of BPm, c_{In}, c_{PAH} and R_{ren} by infusion of oxygenated or desoxygenated blood into the inferior or superior vena cava.
(o) - differences between both modes are significant (2 $p < 0.05$)

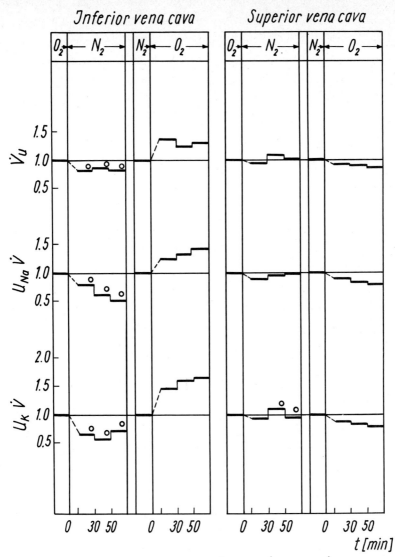

Fig. 3. Mean relatively changes of $\dot{V}_U$, $U_{Na}\dot{V}$ and $U_K\dot{V}$ by infusion of oxygenated or desoxygenated blood into the inferior or superior vena cava.
(o) - differences between both modes are significant $(2\ p < 0.05)$

filtration rate (c_{In}) and renal plasma flow (c_{PAH}). The renal resistance (R_{ren}) was increased (Fig. 2). In the same way a lowered $pO_{2\bar{v}}$ was connected with a decrease of urine volume ($\dot{V}_U$), sodium excretion ($U_{Na}\dot{V}$) and potassium excretion ($U_K\dot{V}$) (Fig. 3).

No significant changes of all of these parameters occurred in the experiments with superior vena cava infusion (Fig. 2 and 3). The infusion into the inferior vena cava in cervical vagotomized cats had no influence on the urine volume and the sodium excretion when the gas composition in the oxygenator was changed.

DISCUSSION

The results show that changes of pO_2 in the central venous region produce an alteration in the urine sodium excretion.

The $pO_{2\bar{v}}$ sensitive structures must be located between the site of the perfusion and the lung capillaries, because the composition of the arterial blood gases remains unchanged.

The location of sensitive structures can only be before the right ventricle, that is, in the area of the vena cavas and the right auricle because comparative changes in the pO_2 of right ventricle resulted from perfusion into the inferior or the superior vena cava. However, only the perfusion into the inferior vena cava resulted in changes in the electrolyte balance.

The results in few vagotomized animals showed no changes in the electrolyte balance when the gas composition in the oxygenator was changed. It is possible that the vagus may be the afferent pathway but more investigations will be necessary.

Alterations of mixed venous pO_2 induce variations of renal excretion function, similar as in heart failure, exercise and volume expansion.

Hormonal Regulation of Sodium Excretion,
B. Lichardus, R.W. Schrier and J. Ponec, eds.
© 1980 Elsevier/North-Holland Biomedical Press

THE INFLUENCE OF MIXED VENOUS pO_2 VARIATIONS ON SODIUM HANDLING
- INVESTIGATIONS ON THE EFFERENT PATHWAY

BERT FLEMMING, DIETER ROLOFF, JOSE A. MENENDEZ
Institute of Physiology, Humboldt University, Hessische Str. 3/4
1040 Berlin, GDR

INTRODUCTION

In previous experiments we have demonstrated that an alteration of mixed venous pO_2 is followed by changes of renal
function.

After decrease of mixed venous pO_2 the renal sodium excretion
is lowered, while an increase of this pO_2 is accompanied with a
rise of renal sodium excretion. Under conditions of alterations
of mixed venous pO_2, i.e. heart failure, and volume expansion,
it is suggested and described that the renal responses are
mediated by a humoral factor.

The purpose of this work was to examine the participation of
an humoral factor in the efferent way in the above described
phenomenon.

METHODS

The acute experiments were performed in chloralose-urethane
anaesthetized cats. The alteration of mixed venous pO_2 was induced, as previously described, by assistance of an oxygenator in
a veno-venous bypass. The blood from the oxygenator was infused
into the inferior vena cava. The gas mixture in the oxygenator
was changed from 95 % O_2 and 5 % CO_2 to 95 % N_2 and 5 % CO_2 or
back for one hour in each case.

Beside the normal renal parameters the sodium lost of cats
own erythrocytes after incubation in LiCl-solution and the Na^{22}
influx were determined.

Blood was obtained every 20 min from a. femoralis. Isotonic
solution with Na^{22} was given to whole blood and incubated and
shaked (38 $^{\circ}$C, 1 h). The Na^{22} activity in the erythrocytes and

106

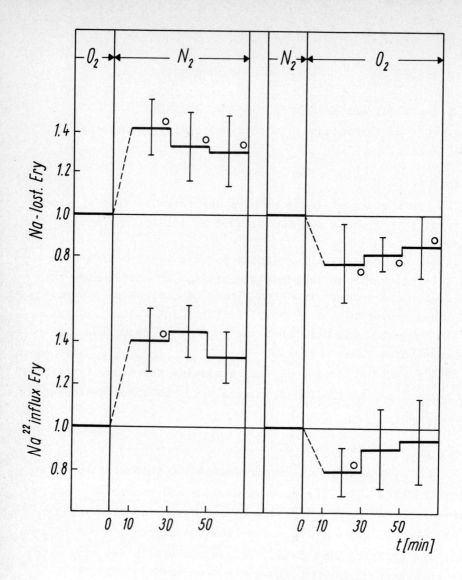

Fig. 1. Mean relatively changes of Na-lost of cat red blood
cells in a Na-free solution and Na^{22} influx into the cat red
cells after alteration of mixed venous pO_2.
O_2 = high pO_2 in the oxygenator
N_2 = high pN_2 in the oxygenator
o = differences between both changes of the pO_2 are
significant (2 p < 0.05)

in the plasma was determined before and after incubation.

For the determination of the sodium lost blood was centrifugated (20 000 g, at 4 $^{\circ}$C) and the plasma and buffy coat were removed. The erythrocytes were diluted with isotonic LiCl Ringer-solution. The first part of this suspension was immediately centrifugated, the second part after incubation (38°C, 1 h). The sodium concentration of the red blood cells and the supernatants were measured before and after incubation.

Normal unhydrated anaesthetized rats were used for bioassay. The urine, collected by bladder catheter into tared plastic tubes over 20 min periods, was analysed for sodium concentration. The native cat plasma was injected every 20 min into the jugular vein of rats.

RESULTS

The sodium lost of cats own red blood cells in a LiCl-solution and the influx of Na^{22} were increased after the lowering of mixed venous pO_2 (95 % N_2 into the oxygenator). After the changing of the gas mixture in the oxygenator the sodium lost and the Na^{22} influx of the red blood cells were decreased. The differences of these parameters by changes of mixed venous pO_2 are significant (Fig. 1).

The sodium concentration of urine (U_{Na}) and the sodium excretion ($U_{Na}\dot{V}$) in the cats reacted in the same manner as previously described (Fig. 2, Fig. 3). The sodium concentration of urine and the renal sodium excretion of the rat decreased after donation of plasma taken from cats during a low mixed venous pO_2. After elevation of mixed venous pO_2 in the cats the injection of cat's plasma to rats induced an increase of urine sodium concentration and renal sodium excretion. These reactions we have observed in all cases.

The urine volume in cats and rats did not show any dependence on the mixed venous pO_2.

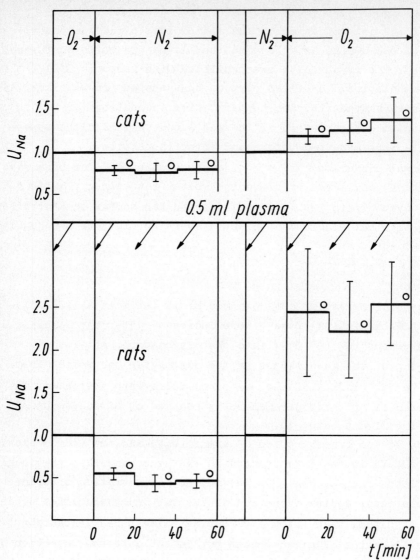

Fig. 2. Mean relatively changes of urine sodium concentration
(U_{Na}) in cats and rats.
The mixed venous pO_2 in cats was changed (O_2, N_2)
⟋ plasma was given from cats to rats
o = differences between both modes are significant (2 $p < 0.05$)

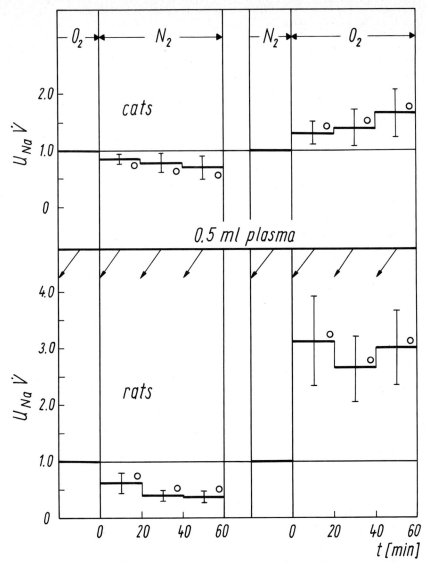

Fig. 3. Mean relatively changes of renal sodium excretion
(U$_{Na}$V̇) in cats and rats.
The mixed venous pO$_2$ in cats was changed (O$_2$,N$_2$)
↗ plasma was given from cats to rats
o = differences between both modes are significant (2 p < 0.05)

TABLE 1

THE ABSOLUTE BASIC VALUES

The mean basic values to which the other ones are related after changing the $pO_{2\bar{v}}$

Parameter	cats		rats	
	O_2-N_2 [a]	N_2-O_2 [b]	"O_2-N_2"	"N_2-O_2"
Na-lost$_{Ery}$	0.24	0.37	–	–
Na^{22}-Influx$_{Ery}$	0.73	1.60	–	–
U_{Na} (mmol/l)	20.5	21.3	5.4	3.1
$U_{Na}\dot{V}$ (µmol/min)	17.5	15.2	0.201	0.077

DISCUSSION

From the results we can conclude that the alterations of mixed venous pO_2 induced the releasing of an humoral factor. This humoral factor influenced the sodium metabolism of the red blood cells and induced in a bioassay on rats the same reactions of renal sodium excretion as in the donator cats. By reason of the specific properties of cat red blood cells, that means no or very small activity of Na-K-ATPase, we suggested that the humoral factor alters the membrane permeability for sodium. The origin and the nature of this humoral factor are unknown.

HYPOPHYSEAL HORMONES

Hormonal Regulation of Sodium Excretion,
B. Lichardus, R.W. Schrier and J. Ponec, eds.
© 1980 Elsevier/North-Holland Biomedical Press

EFFECT OF CALCIUM TRANSPORT INHIBITORS ON RENAL HEMODYNAMICS AND
ELECTROLYTE EXCRETION IN THE DOG

H. LAWRENCE McCROREY, TOMAS BERL, THOMAS J. BURKE, ANTOINE deTORRENTE,
ROBERT W. SCHRIER
Department of Medicine, University of Colorado Health Sciences Center,
4200 East Ninth Avenue, Denver, Colorado 80262, U.S.A.

INTRODUCTION

The clinical observation of marked polyuria associated with hypercalcemia,
together with early in vivo experiments in which the infusion of calcium salts
produced a natriuresis[1,2], suggest a relationship between calcium and sodium
transport. In general, these findings have supported the view that hypercalcemia decreases sodium reabsorption, probably in the proximal tubule. In
direct contrast, in vitro evidence derived from studies in various epithelial
membranes has been consistent with the view that increased cytosolic calcium
inhibits the rate of sodium transport[3,4]. The present study was undertaken in
order to investigate this possible relationship between calcium and sodium
transport in vivo, in an animal model not requiring calcium infusion. Two
drugs, verapamil[5] and proadifen[6], which inhibit intracellular transport of
calcium, were employed. Our results reveal that the infusion of these drugs
into the renal artery of the anesthetized dog results in a marked increase in
sodium excretion. This natriuresis could be dissociated from changes in
glomerular filtration rate (GFR) and renal blood flow (RBF), thus indicating a
direct tubular effect of these agents to inhibit cellular sodium transport.
Assessment of this effect by free water clearance techniques and micropuncture
studies suggest a site of action in the proximal tubule.

MATERIALS AND METHODS

Mongrel dogs of either sex weighing between 18 and 36 kg were anesthetized
with intravenous pentobarbital (30 mg/kg), intubated, and ventilated with a
Harvard respirator. Polyethylene catheters were placed in both ureters and
renal veins. One renal artery was isolated for placement of a 25-gauge
needle. In animals whose renal perfusion pressure was controlled, a Blalock
clamp was placed around the aorta above the origin of the renal arteries.
Catheters were placed in the femoral artery (and, in some cases, the brachial
artery) for continuous measurement of arterial pressure via a Statham

transducer. After surgery, fluid losses were replaced by the infusion of isotonic saline. In some dogs an additional infusion of 2.5% dextrose in water was administered in order to establish a water diuresis. Experiments were started 1-2 hours after commencing the infusion and after urine flow had stabilized. Throughout the experiments, urine was collected separately from each kidney at 5-10 minute intervals. Arterial and renal venous blood samples were collected at alternate collections of urine. Standard clearance techniques were utilized to measure GFR, RBF, solute excretion rate, and free water clearance from each kidney.

The following five groups of experiments were performed:

Group I. Intrarenal verapamil (n=5). After the collections of 3-4 control periods, verapamil (α-isoproply-α-[(N-methyl-N-homoveratryl)-α-aminopropyl]-3,4-dimethoxyphenylacetonitril HCl) (Knoll Pharmaceutical Co., Whippany, NJ)[5] was infused into one renal artery at a rate of 0.005 mg/kg/min. Preliminary studies revealed that this dose of verapamil causes unilateral renal but no systemic effects. After a 20 minute equilibration period, three 5 minute experimental periods were collected. The infusion of verapamil was then discontinued, and after another 20 minute equilibration, post-control periods were collected.

Group II. Intrarenal proadifen (n=4). The experimental protocol employed in these animals was identical to that in Group I with the exception that the intrarenal infusion employed was with Proadifen-SKF 525 (2-diethylaminoethyl-2,2-diphenylvalerate HCl) (Smith, Kline and French Labs., Philadelphia, PA)[6] at a rate of 0.375 mg/kg/min.

Group III. Intrarenal verapamil in vasodilated kidneys (n=8). The experimental protocol employed was the same as that described in Group I. However, in these animals, a suprarenal clamp was used to reduce renal perfusion pressure to between 90 and 110 mmHg in order to vasodilate the kidney by autoregulation prior to verapamil administration. The perfusion pressure was maintained constant by adjustment of the clamp throughout the experiment.

Group IV. Intrarenal verapamil in dogs undergoing a water diuresis (n=12). In these animals, experiments were started only after a stable water diuresis (urinary osmolality below 100 mOsm/kg H_2O) was established. The control period was followed by the intrarenal infusion of verapamil as described above.

Group V. Micropuncture studies (n=6). Recollection micropuncture studies were performed before and during verapamil infusion into the left renal artery. Small droplets of Sudan black stained mineral oil were injected into random proximal tubules; as these droplets traversed the last visible proximal segment on the surface of the kidney a small oil droplet was placed in the interstitium next to this segment to permit future localization. At least 40 minutes were allowed to elapse before initial collections were performed. Tubular fluid (TF) and plasma (P) samples were obtained simultaneously. TF and P samples were analyzed for inulin concentration. Comparison of TF/P inulin ratios were made between control collections and recollections obtained approximately 15-30 minutes after initiating verapamil infusion, a time when urine flow rate had increased.

RESULTS

   Group I. Effect of intrarenal verapamil in hydropenic dogs (n=5). Renal arterial infusion of verapamil at a dose that exerted no detectable effect on the function of the contralateral kidney increased renal blood flow (314$\pm$71 to 365$\pm$75 ml/min, p<.05) but glomerular filtration rate was unaltered. This vasodilatation was associated with a reversible diuresis (1.23$\pm$0.43 to 3.04$\pm$0.21 ml/min, p<.05) and natriuresis (100$\pm$27 to 357$\pm$105, p<.05).

   Group II. Effect of intrarenal proadifen in hydropenic dogs (n=4). These effects of verapamil were duplicated by the intrarenal infusion of a chemically-dissimilar blocker of cellular calcium transport, proadifen. With this agent, urine flow increased from 1.07$\pm$0.18 to 3.27$\pm$0.76 ml/min (p<.05). Likewise, a marked natriuresis ensued as mean urinary sodium excretion increased from 143.0$\pm$32.0 to 408.5$\pm$115.5 μEq/min (p<.05). As was the case with verapamil, proadifen increased renal blood flow while glomerular filtration rate was unaltered. The contralateral kidney displayed none of these changes in renal function.

   Group III. Effect of intrarenal verapamil in hydropenic dogs with vaso-dilated kidneys (Figures 1 and 2) (n=8). In an attempt to dissociate the renal vasodilatory effect of verapamil from the effects on renal electrolyte excre-tion, renal perfusion pressure was lowered by means of an adjustable aortic clamp in order to vasodilate the kidney maximally prior to verapamil adminis-tration. As is shown in Figure 1, the employed maneuver prevented an increase in renal blood flow following the administration of the agent (255.1$\pm$26.8 before and 247.5$\pm$16.1 ml/min after verapamil). Likewise, renal vascular resistance remained unaltered (0.49$\pm$0.07 to 0.45$\pm$0.02 mmHg/ml/min). Despite the absence of any changes in renal hemodynamics, the administration of verapamil significantly and reversibly increased urine flow (Figure 2) (0.54$\pm$0.11 before, 1.46$\pm$0.16 during, p<.001, and 0.46$\pm$0.12 ml/min, p<.001, after verapamil). Likewise, sodium excretion also increased from 73.0$\pm$12.0 to

116

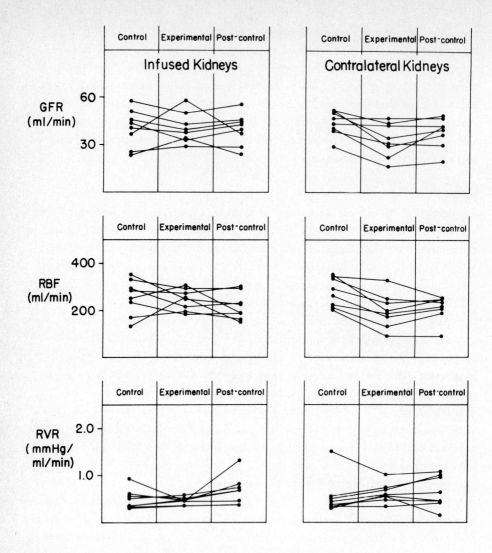

Fig. 1. Effect of intrarenal verapamil on renal blood flow and renal vascular resistance in dogs with vasodilated kidneys. In this setting neither renal blood flow nor renal vascular resistance were altered.

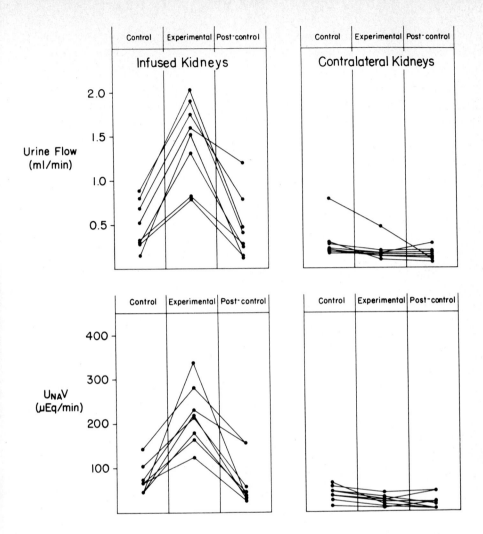

Fig. 2. Effect of intrarenal verapamil on urine flow and sodium excretion in dogs with vasodilated kidneys. Note that despite the absence of changes in renal hemodynamics (Figure 1) the drug reversibly increased both urine flow and sodium excretion.

217.5+24.0 µEq/min (p<.001) and returned to 66.8+19.6 µEq/min (p<.001) when the infusion was discontinued. As shown in the right panel of the figure, the contralateral kidney remained unaltered.

Group IV. Effect of intrarenal verapamil in dogs undergoing a water diuresis (Figure 3). In order to gain some insight into the possible localization of the effect of verapamil on sodium reabsorption studies were performed in dogs undergoing a water diuresis. In these animals, verapamil produced a significant increase in fractional distal delivery as estimated from changes in fractional water excretion from 12.72+0.92 to 15.67+1.19% (p<.01). However, as can be seen in Figure 3, the fractional free water clearance (C_{H_2O}/GFR) as a function of fractional delivery (as estimated by $C_{H_2O}/GFR + C_{Na}/GFR$) appeared to be unaltered by verapamil administration, i.e., the slopes of the regression lines were not significantly different. These results therefore suggested an effect of verapamil to decrease proximal but not distal tubular sodium reabsorption.

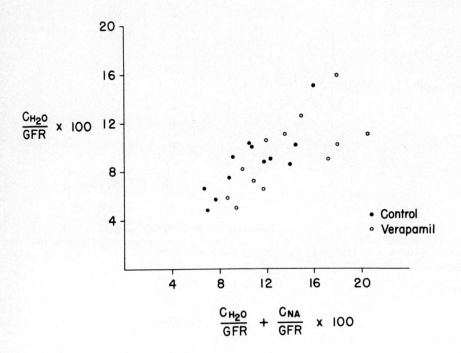

Fig. 3. Effect of verapamil on fractional free water clearance versus a function of fractional delivery. Note that control (closed circles) and verapamil treated kidneys (open circles) are indistinguishable.

Group V. Micropuncture studies (Figure 4). In order to ascertain more directly the specific nephron segment responsible for our observation micro-puncture studies were undertaken. Figure 4 demonstrates the collection-recollection values for TF/P inulin ratios in this study. Fractional reab-sorption fell from a mean of 33% to 21% as mean TF/P inulin ratios decreased from 1.49 ± 0.05 to 1.27 ± 0.04 ($p<.01$). Concomitant with this decrease in proximal fractional reabsorption was an approximate doubling of both urine flow rate from 0.62 ± 0.15 to 1.22 ± 0.26 ml/min ($p<.05$) and sodium excretion from 107 ± 20 to 215 ± 34 µEq/min ($p<.05$). In these studies neither glomerular filtra-tion rate nor para-aminohippurate clearance changed significantly; glomerular filtration rate averaged 24.3 ± 6.2 ml/min before and 26.4 ± 6.3 ml/min during verapamil; para-aminohippurate clearance averaged 105 ± 17 ml/min before and 111 ± 20 ml/min during verapamil.

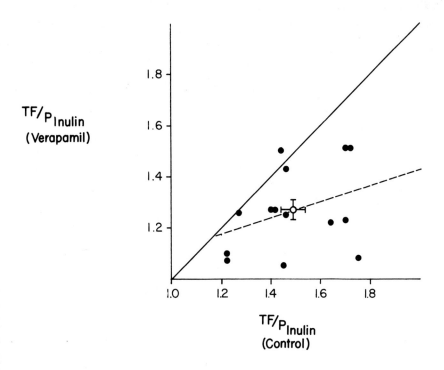

Fig. 4. TF/P inulin ratios before (Control) and during verapamil are demon-strated. The mean value ($\pm$SE) is noted by the open circle. Most values fall below the line of identity.

120

SUMMARY

In the present study verapamil, an inhibitor of cellular calcium uptake, was found to decrease tubular reabsorption primarily in the proximal portion of the nephron. This effect was dissociated from changes in either glomerular filtration rate or renal blood flow. Moreover, this effect of verapamil could be mimicked by a chemically dissimilar inhibitor of calcium membrane transport, proadifen. These findings suggest an important link between cellular calcium movement and tubular sodium reabsorption.

REFERENCES

1. Wolf, A.V., et al. (1949) Am. J. Physiol., 158, 205-217.
2. Levitt, M.F., et al. (1958) J. Clin. Invest., 37, 294-305.
3. Weismann, W., et al. (1977) J. Clin. Invest., 59, 418-425.
4. Grinstein, S., et al. (1978) J. Membrane Biol., 40, 261-280.
5. Rasmussen, H., et al. (1977) Physiol. Rev., 57, 421-508.
6. McMurtry, I.F., et al. (1976) Circ. Res., 38, 99-104.

Hormonal Regulation of Sodium Excretion,
B. Lichardus, R.W. Schrier and J. Ponec, eds.
© 1980 Elsevier/North-Holland Biomedical Press

EFFECT OF OXYTOCIN ON RENAL FUNCTION IN CONSCIOUS BRATTLEBORO HOMOZYGOUS RATS.
A MODEL FOR STUDYING RENAL REGULATION BY HORMONES

MIKLOS GELLAI, FREDERICK T. LAROCHELLE, JR., HEINZ VALTIN
Department of Physiology, Dartmouth Medical School, Hanover, N.H. 03755, U.S.A.

INTRODUCTION

Despite a considerable amount of work, both in man[1,2] and in laboratory animals[3,4,5,6], the possible influences of oxytocin on various renal functions remain unclear. Depending on the study cited, oxytocin may or may not play a role in the maintenance of glomerular filtration rate (GFR) and renal plasma flow (RPF), and it may have diuretic or antidiuretic as well as natriuretic effects[7]. Two facets of prior work make interpretation of the results diffi-cult: Usually very high doses of oxytocin were given, and most of the experi-ments were conducted under anesthesia, which depresses renal hemodynamics[8].

The development by us of an experimental model that permits measurement of renal functions in trained, conscious rats[9] has enabled us to test the effects of oxytocin in the absence of anesthesia and to correlate changes in renal excretory functions with simultaneous changes in GFR and RPF. Furthermore, by applying a new procedure for extracting neurohypophysial hormones from plasma[10], we have been able to determine the plasma concentrations of oxytocin that resulted from our infusions. And finally, by using Brattleboro homozy-gotes, which almost certainly cannot synthesize any vasopressin[11], we have been able to rule out any influence of that other neurohypophysial hormone in the changes that we have observed.

The experiments that we describe in this report seem particularly apt for this symposium, for any explanation of a regulatory role of hormones in the urinary excretion of sodium must take into account simultaneously induced alterations in renal hemodynamics.

MATERIALS AND METHODS

Animal model. Brattleboro homozygotes with hereditary hypothalamic diabetes insipidus (DI rats)[11] were used; they were of both sexes and weighed 200-240 g. They were prepared surgically and accustomed to the restraining cage (Fig. 1b) 4 to 7 days prior to running an experiment[9]. Indwelling tygon catheters were placed in the descending aorta for monitoring of pressure and sampling of blood (Fig. 1a); in the superior vena cava for infusion of polyfructosan (Inutest)

122

and para-aminohippuric acid (PAH); and (in 8 of the 16 rats studied) in the left renal vein to gauge the renal extraction of PAH (Fig. 1a). A cannula of silastic-covered stainless steel[9] was tied into the bladder.

(a)

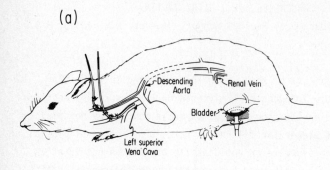

Fig. 1. (a) Diagram of the preparation, showing location of catheters and cannula, which are placed under ether anesthesia at least 4 days prior to running an experiment. (b) A rat in the plastic restraining cage during the course of an experiment. The animal's tail is visible at the left. The key to the various instruments is given in reference 9, from which both illustrations were adapted; the instruments used will vary with the type of experiment that is being run.

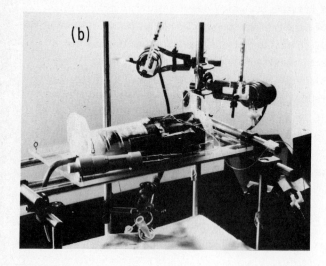

During an experiment, the animal remained quietly in a plastic restraining cage (Fig. 1b), and its systemic blood pressure and heart rate were recorded continuously. Inutest, PAH, synthetic oxytocin (Vega Biochemicals, Tucson, ARIZ; concentrations corrected for peptide content[12]) and 1/4-strength Ringer's solution were delivered into the superior vena cava by means of a three-branched catheter especially constructed by us. The rate of infusion was adjusted to approximate the rate of urine flow, so that the weight of an animal did not change significantly during the course of an experiment. Inutest and PAH, 1/4 strength Ringer's, and oxytocin were delivered from separate reservoirs to permit regulation of the substances independently as the rate of infusion was altered.

   Radioimmunoassay (RIA) for oxytocin. In the two protocols (8 experiments each) where oxytocin was infused to attain a steady state (Fig. 3a and b) a 1 ml sample of blood was collected at the end of 60 minutes of infusion. Oxytocin was extracted from this sample using octadecasilyl-silica (C18 Sep-Paks, Waters Assoc., Milford, MA), by a method recently described for vasopressin[10]. The RIA for oxytocin is similar to one used by us for vasopressin[12]. Synthetic oxytocin (Vega) was used for standards (corrected for peptide content[12]) and for radioiodination. The antiserum (B3P) was generated by us; its cross-reactivity with either arginine-vasopressin or arginine-vasotocin is less than 1:10,000. The sensitivity of the RIA is 1.25 pg/ml of plasma when 0.5 ml of plasma is extracted.

RESULTS AND DISCUSSION
   Dose-Response with bolus injections. Antidiuretic dosages of oxytocin were explored by delivering bolus injections of 100 μl containing different amounts

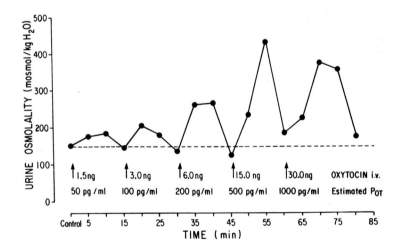

Fig 2. Dose-responses to intravenous (i.v.) bolus injections of synthetic oxytocin in an unanesthetized, trained Brattleboro homozygote (DI rat). The graph shows the exact time-course in a single animal. Plasma concentrations of oxytocin (P_{OT}) were estimated using a volume of distribution for the bolus equal to 15% of body weight.

of oxytocin. Initial injections (not shown in Fig. 2) of 0.03, 0.06, 0.15,
0.3, and 0.6 ng had no antidiuretic effect in DI rats. The threshold dose was
1.5 ng, and responses to progressively higher dosages are shown in Figure 2.
The graph gives results of consecutive, 5-minute urine collections; the rapid
return to baseline values as well as the relatively stable baseline emphasize
the suitability of the unanesthetized, trained Brattleboro homozygote for the
bioassay of antidiuretic substances. The plasma concentration of oxytocin in
the exploratory experiments was estimated using a volume of distribution for
oxytocin of 15% of body weight; the approximate correctness of the estimate
was confirmed in subsequent experiments. The plasma level of oxytocin in
Brattleboro homozygotes eating and drinking ad lib is roughly 10 pg/ml of
plasma[13]. Thus, the threshold concentration for an antidiuretic effect is
well above the usual normal level (Fig. 2), and a maximal antidiuretic effect
appears to occur at a concentration of about 500 pg/ml.

Sustaining infusions. In order to determine whether a steady antidiuretic
effect of oxytocin is accompanied by changes in renal hemodynamics, we infused
oxytocin intravenously at a constant rate calculated to achieve a plasma concentration between 200 and 500 pg/ml (Fig. 3a). Following 3 10-minute control
collections, 8 DI rats (4 female, 4 male) were given oxytocin at a rate of
2,500 pg/min·100 g body weight (BW) for one hour; at the end of this infusion,
the measured plasma concentration for oxytocin was 327 ± 29 pg/ml (Mean ± SEM).
As is shown in Figure 3a, this concentration decreased urine flow and increased
urine osmolality significantly. Urine was hypertonic to plasma after 10 minutes of infusion, and it rose to a mean peak osmolality of nearly 500 mOsm/kg
H_2O. Fractional excretion of sodium increased slightly but significantly,
from about 1% of the filtered load to a little more than 2% of that load. RPF
decreased initially (although not significantly) and then returned to the
control value. GFR did not change significantly during the first 30 minutes
of infusion but then rose significantly, by as much as 25% over the control
level (from about 820 to 1,030 µl/min·100 g BW). Neither this high dose of
oxytocin nor the lower dose (see next paragraph) altered systemic blood
pressure or heart rate.

We next wished to know whether oxytocin would similarly increase GFR when
it occurs at lower plasma concentrations -- the kind of levels that are seen
during certain states, such as mild volume contraction[13]. A second group of
8 DI rats (4 females, 4 males) was therefore infused with oxytocin at a rate
of approximately 250 pg/min·100 g BW, which led to a mean measured plasma concentration of 46 ± 5 pg/ml. Note first of all (Fig. 3b) that the average GFR

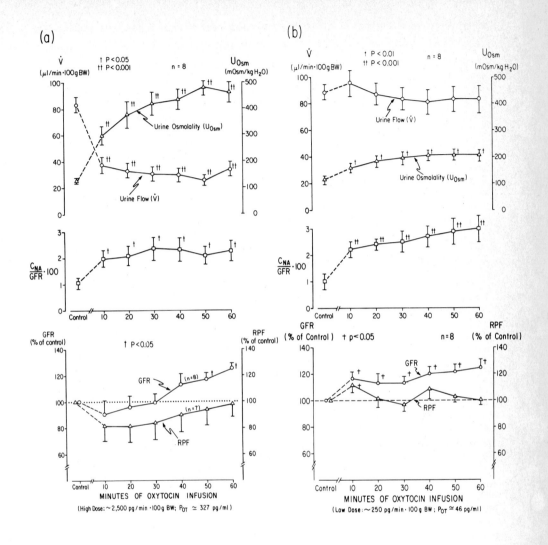

Fig. 3. Changes in urine flow ($\dot{V}$), urine osmolality (U_{Osm}), percent of filtered sodium excreted ($C_{Na}/GFR·100$), glomerular filtration rate (GFR) and renal
plasma flow (RPF) in DI rats in response to infusions of oxytocin at a high
(a) and a low (b) dose. Plasma concentrations of oxytocin (P_{OT}) were determined by radioimmunoassay. P-values refer to comparisons with control. BW =
body weight.

rose by as much with the low as with the high dose of oxytocin (from about 860
to 1,090 µl/min·100 g BW); RPF did not change significantly except at 10 minutes
after the onset of infusion. As could be anticipated from the results shown in
Figure 2, the infusion of oxytocin at the low dose (Fig. 3b) increased urine

osmolality very slightly. This increase was not associated with a significant reduction in urine flow, and the rise in osmolality could in fact be accounted for fully by the increased excretion of sodium (and presumably chloride). The natriuretic effect of oxytocin was more striking at the low than at the high dose of the hormone, with the fractional excretion of sodium rising from 1% of the filtered load to 3% of that load (Fig. 3b). Although the greater natriuretic effect is not so apparent when expressed as fractional excretion, it amounts to a 50 % increase in absolute excretion (from approximately 2.8 to 4.2 μEq/min· 100 g BW) over the value seen during the infusion of the high dose.

Three differences between the high dose and low dose of oxytocin are apparent from a comparison of Figure 3a with 3b: (1) the high dose has a clear anti-diuretic effect that resembles the response to vasopressin; (2) the low dose causes more natriuresis; and (3) the high dose tends to lower RPF more than the low dose. These effects may well be interrelated.

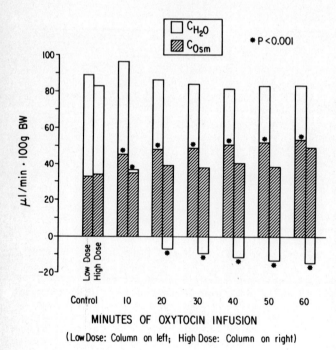

Fig. 4. Bar graphs re-presenting the equation, $C_{H_2O} = V - C_{Osm}$. The low dose and high dose of oxytocin are the same as given in Figures 3b and 3a, respectively. P-values refer to a comparison with control, and the asterisks are given for osmolal clearance (C_{Osm}) at low dose and free water clearance (C_{H_2O}) at high dose only; not indicated is the fact that the decreases in C_{H_2O} at the low dose were also statistically significant except at the 10-minute point. BW = body weight.

The mechanism(s) by which the two dosages of oxytocin influence urine flow and urine osmolality may be partly deduced from Figure 4. Inasmuch as $C_{H_2O} = \dot{V} - C_{Osm}$, the height of each column in that figure represents urine flow ($\dot{V}$)

-- except that in the case of a negative free water clearance (C_{H_2O}), C_{H_2O} must be subtracted from the shaded column in order to derive $\dot{V}$. It can thus be seen at a glance that the low dose of oxytocin (the left column in each pair) did not alter urine flow. Yet, this dose significantly increased osmolal clearance (C_{Osm}) and thereby the urine osmolality (Fig. 3b). In turn, the increase in C_{Osm} can be fully accounted for by the increased excretion of sodium (Fig. 3b) and its accompanying anion, mainly Cl^-. We cannot tell, from the present data, whether the natriuretic effect results mainly from the increased filtered load of NaCl or from some direct effect of oxytocin on tubular function. The latter could take the form of either an inhibition of NaCl reabsorption, possibly in the ascending limbs of Henle, or a slight increase in the water permeability of the distal nephron, or a combination of the two. Either or both effects could account for the decrease in C_{H_2O} that was seen with the low dose, the first effect by decreasing the generation of free water, the second by slightly augmenting its reabsorption.

On the other hand, the results with the high dose (right column of each pair in Figure 4) -- with a striking decline in C_{H_2O} from a positive to a negative value -- could be due mainly or solely to an augmentation of the water permeability of the distal nephron, similar to the effects of oxytocin on anuran membranes[14,15]. The lesser increase of NaCl excretion with the high dose, despite a similar rise in GFR (Fig. 3, 40-60 minutes), must mean that this dose somehow inhibited reabsorption of $Na^+(Cl^-)$; this conclusion is also inherent in the first 30 minutes of infusion (Fig. 3a), when fractional excretion of Na^+ increased without a change in GFR. The present experiments do not tell us by what mechanism(s) this inhibition occurred.

SUMMARY

The effects of oxytocin on renal function were ascertained in conscious, trained Brattleboro homozygotes (DI rats) at two levels of the hormone: a high dose seen in states such as coitus, parturition, and lactation[16]; and a low dose seen in animals eating and drinking ad lib or in mild volume contraction[13]. An antidiuresis, resembling that seen with the administration of vasopressin, was seen only with the high dose, whereas the natriuresis was more striking with the low dose. Both doses led to significant increases in GFR (but not of RPF), to approximately 125% of the control value. We emphasize that these results were obtained in DI rats and that the possible modulating influences of endogenous vasopressin, especially on renal hemodynamics, need still to be determined.

128

ACKNOWLEDGMENTS

This work was supported in part by Research Grants AM-08469 and HD-12123, National Research Service Award AM-07301, and Basic Research Support Grant 5S07-RR-05392 -- all from the National Institutes of Health, U.S. Public Health Service. Assistance from the Charles H. Hood Foundation is also gratefully acknowledged.

REFERENCES

1. Cross, R.B., Dicker, S.E., Kitchin, A.H., Lloyd, S. and Pickford, M. (1960) J. Physiol., 153, 553-561.

2. Abdul-Karim, R. and Assali, N.S. (1961) J. Lab. Clin. Med., 57, 522-532.

3. Heller, H. and Stephenson, R.P. (1950) Nature (London), 165, 189.

4. Gyermek, L. and Fekete, G. (1955) Experientia, 11, 238-239.

5. Brooks, F.P. and Pickford, M. (1958) J. Physiol., 142, 468-493.

6. Chan, W.Y. and Sawyer, W.H. (1961) Am. J. Physiol. 201, 799-803.

7. Thorn, N.A. (1968) In Handbook of Exp. Pharmacology. Vol. 23: Neuro-hypophysial Hormones and Similar Polypeptides, edited by B. Berde, Springer-Verlag, Berlin, pp. 372-442.

8. Gellai, M. and Valtin, H. (1980) In Proc. XXVIII Int. Cong. Physiol. Sci., edited by L. Takács, Hung. Acad. Sci., Budapest (in press).

9. Gellai, M. and Valtin, H. (1979) Kidney Int., 15, 419-426.

10. LaRochelle, F.T., Jr., North, W.G. and Stern, P. (1980) Pflügers Arch. Eur. J. Physiol. (in press).

11. Valtin, H. (1977) In Disturbances in Body Fluid Osmolality, edited by T.E. Andreoli, J.J. Grantham, and F.C. Rector, Jr., Am. Physiol. Soc., Bethesda, pp. 197-215.

12. North, W.G., LaRochelle, F.T., Jr., Haldar, J., Sawyer, W.H. and Valtin, H. (1978) Endocrinology, 103, 1976-1984.

13. LaRochelle, F.T., Jr., Gellai, M. and Edwards, B.R. (1980) The Physiologist (in press).

14. Sawyer, W.H. and Schisgall, R.M. (1956) Am. J. Physiol., 187, 312-314.

15. Chevalier, J., Bourguet, J. and Hugon, J.S. (1974) Cell Tissue Res., 152, 129-140.

16. Tindal, J.S. (1974) In Handbook of Physiology. Section 7: Endocrinology. Vol. IV, Part 1: The Pituitary Gland and Its Neuroendocrine Control, edited by E. Knobil and W.H. Sawyer, Am. Physiol. Soc., Washington, D.C., pp. 257-267.

Hormonal Regulation of Sodium Excretion,
B. Lichardus, R.W. Schrier and J. Ponec, eds.
© 1980 Elsevier/North-Holland Biomedical Press

SODIUM METABOLISM IN RATS WITH HEREDITARY DEFECT OF VASOPRES-
SIN SYNTHESIS

HELENA DLOUHÁ, JIŘÍ KŘEČEK, JOSEF ZICHA
Institute of Physiology, Czechoslovak Academy of Sciences,
Prague

As reported in this Symposium in an other paper of our wor-
king group, a clear cut hypernatremia was observed in Wistar
rats drinking hypertonic NaCl solution from prepuberty. Only
very moderate sodium concentration elevation was observed in
rats drinking hypertonic saline only from adulthood[1].

Several authors demonstrated a higher plasma Na^+ concentration in homozygous Brattleboro rats with hereditary diabetes
insipidus of hypothalamic origin in comparison with their vasopressin producing heterozygous littermates. This difference
was observed under the conditions of normal salt intake[2,3,4,5],
but it was brought into prominence by replacing water for 0.6%
NaCl solution as drinking fluid[5]. The osmoregulatory system
neurohypophysis-kidney commes into full function in rats only
several weeks after birth[6]. Hypernatremia in rats drinking salt
solution from youth could be, therefore, caused by low efficiency of this osmoregulatory system.

To test this hypothesis experiments were undertaken in homozygous Brattleboro rats in which vasopressin is absent not only
in young age but in adulthood as well. 0.6% NaCl solution was
used as drinking fluid because rats with diabetes insipidus
are unable to survive the consumption of hypertonic saline[5].

In the first experiment 6 groups of Brattleboro rats were
studied: homozygots and heterozygots drinking water, homozygots
and heterozygots drinking 0.6% NaCl solution from the 5th week
of age and homozygots and heterozygots drinking 0.6% NaCl solution from the 12th week of age. At the age of 22 weeks Na^+
concentration was determined in the blood plasma in all experimental groups. Tab. 1 illustrates the results of this experiment.

TABLE 1

BLOOD PLASMA Na$^+$ CONCENTRATION

Effect of drinking saline from the 5th or 12th week of age in Brattleboro rats aged 22 weeks. Concentration in meq/l.

Drinking fluid	Homozygots	Heterozygots
Water	141.3 ± 0.86 (48)	145.2 ± 2.74 (15)
0.6% NaCl from 5th week	171.8 ± 4.20^{abc} (9)	159.6 ± 3.42^{bc} (17)
0.6% NaCl from 12th week	147.4 ± 1.66^{ac} (11)	130.0 ± 2.06^{c} (16)

[a] Significantly different from Heterozygots ($p < 0.05$)
[b] Significantly different from 0.6% NaCl from 5th week ($p < 0.01$)
[c] Significantly different from Water ($p < 0.01$)
In parentheses: number of animals

A distinct difference in plasma Na$^+$ concentration was observed between saline drinking homozygots and heterozygots. Nevertheless, there was also difference between rats drinking saline from youth or from adulthood independent on the genotype of Brattleboro rats. It could be concluded that the absence of vasopressin is connected with a limited capacity to keep normal plasma Na$^+$ concentration but the extremely high plasma Na$^+$ concentration in rats drinking saline from youth has to be attributed to an other contributing cause.

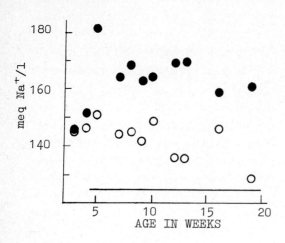

Fig. 1. Plasma Na$^+$ concentration in homozygous ● and heterozygous ○ Brattleboro rats drinking 0.6% NaCl solution from the 5th week of age as indicated by the horizontal line.

As shown in Figure 1 this hypernatremia developed in a few days after the onset of saline drinking and it is maintained till the adulthood. In this way, sodium might be more accumulated in the body of homozygots drinking saline from youth than of those consuming salt only in adulthood. In accordance with

TABLE 2

URINE AND SODIUM EXCRETION AND URINARY SODIUM CONCENTRATION
Urine sampled for 24 hours of food and water deprivation. Effect of drinking 0.6% NaCl solution from the 5th week of age in homozygots and heterozygots and from the 12th week in homozygots aged 22 weeks.

Drinking fluid	V $ml.100g^{-1}.24h^{-1}$	U_{Na} meq/l	$U_{Na}.V$ $\mu eq.100g^{-1}.24h^{-1}$
	Homozygotes		
Water	6.28 ± 0.35^a (9)	56.3 ± 3.07^a (9)	549.1 ± 24.3^a (9)
0.6% NaCl from 5th week	10.30 ± 0.95^{ac} (6)	149.3 ± 8.26^c (6)	$1538,2\pm167.3^{ac}$ (6)
0.6% NaCl from 12th week	11.60 ± 1.05^c (10)	98.3 ± 3.07^{bc} (10)	1127.0 ± 88.3^{bc} (10)
	Heterozygotes		
Water	1.40 ± 0.18 (6)	112.6 ± 7.66 (6)	276.0 ± 33.3 (6)
0.6% NaCl from 5th week	3.38 ± 0.25^c (6)	138.8 ± 8.06 (6)	440.5 ± 15.5^c (6)

Footnotes see Table 1

this assumption were data obtained from the experiment in which urine excretion, sodium excretion and urinary Na^+ concentration were estimated in adult Brattleboro rats (age 22 weeks) drinking 0.6% NaCl solution either from the 5th or from the 12th week of age. Urine was sampled for 24 hours in the course of which the animals were deprived of food and drinking fluid. Of course, both the water and sodium excretion were higher in homozygotes than in heterozygotes and sodium loss was greater in rats consuming saline than in those drinking water but in homozygotes the sodium loss was significantly higher in the group with saline intake from youth, while no dependence on the onset of saline drinking was observed in urine flow (Tab. 2).

In order to specify the age till which the rats have to be-gin to consume saline for keeping in adulthood the pattern of sodium excretion observed in rats drinking saline from the 5th week, two additional groups of homozygous Brattleboro rats were included into experiment: one of them was formed of rats drin-king 0.6% saline from the 6th week, the other one of rats drin-king it from the 8th week. At the age of 22 weeks urine excre-tion was measured (Tab. 3). No difference was found in urine flow in dependence on the age at which saline drinking begun.

TABLE 3
URINE FLOW, SODIUM EXCRETION AND URINARY SODIUM CONCENTRATION IN THE COURSE OF 24 h FOOD AND FLUID DEPRIVATION IN ADULT RATS DRINKING 0,6% NaCl SOLUTION FROM DIFFERENT AGES

Drinking 0.6% NaCl from the age of	V $ml.100g^{-1}.24h^{-1}$	U_{Na} meq/l	$U_{Na}.V$ $\mu eq.100g^{-1}.24h^{-1}$
5 weeks	$10.30^{\pm}0.95$ (6)	$149.3^{\pm}8.26^{b}$ (6)	$1538.2^{\pm}163.30^{b}$ (6)
6 weeks	$11.64^{\pm}0.50$ (5)	$132.4^{\pm}3.66^{b}$ (5)	$1554.0^{\pm}103.60^{b}$ (5)
8 weeks	$11.20^{\pm}1.20$ (6)	$117.7^{\pm}6.56^{a}$ (6)	$1315.1^{\pm}156.36$ (6)
12 weeks	$11.60^{\pm}1.05$ (10)	$98.3^{\pm}3.07$ (10)	$1127.2^{\pm}88.3$ (10)

[a] Significantly different from the week 5 and 12 ($p < 0.02$)
[b] Significantly different from the week 12 ($p < 0.05$)

On the other hand, a gradual decrease with the age of the out-set of saline intake was observed in sodium excretion and, name-ly, in urinary sodium concentration. Highest values were obser-ved in rats consuming saline from the 5th week. The low concen-tration found in the group drinking saline only in adulthood was not attained even in rats in which saline consumption star-ted at the age of 8 weeks.

Puberty is set in at the age of 6 - 9 weeks in rats[7]. At that age the mechanisms of both the salt consumption[8] and

the sodium excretion[9] mature and the distribution of single
nephron glomerular filtration rate (SNGFR) which is shifted in
the direction of deeper nephrons in young rats,reaches the adult

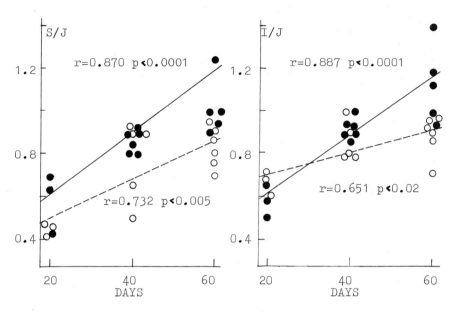

Figure 2. Single nephron glomerular filtration rate in homozy-
gous ● and heterozygous ○ Brattleboro rats at different ages.
S/J - ratio of SNGFR by superficial to juxtamedullary nephrons,
I/J - ratio of SNGFR by intercortical to juxtamedullary nephrons.
Abscissa: age of rats

pattern[10]. Data were reported suggesting a role of SNGFR in sodium excretion[11,12]. Therefore, SNGFR distribution was estimated
in developing Brattleboro rats. Baines[12] modification of Hansen[13] method was used and ratios of superficial to juxtamedullary (S/J), superficial to intercortical (S/I) and intercortical to juxtamedullary (I/J) nephrons SNGFR were determined.
As shown in Figure 2 no substantial difference was observed
in the development of S/J and I/J SNGFR ratios between homozygous and heterozygous Brattleboro rats and the observed values
are in good accordance with data found earlier in Wistar rats[10].
    Baines[12] first reported that the effect of salt intake on
the SNGFR distribution is well expressed only in rats of low
body weight, i.e. in young animals. In Brattleboro rats and

in Wistar strain as well SNGFR distribution develops until the
sexual maturity is reached. The particular adaptibility of
young rats to increased salt intake, demonstrated in the present paper is limited to the age period of prepuberty and puberty. Therefore, it could be possible that SNGFR distribution
might play some role in this particular adaptibility.

REFERENCES

1. Křeček, J. (1980) A contribution in this volume
2. Valtin, H. and Schroeder, H. A. (1964) Am. J. Physiol. 206
   425 - 430
3. Gross, F. et al. (1972) Circul. Res. 30 and 31, 173 - 181
4. Friedman, S. M. and Friedman, C. L. (1965) Canad. J. Physiol.
   Pharmacol. 43, 699 - 705
5. Hall, C. E. et al. (1973) Texas Rep. Biol. Med. 31, 471-487
6. Dlouhá, H. et al. (1976) Experientia 32, 59 - 60
7. Ramírez, V. D. (1973) Handbook of Physiology 7, II, Female
   Reproduction. Am. Physiol. Soc. Washington, pp 1 - 28
8. Křeček, J. et al. (1972) Physiol. Behav. 8, 183 - 188
9. Bengele, H. H. and Solomon, S. (1974) Am. J. Physiol. 227,
   364 - 368
10. Dlouhá, H. et al. (1976) Pflügers Arch. 336, 277 - 279
11. Horster, M. and Thurau K. (1968) Pflügers Arch. 301, 162 -
    181
12. Baines, A. D. (1973) Am. J. Physiol. 224, 237 - 244
13. Hansen, O. E. (1963) Proc. Int. Congr. Nephrol. Prague,
    pp 527 - 529

Hormonal Regulation of Sodium Excretion,
B. Lichardus, R.W. Schrier and J. Ponec, eds.
© 1980 Elsevier/North-Holland Biomedical Press

NATRIURETIC EFFECT OF NEUROHYPOPHYSIAL HORMONS IN MAMMALS

L.N.IVANOVA,N.N.MELIDI,J.V.NATOCHIN,G.G.FOFANOVA
Institute of Cytology and Genetics,USSR Acad.Sci.Sib.Dept.,
Novosibirsk;Sechenov Institute of Evolutionary Physiology
and Biochemistry, Leningrad (USSR)

Participation of neurohypophyseal hormones in regulation of
the sodium excretion remains disputable.Hormone-induced natriuresis itself and the mechanism of its development are the subject of controversy.The majority of investigators regard this
natriuresis as a result of hormone indirect effect (Akutsura et
al.[1],Antoniou et al.[2],Fejes-Toth et al.[3], Humphreys et al.[4],
Luke[5]).There is no clarity about the part of nephrone in which
the effect of these hormones develops.Relative role of vasopressin and oxytocin in the development of natriuresis is also
unclear.The present study was undertaken to elucidate the mechanism of the natriuretic effect of neurohypophyseal hormones.

The experiments were performed on conscious dogs with ureters
brought out into the abdominal skin and gastric fistula for
water infusion.The antidiuretic reaction evoked by pituitrin P
injection (50–500μU/kg) was followed by increase in urinary
sodium excretion which is dependent on the dose of the injected
hormone (Table 1-A).The degree of the natriuresis is also determined by the initial urinary sodium excretion: the higher the
initial background, the more pronounced natriuretic reaction
(Table 1-B).When tubular sodium reabsorption is intensive, the
injection of pituitrin is not followed by any significant natriuretic reaction.The magnitude of pituitrin-induced natriuresis depends on the state of hydration of the animal, being more
pronounced in high initial diuresis (Table 1-C).The sensivity
of the kidney to ADH is evidently very important for development of the natriuretic reaction.

The magnitude of pituitrin-induced natriuresis also depends
on the degree of urinary osmotic concentration.A linear positive
correlation exists between the level of urinary osmolality and

TABLE 1

EFFECT OF INTRAVENOUS INJECTION OF PITUITRIN ON RENAL SODIUM EXCRETION IN CONSCIOUS DOGS

Dose of injected hormone (μU/kg)	Initial diuresis (ml/min m^2)	Sodium excretion (μEq/min m^2)		Excreted sodium fraction (% filtered)	
		Initial period	$\Delta U_{Na} V$	Initial period	Δ EF$_{Na}$
A					
50 (3)	7.0 ± 0.1	25 ± 0.1	+35 ± 11	0.28 ± 0.08	+0.22 ±0.11
200 (5)	7.0 ± 1.9	26 ± 7.0	+78 ± 32	0.43 ± 0.15	+0.90 ± 0.63
500 (13)	7.1 ± 0.8	25 ± 11.0	+100± 22*	0.27 ± 0.09	+2.30 ±0.31*
B					
500 (6)	5.2 ± 0.7	2 - 10	+39 ± 4	0.05 ± 0.2	+0.36 ±0.06
500 (5)	8.7 ± 1.6	20 -150	+245± 30**	0.30 ± 1.2	+2.31 ±0.39
C					
500 (4)	1 - 5	25 ± 5	+40 ± 3	0.31 ± 0.11	+0.29 ±0.30
500 (5)	8 -12	51 ± 24	+179± 32**	0.54 ± 0.18	+2.32 ±0.38

Values are means ± SE. Number of observation for each dose is given in parenthes. *P<0.02, **,P<0.002, as compared to the reaction to 50 μU/kg, as

value of natriuresis (r=0.84).

The increase of the renal medullar osmolality under antidiuresis may be one of factors decreasing the sodium reabsorption in collecting tubules.Supposing this, it was interesting to know whether the sodium excretion will change a hypertonic medium is established artificially in collecting tubules by retrograde osmotically active substances infusion (Babics and Renyi-Vamos[6]).Indeed in all experiments retrograde infusion of 1500 mM/l mannitol was followed by increase in urinary sodium excretion(Fig.1).The injection of hypotonic mannitol solution (50 mM/l) had no significant effect on the sodium excretion.

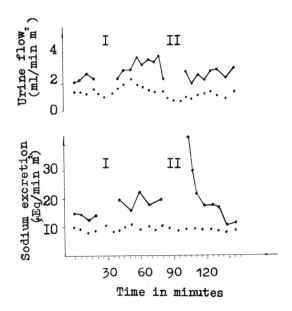

Fig.1.Effects of retrograde mannitol injection on the urine flow and sodium excretion.I − retrograde hypotonic mannitol injection (50 mM/l).II − retrograde hypertonic mannitol injection (1500 mM/l); ↦ − experimental kidney; ··· − control kidney.

138

The determination of the natriuretic effect localization by
the "push flow" method (Aukland and Kjekshus[7]) showed that in
the experimental kidney the synthetic arginin-vasopressin induces a sharp increase in sodium concentration in samples from
distal segment (2-nd and 3-rd portions), whereas the sodium
content in proximal samples (7-th and 8-th urine portions) practically did not differ from analogous control samples.(Fig.2)

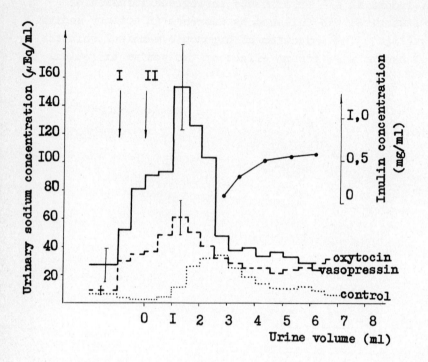

Fig.2.Effects of intravenous injection of arginin-vasopressin
and oxytocin on sodium concentration in urinary samples
obtained by "push flow" method.I - injection of 15 mU vasopressin or 60 mU oxytocin;II - injection of 50 ml 20% mannitol +
+ 100mg inulin.

The observed increase of sodium concentration in distal samples
is not a result of a simple urine concentration due to osmotically free water reabsorption during antidiuretic reaction,
because the ratio U_{Na} experiment/U_{Na} control increased by
approximately 18 times wherease $\frac{U}{P}Cr$ rose only by 6 times
($p < 0.001$).Oxytocin induced small increase in sodium excretion
only in large doses when antidiuretic reaction was followed by
significant increase in the urine osmolality (Fig.2).Oxytocin
did not potentiate natriuretic effect of vasopressin, since the
natriuresis induced by infusion of vasopressin and oxytocin
mixture (169 ± 26 μEq/ml) did not differ from the natriuresis
after injection of arginin-vasopressin alone (153 ± 29 μEq/ml).

Let us consider possible cellular mechanisms of the natriuretic effect.The ADH-induced increase of renal sodium excretion
as it is seen from above mentioned results, can not explained by
a direct hormone inhibiting effect on sodium reabsorption.It is
also well known that in some vertebrates the ADH activates the
sodium transport but not inhibits it (Bentley[8]).The ADH effect
on sodium reabsorption in collecting tubules mediated by increase
of extracellular medium osmolality could depend on increase of
intercellular permeability for sodium flux into the tubular
lumen or on decrease in transcellular sodium transport (Borisova et al.[9]).It was interesting to analyze the possible cause of
decrease in sodium reabsorption with an increase of osmolality -
- whether it depends on the changes in energy supply to the ion
transport, or on the changes in a hyperosmy of the cellular
ionic composition.Under these condition, the energy supply of
cells is evidently ensured by glycolysis, since in dehydration
the glycolysis level in the inner layer of the kidney raises
(Natochin et al.[10]).To counteract the decrease of the cellular
volume the influx of sodium and chloride into the cytoplasm
increases.The amount of osmotically active substances in the
intracellular content rises parralel with the raise of extracellular fluid osmolality which ensures the cellular volume regulation (Morgan[11]).The above gives the basis for the hypothesis
on the possible mechanism of natriuretic effect during ADH in-
jection.The hormone increases the concentration of osmotically

active substances in renal medulla, the concentration of sodium and chloride in cell rises.Under these conditions in order to maintain the cell volume, the effectiveness of pump removing the sodium and chloride from the cell, possibly is decrease temporarily (Natochin[12]).It decrease the transcellular transport which is followed in the kidney by transient natriuresis (Atherton et al.[13]).Another cause might be that during the increase in the intracellular sodium concentration the influx of sodium into the collective tubule cells from the tubular lumen due to the gradient is made difficalt.This is supported by abovementioned data on the dependence of the magnitude ADH natriuretic effect on the basal level of sodium excretion.Under basal conditions, when the influx of sodium into the collecting tubules is large, it is adsorbed by cells, since there is a possibility for sodium influx into the cell due to electrochemical potential gradient. When the renal medullar osmolality is high, the sodium concentration in collecting tubule cells rises, and the influx of sodium into the cell through the luminal membrane becomes therefore difficult.It leads to decrease in sodium reabsorption.

Thus for the development of natriuretic effect of neurohypophyseal hormones a certain physiological dose of hormone and optimum level of hydro- and natriuresis are necessary.Natriuresis develops in the distal parts of tubules and is evidently conditioned not by the direct effect of neurohypophyseal hormones on the cellular systems of sodium reabsorption, but depends on a complex of factors making the sodium reabsorption in renal tubules difficult.One of the causes of natriuretic reaction developing after neurohypophyseal hormones injection is possibly the suppression of the sodium transport by tubular epithelium as a result of the increase in intracellular sodium concentration under the influence of an increasing osmolality in the renal medulla.

REFERENCES

1. Akatsura N.,Moran W.H., Morgan M.L. and Wilson M.F. (1977) J. Physiol., London, 266, 567-586.

2. Antoniou L.D., Burke T.J., Robinson R.R. and Clapp J.R. (1973) Kidney Int., 6, 6-13.

3. Fejes-Toth G., Magyar A. and Walter J. (1977) Am.J.Physiol.: Renal Fluid Electrolyte Physiol., 1, F 416-F 423.

4. Humphreys M.H., Friedler R.M. and Earley L.E. (1970) Am.J. Physiol., 219, 658-665.

5. Luke R.G. (1973) Am. j. Physiol., 224, 13-20.

6. Babics A., Renyi-Vamos F. (1947) Das Lymphagetäsystem der Niere und scine Bedeutung in der Nieren Pathologie und Chirurgie, Budapest,

7. Aukland K. and Kjekshus J. (1966) Am. J. Physiol., 210, 5, 971-979.

8. Bentley P.J. (1971) Endocrines and osmoregulation Springer--Verlag, Berlin-Heidelberg-New York.

9. Borisova S.A., Dubinina N.N., Ivanova L.N., Natochin Yu.V., Sokolova M.M., Shakhmatova E.I. (1971) Fiziol. J. SSSR, 57, 1038-1045.

10. Natochin Yu.V., Babaeva A.Kh.,Serebryakov E.P.,Seferova R. I.,Podsekaeva G.V.,Ivanova O.I., Lavrova E.A.,Manenkova I.D.,Shakhmatova E.I. (1979) Fiziol. J. SSSR, 65, 9, 1329-1333.

11. Morgan T. (1977) Am.J. Physiol., 232, F 117-F 122.

12. Natochin Yu.V., Berger V.Ya., Khlebovich V.V., Lavrova E.A. and Michailova O.Yu. (1979) Comp. Biochem. Physiol., 63A, 115-119.

13. Atherton J.C., Hai M.A., Thomas S. (1969) Pflügers Arch., 310, 281-396.

Hormonal Regulation of Sodium Excretion,
B. Lichardus, R.W. Schrier and J. Ponec, eds.
© 1980 Elsevier/North-Holland Biomedical Press

SODIUM REABSORPTION IN THE SUPERFICIAL PROXIMAL TUBULE AND
PAPILLARY COLLECTING DUCT OF SHAM-OPERATED AND ACUTELY
HYPOPHYSECTOMIZED RATS

J. PONEC[+], K.J. ULLRICH, F. PAPAVASSILIOU
Max-Planck-Institut für Biophysik, Frankfurt/Main, Federal Republik
of Germany, ([+]Institute of Experimental Endocrinology, Center of
Physiological Sciences, Slovak Academy of Sciences, 809 36 Bratislava, Czechoslovakia)

INTRODUCTION

In previous series of experiments, rats in Inactin anaesthesia
2 hours after hypophysectomy /hypox/ excreted significantly less
sodium than the sham-operated ones: 0.03 ± 0.01 /umol Na^+ per min
vs. 0.09 ± 0.02, respectively, both means of $13 \pm$ SE, $P<0.05$. At
the same time the acutely hypophysectomized rats increased excretion of free water as opposite to the sham-operated animals. On
the basis of these and other studies[1-5] where conservation of sodium in hypophysectomized rats was found, a site in the nephron of
hypophysectomized rats was supposed along which sodium reabsorption
was increased after hypophysectomy.

In the present study we performed measurement of reabsorption
of Ringer's solution in both the proximal convolution and papillary
collecting duct using shrinking split-droplet with simultaneous
perfusion of peritubular capillaries with the same solution. It
was found that volume reabsorption in the proximal tubule was decreased after hypophysectomy while the reabsorption of sodium in
the papillary collecting duct was decreased or abolished even by
sham-operation.

MATERIALS AND METHODS

The experiments were performed on male Wistar rats of the Max-
-Planck-Institute breed, 10-12 weeks of age (150-180 g) for proximal tubules puncture experiments and 6-8 weeks of age (60-80 g)
for collecting ducts puncture experiments. All three experimental

groups in each series were anaesthetized by Inaktin (BYK, FRG) 80-100 mg/kg b.w. and trachea was cannulated soon. The control groups were taken for puncture experiments after a lag time of at least 1 h. In sham-operated and hypophysectomized groups bottom of the skull was cleaned from muscles by a cotton piece through the parapharyngeal approach and the skull was bored with a dental boring instrument shortly to make a shallow hollow to complete the sham-operation or a hole was bored to open the bone below the pituitary. The gland was then sucked out by a vacuum motor pump.

For micropuncture experiments, the rats were placed on automatically heated table. The left kidney was exposed by flank incision, placed in a special kidney cup and superfused by paraffin oil of 37 ^{o}C. The kidney was iluminated by a quartz rod. It was assured that at least 1-hour lag period was allowed between the hypophysectomy and micropunctures.

In the micropuncture experiments the Gerts method[6] was applied.

In proximal tubule micropuncture experiments 3 glass capillaries were used, one for inserting coloured castor oil into a proximal tubule, second to set the split droplet and third for perfusing the peritubular capillaries.

In the collecting duct experiments 2 capillaries were used, one double-barrelled glass capillary of tip diameter of 25-40 um was introduced into the lumen of the collecting duct through ducts of Bellini for 200-300 um to reach a straight unbranched piece of a collecting duct. Coloured castor oil was then injected through one branch of the capillary and split droplet was set through the other. Vasa recta were perfused by the second glass capillary with about 8 um tip diameter as in the proximal puncture experiments[7].

The reabsorption of the droplets in all experiments was registered by an automatic Robot 36M Camera timed by a Robot Ia regulation circuit. The camera was mounted on a double stereomicroscope (Wild, Heerbrugg, Switzerland). Microphotographs were taken in 5 s intervals in proximal tubule experiments and in 10 s intervals in collecting duct experiments. The tubules were photographed until most of the volume was reabsorbed, in cases of standing, not reabsorbed droplets about 10 pictures were taken to assure the observation.

The logarithm of split-droplet length was plotted against time and thus half-time of reabsorption was determined. The data were analysed as described by Gyory["]8. Volume reabsorption J_v per length was calculated as $0.347 \times 2\pi r^2/t_{1/2}$ where r = radius of the tubule and $t_{1/2}$ = reabsorption half-time.

The perfusion of the peritubular capillary started always 2-6 min before the first picture was taken. The fluid used for split droplets and blood capillaries perfusion was always the same: in mmol/l, NaCl 125, $NaHCO_3$ 25, Ca^{2+}-acetate 1.5, Na^+-acetate 1, Mg^{2+}- - acetate 0.5, KH_2PO_4 2, D-glucose 5. It was shown[9] that in the preparation described sodium concentration in the shrinking droplet and blood capillaries perfusate was not different. To assure that also in our collecting duct experiments the not reabsorbed split droplets were not a result of an unisotonic reabsorption, we measured the Na^+ concentration in both the standing droplets and capillary perfusates. In the sham-hypophysectomized rats mean Na^+ concentration in the not reabsorbed droplets was 170.2 ± 3.22 (SE), in blood capillary perfusate samples 160.0 ± 5.43 mmol/l. In the hypophysectomized rats mean Na^+ concentration in the standing droplets was 163.8 ± 5.02 (SE) and in the vasa recta perfusate 149.8 ± 3.97 mmol/l. Determination of the Na^+ concentration in the perfusion fluid taken from the glass vial yielded 160.0 ± 2.05 mmol/l procedured and determined by the same way as the microsamples on a microflamephotometer. No differences between these means are statistically significant. For statistical analysis of all results Student's t-test was used.

RESULTS

The results of micropuncture experiments in the proximal tubule show that volume reabsorption was decreased after hypophysectomy as compared to both control and sham-operated rats (Tab. 1).

As shown in Table 2 reabsorption half-time was prolonged and volume reabsorption was decreased in the papillary collecting duct of rats after either sham-hypophysectomy or hypophysectomy.

146

TABLE 1

REABSORPTION HALF-TIME, $t_{1/2}$ [s] AND VOLUME REABSORPTION IN THE PROXIMAL TUBULE J_v $[10^{-7} \ (cm^3 \ cm^{-1}) \ s^{-1}]$. MEANS $\pm$ SE

	I Control n=13[a]	II Sham-hypox n=11	III Hypox n=9	Significance I:II	I:III	II:III
$t_{1/2}$	18.14 $\pm$ 0.80	16.92 $\pm$ 0.83	17.13 $\pm$ 0.75	ns	ns	ns
J_v	3.35 $\pm$ 0.09	3.40 $\pm$ 0.13	2.90 $\pm$ 0.21	ns	P<0.05	P<0.05

[a] n=number of punctures. In all 3 groups together 16 rats were used.

TABLE 2

REABSORPTION HALF-TIME $t_{1/2}$ [s] AND VOLUME REABSORPTION IN THE PAPILLARY COLLECTING DUCT J_v $[10^{-7} \ (cm^3 \ cm^{-1}) \ s^{-1}]$. MEANS $\pm$ SE

	I Control n=13[c]	II Sham-hypox[a] n=7	III Hypox[b] n=17	Significance I:II	I:III	II:III
$t_{1/2}$	65.79 $\pm$ 5.90	111.54 $\pm$ 12.25	136.31 $\pm$ 9.97	P<0.001	P<0.001	ns
J_v	1.60 $\pm$ 0.09	1.04 $\pm$ 0.13	0.97 $\pm$ 0.13	P<0.001	P<0.001	ns

[a] In the sham-hypox group 7 more droplets were not reabsorbed.
[b] In hypox group 22 more droplets were not reabsorbed.
[c] n=number of punctures. In all 3 groups together 20 rats were used.

On the basis of these results following conclusions were made:
1 Acute hypophysectomy causes inhibition of sodium reabsorption in the proximal tubule. 2 Sodium reabsorption in the papillary collecting duct may be inhibited not only by hypophysectomy but already by surgical preparatory steps to it i.e. parapharyngeal approach to the skull, thus showing potential sensitivity of the method used to some kinds of surgical performance upon the animals.
3 The present results do not allow to explain the increased reabsorption of sodium which manifested itself by decreased renal sodium output following hypophysectomy.

REFERENCES

1.   Lichardus, B. and Ponec, J. (1972) Experientia, 28, 471.

2.   Lichardus, B. and Ponec, J. (1972) Experientia, 28, 1443.

3.   Ponec, J. and Lichardus, B. (1977) Endocr. Exper., 11, 235.

4.   Ponec, J. and Lichardus, B. (1977) Experientia, 33, 685.

5.   Ponec, J., Turek, R. and Lichardus, B. (1978) Nephron, 20, 336.

6.   Gertz, K.H. (1963) Pflügers Arch., 276, 336.

7.   Uhlich, E., Baldamus, C. and Ullrich, K.J. (1969) Pflügers
     Arch., 308, 111.

8.   Gyóry, A.Z. (1971) Pflügers Arch., 324, 328.

9.   Ullrich, K.J. and Papavassiliou, F.(1979) Pflügers Arch.,
     379, 49.

Hormonal Regulation of Sodium Excretion,
B. Lichardus, R.W. Schrier and J. Ponec, eds.
© 1980 Elsevier/North-Holland Biomedical Press

THE EFFECT OF BOVINE GROWTH HORMONE ON RENAL WATER AND ELECTROLYTE EXCRETION IN THE DOG

JÁNOS FILEP, GÉZA FEJES-TÓTH and TIBOR ZAHAJSZKY
Departemant of Physiology, Semmelweis University Medical School,
Budapest 8 POB 259, H-1444 Hungary

INTRODUCTION

It has long been known that adenohypophyseal hormones are involved in the regulation of salt- and water balance[1]. Initially interest was mainly focused on growth hormone[2,3] but after the discovery that prolactin is an osmoregulatory hormone in some lower animals /c.f. Horrobin/[4] growth hormone has received relatively little attention. Even the scant reports on the effect of growth hormone on water and electrolyte excretion are controversial with both decrease[5,6,7] and increase[8,9] being reported. Since adenohypophyseal hormone preparations are frequently contaminated with vasopressin[9,10] the present study was undertaken to study the renal effects of a vasopressin-free growth hormone preparation.

MATERIALS AND METHODS

Experiments were carried out on 12 female conscious mongrel dogs weighing 10-18 kg. An episiotomy was performed on all dogs. Water diuresis was achieved by gavage giving the animals 70 ml/kg of tap water and subsequent doses equaling the volume of urine excreted. Urine was collected through a self-retaining bladder catheter. When urine flow rate had stabilized the experiment was begun with two consecutive urine collection periods of 15 min each. Immediately after the second clearance period 100 µg/kg bovine growth hormone /bGH/ was given intra-venously. This was followed by two 10 min and four 15 min clearance periods. The third and fourth 15 min peroids were considered as recovery periods. Cardiac output and intracortical blood flow were measured by radioactive microspheres[11].

Purified bovine growth hormone /NIH-GH-B 18/ was obtained from National Institute of Arthritis and Metabolic Disease.

It was further purified by gel-filtration on a Sephadex G-25 column. In three occasions tritiated lysine-vasopressin was used to monitor the effectiveness of the separation of bGH from vasopressin.

Student's t test for paired data was used for statistical analysis.

RESULTS

In order to eliminate a possible vasopressin contamination the bGH preparation was submitted to gel-filtration. Fig. 1. shows a representative chromatogram for the purification of bGH. As can be seen vasopressin eluted far beyond the internal volume of the column and is practically completely separated from the high molecular weight fraction. Pooled bGH fractions contained less than 1/50000th of the radioactivity that was applied to the column.

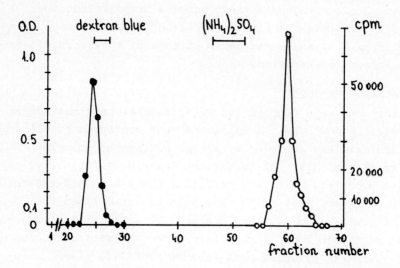

Fig.1. Chromatographic pattern of bGH admixed with tritiated vasopressin. A 1.1x138 cm Sephadex G-25 column was loaded with 1.2 ml of solution containing 10 mg of bGH and 0.5 nmole of tritiated lysine-vasopressin, followed by washing with 50 mM ammonium carbonate /pH 9/, 2.4 ml fractions were collected. Absorbance 280 nm / ● / and radioactivity / o / were plotted as the functions of elution volume.

Table 1. summarizes the data on water and electrolyte excretion. As can be seen bGH significantly reduced urine flow.
Although urine osmolality increased by 90 % after bGH administration it still remained markedly hypotonic. A small but statistically significant increase in sodium and potassium excretion was observed.

TABLE 1
EFFECT OF BOVINE GROWTH HORMONE ON WATER AND ELECTROLYTE
EXCRETION

n=12	control	bGH	recovery
Urine flow [ml/min/100 g kidney]	9.3 ± 0.6	4.4 ± 0.7 $p < 0.001$	8.4 ± 0.6 $p < 0.01$
Urinary osmolality [mOsm/l]	49 ± 4	99 ± 11 $p < 0.001$	47 ± 3 $p < 0.001$
Free water clearance [ml/min/100 g kidney]	7.7 ± 0.5	2.4 ± 0.8 $p < 0.001$	7.0 ± 0.5 $p < 0.01$
Urinary sodium excretion [μeq/min/100 g kidney]	61.9 ± 17.5	114.1 ± 32.0 $p < 0.05$	68.6 ± 19.9
Urinary potassium excretion [μeq/min/100 g kidney]	29.7 ± 4.9	38.3 ± 6.3 $p < 0.01$	23.4 ± 3.4 $p < 0.01$

Values are mean $\pm$ SE. The p values in recovery period column
refer to a comparision with bGH period.

BGH-induced changes in water and electrolyte excretion
occured in the absence of changes in cardiac output, mean arterial pressure, heart rate, renal blood flow, glomerular filtration rate and filtration fraction / Table 2. /.

Percent distribution of blood flow to the four cortical
zones / Z_1-Z_4 / also remained practically unchanged / Z_1 from
33.8 ± 4.4 % to 34.1 ± 2.6 %, Z_2 from 30.6 ± 2.9 to 32.0 ± 3.2 %,
Z_3 from 22.4 ± 2.4 % to 21.7 ± 1.8 % and Z_4 from 13.2 ± 3.0 % to
12.1 ± 2.0 % /.

Hematocrit, plasma sodium, potassium and osmotic concentrations were unaltered during all experiments.

TABLE 2
THE HEMODYNAMIC EFFECTS OF BOVINE GROWTH HORMONE

n=7	control	bGH
Mean arterial pressure [mmHg]	109 ± 8	108 ± 7
Heart rate [1/min]	110 ± 5	103 ± 8
Cardiac output [ml/min/kg b.w.]	183 ± 20	187 ± 27
Renal blood flow [ml/min/100 g kidney]	483 ± 41	441 ± 38
Glomerular filtration rate [ml/min/100 g kidney]	92 ± 9	95 ± 7
Filtration fraction	0.30 ± 0.03	0.34 ± 0.03

Each value represents the mean $\pm$ SE.

DISCUSSION

An unresolved controversy exists around the renal effects of growth hormone. In the 1950s several observations showed that the administration of growth hormone results in decreased sodium and potassium excretion without any considerable change in water excretion[2,3]. Similar results were obtained by a number of subsequent investigators but an antidiuretic effect was also observed[5,6,7]. However, other authors either failed to demonstrate decreased sodium[8,12] or potassium[6,12] excretion or observed increased electrolyte[9] and water excretion[8]. Still in other studies a biphasic effect was seen: initial natriuresis followed by sustained sodium retention[13] or the reverse[14].

Part of this unusual confusion may be attributed to species differences and to the use of different growth hormone preparations under different experimental conditions. Furthermore, it has been suggested that the renal effects of several growth hormone preparations might be related to their vasopressin contaminations[9,10,15]. In the present study fractions coinciding

with the peak of vasopressin contained some antidiuretic
activity / approximately 10 mU/mg protein applied to the column / indicating that NIH-GH-B 18 is also contaminated with
vasopressin. Although, this relatively small vasopressin contamination could be practically completely removed by gel-
filtration other impurities with higher molecular weights may
be eluted together with growth hormone. Known contaminants of
NIH-GH-B 18 are prolactin / less than 0.5 IU/mg /, thyroid stimulating hormone / less than 0.05 USP units/mg / and luteinizing
hormone / less than 0.025 NIH-LH-S1 units/mg /. However, it is
not possible to account for the observed antidiuretic effect by
these minor contaminations since probably none of these adenohypophyseal hormones exerts any renal effect in the dose that
was present in the bGH preparation. Of course, the possibility
that some as yet unidentified impurity in the high molecular
weight fraction may have antidiuretic and saluretic activity is
not excluded. Even so it is reasonable to assume that the renal
effects of the present bGH preparation can be attributed to
growth hormone itself, or to one of its metabolities and that
it exerts its effect by a direct tubular mechanism and not by
altering renal hemodynamics.

ACKNOWLEDGEMENTS

   The growth hormone preparation was generously supplied by
National Institute of Arthritis and Metabolic Disease.
   We are grateful to Dr. Gy. Kéry, First Department of
Biochemistry, Semmelweis University Medical School for providing
tritiated lysine-vasopressin.

REFERENCES
1. Hann, F. (1918) Frankfurt Ztschr.f.Path., 21, 337-345.
2. Stein, J.D.,Jr., Bennett, L.L., Batts, A.A. and Li, C.H.
    (1952) Am.J.Physiol., 171, 587-591.
3. Whitney, J.E., Bennett, L.L. and Li, C.H. (1952) Proc.Soc.
    Exp.Biol.Med., 79, 584-587.
4. Horrobin, D.F. (1975) Fluid and electrolyte metabolism, In:
    Prolactin 1975, Eden Press, Montreal, pp. 114-119.
5. Bieglieri, E.G., Watlington, C.O. and Forsham, P.H. (1961)
    J.Clin.Endocrinol.Metab., 21, 361-370.

6. Croxatto, H., Labarca, E., Swaneck, G. and Garfias, P.
    (1966) Am.J.Physiol. 211, 588-592.

7. Lockett, M.F. and Nail, B. (1965) J.Physiol.London, 180,
    147-156.

8. Henderson, I.W. and Balment, R.J. (1975) J.Endocrinol.,
    67, 60P-61P.

9. Rabkin, R., Epstein, S. and Swann, M. (1975) Horm.Metab.Res.
    7, 139-142.

10. Baumann, G., Rayfield, E.J., Rose, L.I., Williams, G.H. and
    Dingman, J.F. (1972) J.Clin.Endocrinol., 34, 801-804.

11. Fejes-Tóth, G., Fekete, A. and Walter, J. (1978) Pflügers
    Arch., 376, 67-72.

12. Gershberg, M. (1960) J.Clin.Endocrinol.Metab., 20, 1107-1119.

13. Lockett, M.F. (1965) J.Physiol.London, 181, 192-199.

14. Ludens, J.H., Bach, R.R. and Williamson, H.E. (1969)
    Proc.Soc.Exp.Biol.Med., 130, 1156-1158.

15. Leichter, S.B. and Chase, L.R. (1975) Biochim.Biophys.Acta,
    399, 291-301.

Hormonal Regulation of Sodium Excretion,
B. Lichardus, R.W. Schrier and J. Ponec, eds.
© 1980 Elsevier/North-Holland Biomedical Press

THE EFFECTS OF OVARIAN STEROIDS ON SODIUM EXCRETION IN SHEEP

A.R. MICHELL and D. NOAKES
Departments of Physiology and Obstetrics, Royal Veterinary College,
Royal College Street, London NW1 0TU, England.

INTRODUCTION

These experiments began with the observation that voluntary sodium intake
in sheep was high during the luteal phase of the reproductive cycle and lowest
at oestrus[1]. The obvious explanation, namely that the changes compensated for
salt retention at oestrus and salt loss during the luteal phase, proved in-
correct; the time of maximal sodium excretion was at oestrus[2]. This was very
surprising since the natriuretic effect of progesterone is well known[3] and
the general view that oestrogens cause renal sodium retention has existed for
over 40 years[4,5,6]. Indeed this retention has recently been implicated as a
factor likely to contribute to contraceptive hypertension[7].

Since food and water intake fall at oestrus, the pattern of excretion could
well be dictated by factors other than hormonal changes and the unexpected
results might thus be explained. It nevertheless seemed desirable to clarify
the effects of ovarian steroids on renal function in sheep. As a first step
we examined the effects of oestrogen and progesterone injections on daily
electrolyte excretion in conscious sheep.

METHODS

The animals were ovariectomised Finnish Landrace ewes and their feeding,
management, housing and the relevant analytical procedures have been described
previously[2,8,9]. Each experiment was performed in two stages with 3 control
sheep and 3 experimentals in each stage. Each sheep served once as a control
and once as an experimental, therefore the control and experimental groups
comprised the same 6 sheep.

The effect of intramuscular injections of oestrogen was examined at separate
dose levels of 20, 30 and 60 μg daily and that of progesterone at 10 mg daily[9].
In some experiments the sheep were allowed free access to a 40 mM sodium
bicarbonate solution in order to produce higher levels of sodium intake. The
effect of each hormone was also examined after priming with a course of the
other hormone i.e. oestrogen 48 hours after 6 days of progesterone and
progesterone 48 hours after 2 days of oestrogen. Control sheep received

injections of solvent.

The initial experiments, with 20 and 30 μg of oestrogen daily for 3 days, produced similar results and the data are therefore pooled. The experiments with oestrogen following progesterone and with high-dose oestrogen (both on high sodium intake) involved 4 days of oestrogen treatment instead of three. Progesterone treatment lasted 6 days. The sheep had been accustomed to the management routine for several weeks before the experiments and had been ovariectomised for several months.

Treatment periods are compared with data from the preceding (baseline) and following six days. Results are expressed as means ± S.E.M. and statistical comparisons employ Student's paired t-test.

RESULTS

Effects of oestrogen on sodium excretion

Physiological doses of oestrogen; normal sodium intake. Urinary sodium concentration increased by 157 ± 53% (p<0.05) during oestrogen treatment. Control injections increased sodium concentration by 34% (N/S), probably as a result of a 6% fall in food intake[10]. Food intake fell by 8 ± 2% in oestrogen-treated sheep, fluid intake by 9.6 ± 2.3% and urine output by 10%; despite this, urinary sodium excretion rose from 7.8 ± 1.6 to 16.8 ± 4.7 mmol/day, an increase of 115%. The effect of oestrogen was clearest during the 2nd and 3rd day of treatment when urinary sodium excretion increased by 158% and urine sodium concentration by 205%; control sheep showed values 30% and 32% above baseline at this time.

During the 48 hours after oestrogen treatment, urinary sodium excretion declined sharply to a minimum of 27 ± 5% of baseline levels. This reflected a fall in sodium concentration to 2.7 ± 0.8 mmol/1 (36% of baseline); control sheep had urinary sodium concentrations of 17.1 ± 7.9 mmol/1 at this time, above their baseline value. During the next 2-3 days urinary sodium concentration and excretion returned to the levels seen before oestrogen treatment.

Other treatments. The natriuretic effect of oestrogen was surprising in view of findings in other species. It might have reflected an atypical effect in the absence of progesterone priming or in animals which, compared with man and most laboratory rats, received a very modest (thought adequate) level of dietary sodium (1 mmol/kg bodyweight, approximately). The effect of oestrogen was therefore re-examined in sheep primed with progesterone and on liberal sodium intakes. The effect of supranormal oestrogen doses was also examined, again on liberal sodium intake. The increased sodium intake resulted from the availability of 40 mM sodium bicarbonate solutions, from which the sheep took about 110 mmol/day, thus boosting their total daily intake to about 2.5 mmol/kg.

Among the sheep were 7 which maintained food intakes within 1% of baseline and fluid intakes within 4% of baseline, in spite of oestrogen treatment. Both values were statistically indistinguishable from the baseline readings and less than the reductions of fluid intake (5.5%) in sheep with control injections. Since most sodium intake came from drinking in these experiments it is especially important that intake of sodium solutions fell (by 1%) during oestrogen injection.

Sodium excretion was again increased in both experiments, by a mean of 42.9 ± 15.3 mmol/day (72%) during the 1st 48 hours of oestrogen treatment. During the same period sodium excretion in the 12 control sheep fell by 5%. The natriuretic effect of oestrogen was therefore confirmed in the absence of significant changes of food or fluid intake. By the 3rd day of injection, however, sodium excretion fell below baseline and reached a minimum on the last day of injection and the following day. Sodium excretion had then fallen by 50 ± 9% of its baseline level (p<0.01); it thus falls to a minimum 4-5 days after initiation of oestrogen treatment, whether or not treatment is sustained for four days.

Summary. The effect of oestrogen on sodium excretion in sheep is biphasic; an initial natriuresis is followed by sodium retention. This was true at normal levels of sodium intake (70 mmol/day) and at high levels 180 mmol/day), with or without progesterone priming, and with normal or high oestrogen dosage.

The most striking effect of oestrogen on sodium excretion, however, was seen in faeces, which accounted for 82% of measured sodium excretion in these sheep. Physiological doses of oestrogen increased faecal sodium excretion by 49 ± 10%; two days afterwards it fell to a minimum 17 ± 5% below baseline. Control injections increased faecal sodium excretion insignificantly (8.6 ± 8.6%).

The net effect of oestrogen on sodium excretion was thus to raise it by 61%, mainly through faecal rather than urinary sodium loss. The pattern of loss followed by retention occurred with a similar time scale in both urine and faeces. The results of oestrogen injection, therefore, closely resemble those of natural oestrus in sheep[2].

Effect of oestrogen on urinary potassium excretion.

The effect of oestrogen on urinary potassium excretion was small but highly reproducible. At physiological oestrogen dosage on normal sodium intake, urinary potassium concentration fell by 11%; on higher sodium intake with progesterone priming it fell by 10% and on high sodium intake with high oestrogen dosage it fell by 12%. Combining these results, the fall in urinary potassium concentration was 58.3 ± 14.5 mmol (11.1%; $p<0.02$). After the oestrogen treatment, urinary potassium excretion returned to levels slightly above baseline (106%). In control animals, urinary potassium concentration was stable, being 3% above baseline during and after injections of the oil base.

Effect of progesterone on urinary sodium excretion.

The effect of progesterone on urinary sodium excretion in these experiments is simply summarised; there was none. The results of progesterone and of control injections were identical, whether or not the animal was 'primed' with oestrogen and regardless of whether sodium intake was normal or high.

DISCUSSION

Oestrus in sheep is accompanied by an integrated reduction of body sodium, resulting from reduced food intake, diminished preference for sodium and increased urinary and faecal sodium excretion[2,9]. Neither changes in food intake nor in ovarian steroids explain the changes in sodium preference but the present experiments suggest that oestrogens, as well as changes in food intake[10], independently contribute to the increase in sodium excretion. The effect of oestrogen is, however, biphasic, leading to sodium retention within five days. Sodium retention similarly occurs by the 5th day of the oestrous cycle[2].

A biphasic effect of oestrogens on sodium excretion has also been observed in women, albeit at high dosage[11,12]. More recently, oestrogens have been reported to promote sodium excretion in isolated rabbit kidneys[13]. The majority of experiments with oestrogens, however, indicate that they cause sodium retention in rats, dogs and primates, without causing kaliuresis[5]. In our experiments, the day of minimum urinary sodium concentration did coincide with a peak in potassium concentration. It is interesting that if the experiments had primarily considered the net effect of extended oestrogen treatment (beyond 3 days), the overall result might have appeared to be sodium retention. The normal duration of oestrus in sheep, however, is rather less than 2 days, during which time the predominant effect would certainly be natriuresis.

The natriuretic effect of oestrogen in sheep may involve the distal tubule since it is accompanied by a reduced urinary potassium concentration. It seems unlikely to involve aldosterone, however, since progesterone, a competitive antagonist, failed to affect sodium excretion in these animals despite the dose being at the high end of the physiological range[9]. During the natural cycle too, there is no natriuresis during the luteal phase[2].

The pattern of reabsorbtion and secretion of potassium within the nephron may not be the same in sheep as in more familiar experimental animals such as dogs or rats. The dietary intake of potassium is so large that it is comparable with the daily filtered load, moreover sheep show considerable ability to tolerate even higher levels of potassium[14]. This response does not depend on aldosterone alone[15], indeed despite their low dietary sodium and very high potassium intake, sheep have lower aldosterone secretion rates and plasma levels than humans on comparable salt intakes[16]. Recent data support the existence of important differences in the renal handling of potassium in sheep[17].

If the natriuresis is a direct effect of oestrogen, rather than one mediated by aldosterone, there are two important implications. Firstly, it would seem necessary to assume that oestrogens had more widespread effects on electrolyte balance in view of the changes in faecal sodium. In fact observations of mixed salivary Na/K during the 20 μg oestrogen treatment showed that this ratio also rose; extrarenal mechanisms have been implicated in oestrogen-induced oedema[5]. Secondly, histological evidence in rats suggests that the clearest renal effects of oestrogens are those in the proximal tubule[2,18]; if so, the fall in urinary potassium excretion alongside increased distal delivery of sodium would be very surprising. On the other hand the low aldosterone levels in sheep suggest either that their kidneys are more sensitive to it or that they are more reliant on other means of regulating renal sodium excretion. This would be consistent with the lack of effect of progesterone seen here, although sheep are not unique in this respect[6].

Many workers studying the effects of oestrogen on urinary sodium excretion disregard the possibility that they are secondary to changes in food and water intake; others, however, have concluded from experiments in rats that oestrogens have no effects on excretion except those mediated by changes in intake[19,20]. The present experiments clearly show that, in sheep at least, oestrogens have effects on renal and faecal sodium excretion which are independent of changes in food and fluid intake.

Perhaps the most surprising aspect of the data is the fact that renal changes were the minor aspect of sodium excretion; most of the excreted sodium appeared in faeces and changes in faecal sodium were as swift and pronounced as those in urine. Like all herbivores, sheep have adapted to diets relatively low in sodium yield but adequate, nevertheless, to meet their very small obligatory sodium loss. For these animals, therefore, obtaining sodium is a crucial step in regulating body stores and their position contrasts sharply with humans or laboratory rats which routinely consume sodium in twenty- and thirty-fold excess of their nutritional requirements[21,22].

Among species with exorbitant sodium intake it seems natural that the emphasis should lie with the excretion of excess salt and its curtailment during temporary shortage i.e. with the kidney. Certainly the preponderance of research in such species has led to an almost complete preoccupation with the kidney as the regulator of sodium balance. It seems equally plausible that in species subsisting on marginal sodium intakes, the emphasis lies instead with behavioural mechanisms for seeking salt and physiological mechanisms for regulating its efficient intestinal absorbtion.

The sheep in these experiments were on liberal sodium intakes compared with sheep at pasture, so they excreted the excess in faeces, nevertheless obligatory faecal sodium loss is small. Thus faecal sodium excretion does not invariably exceed urinary sodium excretion in sheep; the interesting thing is that it can, in perfectly healthy animals. This finding was not limited to these sheep[23]. The horse, again a herbivore, similarly eliminates more sodium in faeces than urine and in many circumstances normal cattle do the same[24,25]. It is interesting that Aitken[25] cites a study in which high salt intake suppressed faecal sodium excretion in horses. A reasonable and testable speculation would be that regulation of sodium exchange in the gut involved a large obligatory absorbtion and a small regulatory secretion which is suppressed in individuals or species on extremely high salt intakes. This would explain the observation that sheep on sodium intakes above 300 mmol/day reduce their faecal sodium content[26].

The influence of the gut on sodium excretion may not be confined to faecal loss; in some species it may also influence renal sodium excretion[27,28], although the data, particularly in dogs remain conflicting[29]. Splanchnic receptors may also play a part in the behavioural control of sodium ingestion[30]. Bearing in mind that liberal salt intake is a relatively recent feature of evolution in man[31] and the laboratory rat, further study of the larger and more 'exotic' species may provide a useful perspective in understanding the physiology of body sodium.

CONCLUSION

When we began this work we were confident that the kidney dominated the physiological regulation of body sodium in sheep and that its ability to retain salt was enhanced by oestrogen and diminished by progesterone. None of these assumptions survived the experiments. Instead, we found no response to progesterone, a biphasic response to oestrogen dominated by natriuresis, and a pattern of sodium excretion in which urinary changes were overshadowed by those in faeces.

ACKNOWLEDGEMENT

We would like to thank Mrs. Elizabeth Taylor and Mrs. Edna Gordon for their enormous help in performing and presenting these experiments.

REFERENCES

1. Michell, A.R. (1975) Physiol. Behav, 14, 223-226.

2. Michell, A.R. (1979) Q.J.Exp.Physiol., 64, 79-88.

3. Landau, R.L. (1973) In: Handbook of Physiology, Section 7 Volume III, Part I, Endocrinology (Female Reproductive System). Ed. R.O. Greep. pp.573-589. Washington, D.C.: American Physiological Society.

4. Thorn, G.W., Nelson, K.E. & Thorn, D.W. (1938) Endocrinology, 22, 155-163.

5. Christy, N.P. & Shaver, J.C. (1974) Kidney Int., 6, 336-376.

6. Lindheimer, M.D. & Katz, A.I. (1977) Ann.Rev.Physiol., 39, 97-134.

7. Crane, M.G. & Harris, J.H. (1978) Am.J.Med.Sci., 276, 33-55.

8. Michell,A.R. (1979) Br.Vet.J., 135, 294-296.

9. Michell, A.R. (1980) Q.J.Exp.Physiol., 65, 27-36.

10. Michell, A.R. (1980) Proceedings, XXVIIth International Congress of Physiological Sciences, Budapest: Extracellular Volume Control.

11. Katz, F.H. (1969) In: Metabolic Effects of Gonadal Hormones & Contraceptive Steroids, Eds. H.A. Salahanick, D.M. Kipnis et al. pp.441-446. New York: Plenum.

12. Preedy, J.R.K. (1969) See 11: pp.422-423.

13. Pellanda, E.B. (1975) Annales d'Endocrinologie (Paris), 36, 235-230.

14. Warner, A.C.I. & Stacy, B.D. (1972) Q.J.Exp.Physiol., 57, 89-102

15. Beal, A.M., Budtz-Olsen, O.E., Clark, R.C., Cross, R.B. & French, T.J. (1975) Q.J.Exp.Physiol., 60, 207-221.

16. Coghlan, J.P. & Scoggins, B.A. (1967) J.Clin.Endoc.Metab., 27, 1470-1486.

162

17. Rabinowitz, L.J., & Gunther, R.A. (1978) Am.J.Physiol., 234, F371-376.

18. Schreiber, J.T. & Danner, K.G. (1978) Cell & Tiss.Res., 192, 527-549.

19. Thornborough, J.R. & Passo, S.S. (1975) Endocrinology, 97, 1528-1536.

20. Nocenti, M.R. & Cizek, L.J. (1964) Am.J.Physiol., 206, 476-482.

21. Michell, A.R. (1978) Perspect.Biol.Med., 21, 335-347.

22. Michell, A.R. (1980) Lancet 1, June 21st.

23. Dewhurst, J.K., Harrison, F.A. & Keynes, R.D. (1968) J.Physiol., 195, 609-621.

24. Tasker, J.B. (1967) Cornell Vet., 57, 648-657.

25. Aitken, F.C. (1976) Sodium and Potassium in Nutrition of Mammals. pp.142-146. Farnham Royal, Bucks, U.K.: Commonwealth Agricultural Bureaux.

26. Michell, A.R. (1977) Br.vet.J., 133, 245-257.

27. Lennane, R.J., Carey, R.M., Goodwin, T.J. & Peart, W.S. (1975) Clin. Sci.Mol.Med., 49, 437-440.

28. Carey, R.M., Smith, J.R. & Ortt, E.M. (1976) Am.J.Physiol., 230, 1504-1508.

29. Hanson, R.C., McLane-Vega, L.A., Childers, J.W., Gleason, S.D. & Schneider, E.G. (1980) Am.J.Physiol., 238, F112-F118.

30. Blake, W.D. & Lin, K.K. (1978) J.Physiol. (Lond.), 274, 129-139.

31. Denton, D.A. (1972) Aust.N.Z.J.Med., 2, 203-212.

Hormonal Regulation of Sodium Excretion,
B. Lichardus, R.W. Schrier and J. Ponec, eds.
© 1980 Elsevier/North-Holland Biomedical Press

RENAL SODIUM EXCRETION IN RATS. EFFECT OF STRUCTURAL MODIFICATION
IN POSITION 2 OF DEAMINO-6-CARBA-OXYTOCIN

JANA ŠKOPKOVÁ, PAVEL HRBAS, TOMISLAV BARTH, MICHAL LEBL,
KAREL JOŠT
Institute of Organic Chemistry and Biochemistry, Czechoslovak
Academy of Sciences, 166 10 Prague 6 (Czechoslovakia)

INTRODUCTION

Some attemps were made to account for the mechanism of renal
natrium excretion. A hypothesis assuming the regulatory action of
a "natriuretic hormone" could explain certain states, whether natural of experimentally evoked. This substance has so far eluded
isolation and characterization and its precise mechanism of action at the molecular level is at present largely unknown. In fact,
it was suggested that oxytocin acts either directly as the natriuretic hormone[1], or indirectly by causing the liberation of another
low molecular weight substance from some intracranial structure,
which is responsible for increasing the rejection fraction of
sodium[2]. While further separation work is under way[3], a program
of studying the structure-activity relation of synthetic oxytocin
analogues is also in progress, aiming at specifying which structural features of the peptide molecule are effectual in producing
a natriuretic response. Chan[4] assumed that modifications in position 4 of the oxytocin molecule could result in natriuretically
potent analogues. This supposition was not confirmed by the experimental data obtained so far, on the contrary, modifications
of the S-S bridge, i.e. carba-substitution, combined with the
replacement of the primary amino group by hydrogen have been
found promisable. Among the analogues of this type, deamino-6-
-carba-oxytocin had the highest natriuretic potency[5]. However, the
higher natriuretic activity was accompanied by increased uterotonic and pressor activites[6]. As it was found that certain modifications in position 2 led to a decrease of the uterotonic and
pressor activities[7,8], further synthetic work was aimed in this
direction. A number of analogues modified in position 2 were

produced; their natriuretic potency and specificity are described
in this paper.

MATERIALS AND METHODS

Oxytocin and its analogues were prepared at the Department of
Organic Synthesis of this Institute. The following analogues were
studied: deamino-6-carba-oxytocin[9], [2-isoleucine]deamino-6-carba-
-oxytocin[10], [2-methionine]deamino-6-carba-oxytocin[10], [2-O-met-
hyltyrosine]deamino-6-carba-oxytocin[10], [2-phenylalanine]deamino-
-6-carba-oxytocin[11], [2-O-ethyltyrosine]deamino-6-carba-oxytocin[11]
[2-p-methylphenylalanine]deamino-6-carba-oxytocin[11],[2-p-benzylo-
xycarbonylaminophenylalanine]deamino-6-carba-oxytocin[11], [2-p-
-ethylphenylalanine]deamino-6-carba-oxytocin[11], [2-p-N,N-dimethyl-
aminophenylalanine]deamino-6-carba-oxytocin[11], [2-p-aminophenyl-
alanine]deamino-6-carba-oxytocin[11], [2-p-nitrophenylalanine]dea-
mino-6-carba-oxytocin[11].

Natriuresis was assayed using a modification of Burn`s test
described elsewhere[12] performed on conscious rats. The compounds
were administered s.c. in doses of 0.2, 1, 5 and 25 ug/kg of body
weight in 1 ml of saline/kg after receiving a water load (4% of
body weight). Urine was collected for 4 hours and the sodium
content was determined by means of a flame photometer. Natriuretic activity was expressed as $U_{Na}V$ (meq/kg of body weight in 4
hours) and its dependence on the peptide dosage was evaluated
statistically.

The uterotonic activity of the compounds was assayed on isolated rat uterine strips according to Holton[13] in Munsick`s modifi-
cation.

RESULTS

The modifications performed in position 2 of deamino-6-carba-
oxytocin can be divided into three groups.

The substitution of tyrosine by phenylalanine, isoleucine and
methionine led to a decrease of natriuretic activity. The analogue
containing phenylalanine in position 2 had the highest natriuretic
activity of this group; it had almost half the natriuretic potency
of deamino-6-carba-oxytocin (Figure 1, Table I).

Substitution of the hydrogen of tyrosine hydroxyl by an alkoxy group. The most active analogue of this group was [2-O-methyl-tyrosine]deamino-6-carba-oxytocin with approximately half the natriuretic activity of deamino-6-carba-oxytocin. The activity abruptly decreased when the size of the substituent was increased; the analogue containing the benzyloxycarbonylamino group was without any activity (Table I).

Substitution of the tyrosine hydroxyl by nitro-, amino-, di-methylamino-, methyl- and ethyl-groups. In this series, the most active analogue was [2-p-methylphenylalanine]deamino-6-carba-oxy-tocin; its activity was even higher than that of the parent mole-cule. The analogue containing an ethyl group was also active, whereas the activity of the other analogues containing polar groups was pronouncedly lower (Table I, Figure 2).

Table I presents the relative natriuretic potency expressed in % of activity of deamino-6-carba-oxytocin and the uterotonic activity.

Natriuresis evoked by the neurohypophysial hormones is a com-plex response involving tubular and vascular components, and there is an ongoing discussion as to whether the natriuretic activity of oxytocin and vasopresin is in direct relation to their pressor-vascular and antidiuretic effects. The synthesis of analogues the activities of which are dissociated can be seen as a pre-requisite for analysing the mechanism of natriuresis evoked by neurohypophysial hormones.

CONCLUSION

The modifications of the oxytocin molecule mentioned in the introduction (i.e. carba substitution and deamination) led to an increase of natriuresis, but also to an increase of the uteroto-nic and pressor activities[6]. The alterations performed in posi-tion 2 of deamino-6-carba-oxytocin suppressed these undesirable effects. All the analogues studied had significantly lower utero-tonic activity (cf Table I). The pressor effect was also decre-ased (with the exception of [2-phenylalanine]deamino-6-carba-oxy-tocin); the analogues studied did not influence the systemic blood pressure [10,11] in doses up to 200 ug/kg of body weight. In the first group of analogues in which the whole amino acid had been substituted, the decrease of these activities was accompanied

166

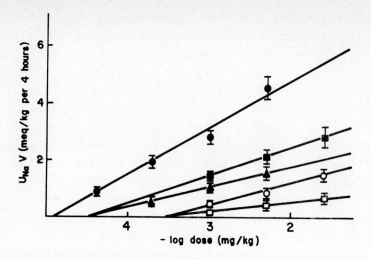

Fig. 1. Log dose - natriuretic response curves for deamino-6-
-carba-oxytocin ● , oxytocin ▲ , [2-phenylalanine]deamino-6-carba-
-oxytocin ■ , [2-isoleucine]deamino-6-carba-oxytocin O and [2-me-
thionine]deamino-6-carba-oxytocin □ .

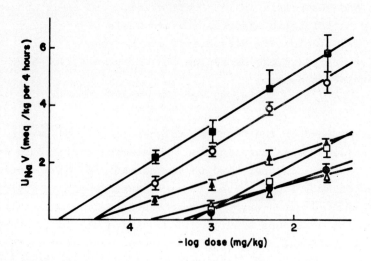

Fig. 2. Log dose - natriuretic response curves for [2-O-methyl-
tyrosine]deamino-6-carba-oxytocin ▲ , [2-p-methylphenylalanine]-
deamino-6-carba-oxytocin ■ , [2-p-ethylphenylalanine]deamino-6-
-carba-oxytocin O , [2-p-aminophenylalanine]deamino-6-carba-oxy-
tocin □ , [2-p-N,N dimethylaminophenylalanine]deamino-6-carba-
-oxytocin ● and [2-p-nitrophenylalanine]deamino-6-carba-oxytocin   .

TABLE I

COMPARISON OF UTEROTONIC AND NATRIURETIC ACTIVITIES OF DEAMINO-
-6-CARBA-OXYTOCIN AND ITS DERIVATIVES

Compound	Natriuretic activity, NA $U_{Na}V$	%	Uterotonic activity, UA I.U./mg	NA/UA ratio
Deamino-6-carba-oxytocin	4.54 ± 0,36*	100	929	0.005
Oxytocin	1.53 ± 0.26	34	450	0.003
[2-Phenylalanine]deamino--6-carba-oxytocin	2.15 ± 0.38	47	75	0.029
[2-Isoleucine]deamino-6--carba-oxytocin	0.87 ± 0.11	19	3.1	0.279
[2-Methionine]deamino-6--carba-oxytocin	0.43 ± 0.07	10	4.7	0.091
[2-O-Methyltyrosine]deamino--6-carba-oxytocin	0.18 ± 0.21	48	3.1	0.694
[2-O-Ethyltyrosine]deamino--6-carba-oxytocin	0.45 ± 0.09	10	< 0.05	9.020
[2-p-Benzyloxycarbonylamino-phenylalanine]deamino-6-car-ba-oxytocin	0.15 ± 0.05	**	0.07	2.086
[2-p-Methylphenylalanine]-deamino-6-carba-oxytocin	4.75 ± 0.48	105	70	0.068
[2-p-Ethylphenylalanine]-deamino-6-carba-oxytocin	3.92 ± 0.18	86	27	0.145
[2-p-Aminophenylalanine]-deamino-6-carba-oxytocin	1.34 ± 0.13	30	< 0.05	26.880
[2-p-N,N-Dimethylaminophe-nylalanine]deamino-6-carba-oxytocin	1.15 ± 0.11	25	< 0.05	23.100
[2-p-Nitrophenylalanine]-deamino-6-carba-oxytocin	1.00 ± 0.14	22	< 0.05	20.060
Controls	0.08			

*Arithmetic mean values ± SE

**The dose-response relation is not statistically significant

with a pronounced decrease of natriuretic activity, as compared with deamino-6-carba-oxytocin. The substitution of hydrogen in the hydroxyl group of tyrosine brought about a further decrease of the uterotonic and pressor activities. The substitution of the whole hydroxyl group of tyrosine resulted in a slight decrease of the uterotonic activity and in a pronounced decrease of the pressor activity (lower than O.2 IU/mg). On the other hand, the natriuretic activity of the ethyl derivate was only slightly lower and that of the methyl derivative was even higher than the parent molecule. The most advantageous ratio of natriuretic and pressor activities, with insignificant pressor activities (O.2 IU/mg) was obtained in the case of [2-p-aminophenylalanine]deamino-6-carba--oxytocin. This group of analogues therefore yielded compounds with specific natriuretic action without systemic pressor activity and with very low uterotonic activity. At present, we do not know whether the analogues change the local hemodynamic parameters in the kidney, which part of the nephron it effects, or to what degree it influences renal Na,K-ATPase. Further studies should decide whether therapeutical application is promissable.

REFERENCES

1. Heller, J. and Pickering, G.W., Eds. (1970) International Encyklopedia of Pharmacology and Therapeutics, Sect. 41, Vol. 1., Pregamon Press, New York, pp. 229-278.
2. Sedláková, E. et al. (1969) Science, 164, 580-582.
3. De Wardener, H.E. (1977) Clin.Sci.Mol.Med., 53, 1-8.
4. Chan, W.Y. (1976) J.Pharmacol.Exp.Therap., 196, 746-752.
5. Machová, A., and Jošt, K. (1975) Endocrinol.Exptl. 9, 269-277.
6. Barth, T. et al. (1973) Europ.J.Pharmacol., 24, 183-188.
7. Jošt, K. et al. (1963) Coll.Czech.Chem.Commun., 28, 1706-1714.
8. Frič, I. et al. (1974) Coll.Czech.Chem.Commun.,39, 1290-1302.
9. Jošt,K. and Šorm, F. (1971) Coll.Czech.Chem.Commun., 36, 234-245.
10. Lebl, M. et al. (1980) Coll.Czech.Chem.Commun., in press.
11. Lebl, M. et al. (1981) Coll.Czech.Chem.Commun., in press.
12. Škopková, J. et al. (1980) Endocrinol.Exptl., in press.
13. Holton, P. (1948) Brit.J.Pharmacol., 3, 328-334.

Hormonal Regulation of Sodium Excretion,
B. Lichardus, R.W. Schrier and J. Ponec, eds.
© 1980 Elsevier/North-Holland Biomedical Press

RENAL SODIUM EXCRETION IN RATS. EFFECT OF AMINO ACID REPLACEMENT
IN POSITION 4 OF THE OXYTOCIN MOLECULE

PAVEL HRBAS, JANA ŠKOPKOVÁ, TOMISLAV BARTH, MICHAL LEBL,
KAREL JOŠT
Institute of Organic Chemistry and Biochemistry, Czechoslovak
Academy of Sciences, 166 10 Prague 6 (Czechoslovakia)

INTRODUCTION

The effect of oxytocin on the excretion of sodium by mammalian
kidneys has been intensively studied lately. The main interest
centers on the investigation of the action mechanisms of oxytocin
on the one hand, and on the determination of the relation between
the primary structure of the hormone or its analogues and sodium
excretion on the other. Several oxytocin analogues with pronounced
natriuretic action have been prepared by modifying positions
2 and 4 (refs. 1,2), position 1 and the disulfide bridge [3, 4]
of the oxytocin molecule. It became apparent that the mentioned
higher natriuretic action of the analogues modified in position 4
was dependent on the experimental arrangement[5-7]. The present
communication deals with the effect of a number of structural
modifications of the parent hormone on its activity to influence
the total sodium excretion of conscious rats with standard 4% water
load.

MATERIALS AND METHODS

Oxytocin and its analogues were prepared at the Department
of Organic Synthesis of this Institute. The following analogues
were tested: deamino-oxytocin[8], 1-carba-oxytocin[9], deamino-1-
carba-oxytocin[10], deamino-6-carba-oxytocin[11], [4-leucine] oxyto-
cin[12], [4-glutamic]acid deamino-1-carba-oxytocin[13], [4-leucine]-
deamino-1-carba-oxytocin[14], [4-isoleucine] deamino-1-carba-oxyto-
cin[14], [4-valine]deamino-1-carba-oxytocin[14], [4-glutamic acid
methyl ester]deamino-1-carba-oxytocin[15], [2-O-methyltyrosine]oxy-
tocin[16], [2-O-methyltyrosine]deamino-1-carba-oxytocin[17], [2-iso-
leucine]deamino-1-carba-oxytocin[17], [2-phenylalanine]deamino-
-1-carba-oxytocin[17], [9-desglycine]oxytocin[18]. Tocinamide[19] was

supplied by Dr.M. Flegel from Léčiva, Prague.

For the determination of the natriuretic activity of oxytocin and its analogues, we used male rats of the Wistar strain, weighing 180-190 g, adapted for one week prior to the experiment to the experimental conditions. The compounds tested were dissolved in physiological saline and administered s.c. in doses of 1-30 ug/kg of body weight after the water load, corresponding to 4% of body weight, had been applied by means of a stomach cathether. The control group of animals was given s.c. injections of saline. The rats were placed in metabolic cages, urine was collected at 30 min intervals for four hours and analysed for the content of sodium. The natriuretic potency was expressed as $U_{Na}V$(meq/kg of body weight in 4 hours). Each group of 5 rats was submitted three times to the experiment and no group received the same compound twice.

RESULTS

The natriuretic effect of the given compounds was determined for a relatively wide range of doses. Table I presents the natriuretic effect of the individual compounds applied in doses of 5 ug/kg of body weight. The natriuretic potency increased when the primary amino group of cysteine in position 1 of the oxytocin peptide chain was substituted by hydrogen (deamino-oxytocin), the sulfur atom was replaced by a methylene group and when the two modifications were combined. The most effective analogues were deamino-1-carba-oxytocin and deamino-6-carba-oxytocin. In the deamino-1-carba-oxytocin series, an estimation was made of the effect of the substitution of the amino acids in position 2 and 4. The substitution of glutamine in position 4 by glutamic acid, glutamic acid methyl ester, isoleucine and valine decreased the natriuretic potency of the resultant analogues to values lower than those of oxytocin. The most significant decrease was caused by the replacement of glutamine with leucine; in the case of oxytocin, sodium excretion decreased by one order of ten and in the case of deamino-1-carba-oxytocin, natriuretic activity was almost eliminated in the range of doses studied. A 50% decrease of natriuretic potency was observed in the case of analogues of deamino-1-carba-oxytocin that had

TABLE I

NATRIURETIC EFFECT OF OXYTOCIN ANALOGUES

Compound	$U_{Na}V$	Activity,%
Oxytocin	1.53	100.0
Deamino-oxytocin	2.02	132.0
1-Carba-oxytocin	2.28	149.1
Deamino-1-carba-oxytocin	3.00	193.8
Deamino-6-carba-oxytocin	4.56	298.0
[4-Leucine]oxytocin	0.19	12.0
[4-Leucine]deamino-1-carba-oxytocin	0.00	0.0
[4-Isoleucine]deamino-1-carba-oxytocin	1.00	65.4
[4-Valine]deamino-1-carba-oxytocin	0.25	16.0
[4-Glutamic acid]deamino-1-carba--oxytocin	0.21	14.0
[4-Glutamic acid methyl]ester deamino--1-carba-oxytocin	0.32	20.8
[2-O-Methyltyrosine]oxytocin	1.56	102.2
[2-O-Methyltyrosine]deamino-1-carba--oxytocin	1.08	70.8
[2-Isoleucine]deamino-1-carba-oxytocin	1.96	128.1
[2-Phenylalanine]deamino-1-carba--oxytocin	2.00	131.3
Tocinamide	0.44	28.7
[9-Desglycine]oxytocin	0.21	13.7

O-methyltyrosine, phenylalanine or isoleucine instead of tyrosine
in position 2. However, the substitution of tyrosine of
oxytocin by O-methyltyrosine did not alter the natriuretic activity. The shortening of the oxytocin peptide chain at the C-ter-
minus decreased the natriuretic potency of the resultant analogue.

CONCLUSION

   The experiments described in this communication help to clarify the relation between the chemical structure and natriuretic
potency of oxytocin analogues. A remarkable decrease of the natriuretic potency was brought about by the substitution of glu-

tamine in position 4 by glutamic acid or by amino acids with hydrophobic side chains; a similar result was obtained when the linear part of the oxytocin molecule was shortened. Although modifications of the amino acid in position 2 did not result in analogues with higher natriuretic activity, several derivatives of deamino-1-carba-oxytocin were obtained that had higher natriuretic activity than oxytocin. The fact that the analogues with modifications in position 2 have relatively high natriuretic effect indicated the possibility of preparing analogues with high specific natriuretic activity. Results of these studies are presented in the following paper.

REFERENCES

1. Chan,W.Y. and du Vigneaud,V. (1970) J.Pharmacol.Exptl.Therap., 174, 541-549.
2. Machová,A. (1971) Physiol. Bohemoslov., 20, 515-520.
3. Chan,W.Y. (1965) Endocrinology, 77, 1097-1104.
4. Machová,A. and Jošt,K. (1975) Endocrinol.Exptl., 9,269-277.
5. Chan,W.Y. (1976) J.Pharmacol.Exptl.Therap., 196, 746-757.
6. Mehta,P.K. et al. (1980) Mineral and Electrolyte Metab., 3, 10-20.
7. Hrbas,P. et al. (1980) Endocrinol.Exptl. in press.
8. du Vigneaud,V. et al. (1980) J.Biol.Chem., 235, PC 64.
9. Jošt,K. et al. (1973) Coll.Czech.Chem.Commun.,38, 1073-1083.
10. Jošt,K. (1971) Coll.Czech.Chem.Commun., 36, 218-233.
11. Jošt,K. and Šorm,F. (1971) Coll.Czech.Chem.Commun.,36,234-245.
12. Hruby,V.J. et al. (1969) J.Biol.Chem., 244, 3890-3894.
13. Lebl,M. and Jošt,K. (1978) Coll.Czech.Chem.Commun.,43,523-524.
14. Lebl,M. et al. (1980) Coll.Czech.Chem.Commun., in press.
15. Lebl,M. et al. (1979) Coll.Czech.Chem.Commun., 44, 2563-2572.
16. Jošt,K. et al. (1963) Coll.Czech.Chem.Commun., 28, 1706-1714.
17. Frič,I. et al. (1974) Coll.Czech.Chem.Commun., 39, 1290-1302.
18. Hlaváček,J. et al. (1979) Coll.Czech.Chem.Commun., 44, 275-278.
19. Zaoral,M. and Flegel,M. (1972) Coll.Czech.Chem.Commun., 37, 1539-1545.

Hormonal Regulation of Sodium Excretion,
B. Lichardus, R.W. Schrier and J. Ponec, eds.
© 1980 Elsevier/North-Holland Biomedical Press

THE NATRIURETIC ACTION OF OXYTOCIN ANALOGUES

ALENA MACHOVÁ

Research Institute for Pharmacy and Biochemistry, U Elektry 8,
194 04 Prague 9, (Czechoslovakia)

INTRODUCTION

The natriuretic action of neurohypophyseal hormones has been
well established and recently reviewed by Walter et al.[1].

We tested two types of structural analogues of oxytocin:

1./ methylderivatives on hydroxyl group of tyrosine, 2-O-methyl-
   tyrosine oxytocin (TMO) and its deamino- analogue (DTMO),
   exhibiting slightly prolonged agonistic and in certain conditions antagonistic action[2]

2./ monocarba-analogues of deaminooxytocin, 1-deamino-carba-1-
   oxytocin (DCOT-1) and 1-deamino-carba-6-oxytocin (DCOT-6),
   which exerted increased and protracted oxytocic activities
   in common assays[3].All these peptides were synthetized in the
   Institute of Organic Chemistry and Biochemistry, Czechoslovak
   Academy of Sciences.

MATERIALS AND METHODS

The experiments were performed in conscious trained male albi-
no rats of Wistar strain, placed in pairs in glass metabolism
cages, either with mild water load - 4 ml/rat -, or with mild
saline load - 5 ml = 750 μmol Na/rat. The tested compounds were
injected subcutaneously; oxytocin (OT) in pharmacological doses
of 0.25, 1.0 and 4.0 μg/kg and the other peptides usually in
theree doses, eliciting comparable diuretic and natriuretic response.

Every analogue, including oxytocin, was tested repeatedly in
separate group of 20 rats and its effect compared not only to
controls, but also to the effect of middle dose of OT, 1 μg/kg.
One single experiment took 5 hours, the urine flow was measured
in one hour intervals and sodium and potassium were determined
in the total urine volume. The statistical significance of differences between was evaluated by analysis of variance with
two-way classification, $p = 0.05$.

RESULTS

In rats under mild water load a significant diuretic response after OT was observed, as depicted in fig. 1. The initial anti- diuretic phase was evident after the highest dose of 4.0 µg/kg. We obtained similar results after all analogues tested, the most marked increase in urine volume having been induced by the hig- hest dose of DCOT-1 (1.0 µg/kg) and the most prolonged initial antidiuresis by the highest dose of DCOT-6 (1.0 µg/kg).

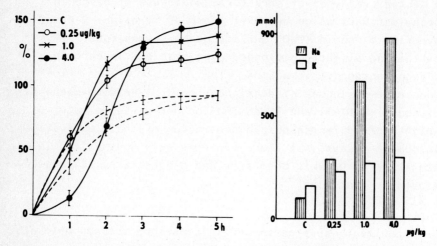

Fig. 1. Cumulative curves of diu- resis after OT in % of given water load.

Fig. 2. Mean values of Na and K excretion after OT in µmol/ 5 h/l pair of rats.

The effect of OT on sodium and potassium excretion is shown in fig. 2. The increase in Na excretion was significant and dose - dependent, and more marked than increase in K excretion, which was significant too. Again was this natriuretic response charac- teristic for all analogues tested, although weaker in case of 2-alkyl derivatives and stronger in case of carba- analogues, as demonstrated in fig. 3.

The ability to excrete the given sodium load after administrat- ion of peptides was studied in rats under mild saline load. In control conditions the animals excreted only about 50 % of the given load, whereas this amount was significantly higher after OT, middle dose caused excretion of the total load, high dose

of greater amount of sodium than was administered - fig. 4.
Even more pronounced effect exhibited DCOT-6, while TMO was
fairly less potent than OT - fig. 5.

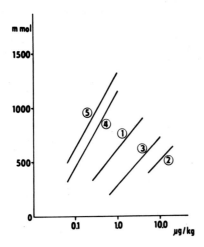

Fig. 3. The relationship between log dose of
peptides and total amount of Na excreted in
umol/5 h/l pair of rats.
1 - OT, 2 - TMO, 3 - DTMO, 4 - DCOT-1, 5 - DCOT-6

CONCLUSION

In our experiments oxytocin tended to be a quite strong natriuretic and diuretic agent. But to detect these activities, the
administration of suitable doses was necessary; after low doses
the effect was significant and after high doses the antidiuresis
prevailed. The same statement applies to the other analogues
tested.

Compared to oxytocin, monocarba-analogues of deaminooxytocin
revealed an increase in all typical activities[3], probably due to
retarded enzymatic degradation of these compounds[4]. According to
our findings their natriuretic potency was enhanced as well, at
least four times or more. This effect, however, should be considered as a reflection of strengthened oxytocin-like action on
renal tubules rather than the specific action of these analogues
themselves.

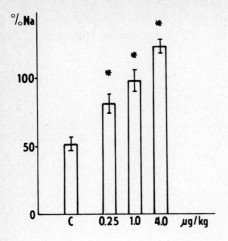

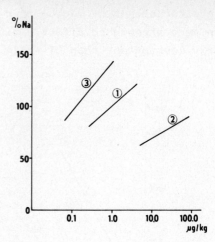

Fig. 4. The excreted amount of
Na in % of Na load after OT.

Fig. 5. The relationship the
log dose of peptides and excreted % of Na load.
1 - OT, 2 - TMO, 3 - DCOT-6

REFERENCES

1. Walter R., Smith C.W., Mehta P.K., Boonjarern B., Arruda J.L.
   A., Kurtzman N.A. (1977) Disturbances on Body Fluid Osmolality, Amer. Physiol. Society, Bethesda, Maryland, pp.1 - 36.

2. Krejčí I., Poláček I., Rudinger J. (1967) Brit. J. Pharmacol.
   30, 506 - 601.

3. Barth T., Krejčí I., Kupková B., Jošt K. (1973) Europ. J.
   Pharmacol. 24, 183 - 188.

4. Suska- Brzezińska E., Fruhaufová L., Barth T., Rychlík I.,
   Jošt K., Šorm F. (1972) Coll. Czechoslov. Chem. Commun. 37,
   2289 - 2294.

PROSTAGLANDINS

Hormonal Regulation of Sodium Excretion,
B. Lichardus, R.W. Schrier and J. Ponec, eds.
© 1980 Elsevier/North-Holland Biomedical Press

THE CONTROL OF SODIUM EXCRETION IN ISOLATED KIDNEYS

A. NIZET

Institute of Medicine, Hôpital de Bavière, Bvd de la Constitution, 66, B 4020, Liège, Belgium.

1. INTRODUCTION

The stability of extracellular space volume requires an accurate adjustment of sodium excretion to slow or fast changes in sodium intake. The most logical way to investigate intrarenal mechanisms susceptible to control sodium excretion is to work with totally isolated kidneys perfused with blood by a pump-oxygenator machine. These experimental conditions eliminate the interference of natriuretic or antinatriuretic hormones of extrarenal origin as well as an eventual nervous control of sodium excretion. Arterial and venous blood pressures are easily controlled. However, some functional disturbances occur in the isolated kidney, and the results obtained with this technique must be appreciated by comparison with these obtained in kidneys transplanted into perfusor animals at equal arterial and venous blood pressures.

2. COMPARATIVE INFLUENCE OF INTRAVASCULAR AND INTERSTITIAL EXPANSION, BLOOD DILUTION, AND NATRIURETIC COMPOUNDS OF EXTRARENAL ORIGIN.

Isolated kidneys increase sodium excretion when isotonic saline is added to the blood ; a direct renal effect of blood dilution on the kidney is demonstrated[1]. The most important dilution indices are the plasma oncotic pressure, the haematocrit and eventually the plasma sodium concentration ; the individual effect of these indices has been evaluated quantitatively in isolated kidneys[2]. The natriuretic response of transplanted kidneys was investigated during isotonic, hypotonic, isooncotic and hyperoncotic intravenous infusions in the dog ; it was found equal to the additive effect of each of these indices[3]. Moreover, the "saline natriuresis" was measured comparatively in isolated and in transplanted dog kidneys ; at equal values of arterial and venous pressures, equal degrees of blood dilution induced equal increases in sodium excretion[4]. An intravascular expansion with blood, excluding blood dilution, induced also a natriuresis in transplanted kidneys ; however, at equal degrees of intravascular expansion, the natriuresis was considerably lesser in these conditions than after equal expansion with saline[5].

Isotonic saline has been infused at a constant flow rate in anaesthetized dogs after transplantation of kidneys into their neck vessels and the natriuretic response of the transplanted kidneys was compared, at constant blood pressure, with extracellular and intravascular expansion and with blood dilution. In these anaesthetized animals, the infused fluid escaped progressively from intravascular space. At the final periods of infusion, the escape became equal to the infusion rate ; haematocrit and plasma proteins concentrations demonstrated no further decrease, and sodium excretion became stable. Thus sodium excretion depended on the rate of blood dilution and not on the degree of total extracellular expansion or of interstitial expansion[6].

These experiments suggest that the "saline natriuresis" is due, for its greatest part, to the direct effect of blood dilution on the kidney. They do not correspond to physiological conditions when the infused volumes of saline are high, however, increases in sodium excretion within the physiological range were detected after moderate blood dilution, exceeding not 2 p.100[7].

It is conceivable that the direct control by the kidney of blood concentration contributes to the constancy of extracellular space volume.

3. INFLUENCE OF DIETARY SODIUM BALANCE ON THE RENAL RESPONSE TO BLOOD DILUTION.

It is well known that ' saline natriuresis' is lesser in sodium-deprived animals. The involvement of intrarenal factors was demonstrated. At identical arterial and venous blood pressures, and at equal levels of blood dilution and of extracellular volume expansion, the sodium excretion in the kidneys of sodium-loaded dogs, transplanted into sodium - deprived perfusors, was as high as in kidneys transplanted into sodium-loaded perfusors[6]. The same observation was made in totally isolated kidneys, following equal dilution of the perfusion blood by isotonic saline ; the response of the kidneys of sodium-deprived dogs was lesser than in the kidneys taken from sodium-loaded donors[4].

The transplantation of sodium-loaded kidneys into sodium-deprived dogs potentiated the response of the kidneys 'in situ', thus demonstrating the release by the kidney of a material which enhances the response to blood dilution[6]. This puts forward the problem of the renal origin of natriuretic compounds.

The decreased sensitivity of the kidneys to blood dilution in a salt-deprived organism represents an additional intrarenal mechanism which contributes to the stability of sodium balance.

4. COMPARISON BETWEEN THE NATRIURESIS AND THE CHANGES IN JEJUNAL
   SODIUM TRANSPORT INDUCED BY BLOOD DILUTION. INFLUENCE OF DIETARY
   SODIUM.

Because of some structural and functional similitudes between the jejunal mucosa
and the proximal tubule, the dog jejunum was used as a model for the investigation of
sodium transport, independent of the changes in glomerular filtration.

It has been demonstrated previously that an intravenous infusion of saline inhibits
sodium and water absorption in the jejunum[8]. The inhibition of sodium absorption was
found lesser in sodium-deprived dogs than in sodium-loaded ones[9]. Moreover, the
inhibition of sodium absorption in the jejunum of sodium-deprived animals was potentiated by transplantation into their neck vessels of the kidneys taken from sodium -
loaded dogs ; the transplantation of the kidneys of sodium deprived animals was
without effect[9]. The differences in net sodium absorption depended on the unidirectional flux of sodium from mucosal to serosal side : this flux was increased in
sodium-deprived dogs and was inhibited by transplantation of sodium loaded kidneys.
Blood dilution increased the flux from serosa to mucosa regardless of the dietary
sodium[9]. The parallelism between the mucosa-to-serosa sodium flux and glucose
absorption suggested the involvement of active transport processes[10].

These similitudes in the response of both organs point to an adjustment of
sodium transport independent of changes in glomerular filtration rate in the kidney.

5. THE INTRARENAL FACTORS POTENTIATING THE RESPONSE   TO BLOOD
   DILUTION.

The above-mentioned experiments show that the direct effect of blood dilution
is modulated by a material present in the kidneys of sodium-loaded animals but not
in the kidneys of sodium-deprived ones, this material being released into the blood.
A 'permissive effect' of a natriuretic hormone on the response to volume expansion
has been suggested[11]. The results summarized here point to a renal origin of this
material. However an accumulation in the kidneys of natriuretic compounds is not
positively excluded[12]. Experimental evidence of a renal origin is presented in
another communication.

An involvement of renal prostaglandins is showed by other experiments. The
potentiation of 'saline natriuresis' by transplantation of the kidneys of sodium-
loaded dogs was not observed if the latter were pre-treated by indomethacin in order
to inhibit prostaglandin synthesis and release[13]. In the same conditions, the inhibition of jejunal sodium absorption was also suppressed (unpublished results).

6. SODIUM EXCRETION AND TUBULO-GLOMERULAR EQUILIBRIUM IN ISOLATED KIDNEYS.

Sodium excretion depends on an equilibrium between the filtered load and the tubular reabsorption. Some mechanisms controlling this equilibrium were demonstrated in isolated kidneys.

Microperfusion and micropunction experiments have given ample evidence of a tubulo-glomerular feedback involving the juxtaglomerular apparatus[14]. There is no agreement as concerns the nature of the "triggering factor" acting at the level of the macula densa (sodium or chloride concentrations, osmolality of tubular fluid ?), and the involvement of the renin-angiotensin system. Species differences are not excluded[15]. This tubulo-glomerular feedback has been demonstrated in isolated , blood perfused dog kidneys[16] ; it represents an autonomous , intrarenal function. Its efficiency is lesser after chronic or acute saline loading[17].

Experiments of another type, performed with isolated kidneys, suggest the existence of a tubulo-glomerular equilibrium which is quantitative, autonomous, and independent of the sodium balance.

The two kidneys of the same pair were perfused independently by two identical pump-oxygenator machines, with identical blood. A load of isotonic saline was added on one side ; on the other side an equal volume of a solution of sodium sulphate was added. This solution contained the same sodium concentration and was adjusted to equal osmolality by addition of mannitol. The urine volume remained equal on both sides despite the inhibition of reabsorption due to the osmotic effect of sulphate. A decrease in glomerular filtration rate equal to the decrease in reabsorption was evidenced, demonstrating an intrarenal tubulo-glomerular equilibrium[18]. Since the experiments were performed in the absence of antidiuretic activity, it may be concluded that the fluid output out of the proximal tubule was unchanged[18]. An identical tubulo-glomerular equilibrium was observed when the tubular reabsorption was reduced by mannitol or by uranyl sulphate.

Many differences exist between this tubulo-glomerular equilibrium, demonstrated in the whole kidney, and the tubulo-glomerular feedback controlled by the juxtaglomerular apparatus. The involvement of "triggering factors" such as sodium or chloride content, or osmolality of distal tubular fluid, was excluded. It was quantitative over a wide range of levels of sodium excretion. Haemodynamic control was not evident. The equilibrium was not altered by an antagonist of angiotensin such as saralasin[18]. Its mechanism is not yet elucidated. Indirect measu-

rements of intratubular pressure suggest that the decrease in glomerular filtration
is due to an increase in intratubular hydrostatic pressure. Since the urine output
did not change, this increase should be explained by an increased intratubular resistance to the fluid flow.

7. GLOMERULO-TUBULAR EQUILIBRIUM AND SODIUM EXCRETION

   A reduction of tubular reabsorption induces a natriuresis provided that there is
no compensatory decrease in the filtered load. A readjustment of the equilibrium is
required. In the case of 'saline natriuresis' it has been well demonstrated that a
decrease in haematocrit and in plasma protein concentration decreases tubular reabsorption and increases the glomerular filtration. Recent experiments, performed
with transplanted kidneys, show that intrarenal mechanisms control the changes
in tubulo-glomerular equilibrium according to the dietary sodium balance. The natriuresis induced by saline infusion was compared in three series of experiments :
a) sodium-loaded perfusor and kidney donor ; b) sodium-deprived perfusor and
kidney donor ; c) sodium-deprived perfusor, sodium-loaded kidney donor[12]. The
dogs were given frusemide, the urine was reinjected into a vein. Plasma renin
activity was measured in the arterial and venous blood from the transplanted
kidneys and the release of renin by the latter was measured. As observed previously,
the saline natriuresis was lesser in the sodium-deprived kidneys transplanted into
sodium-deprived perfusors, but it was high in sodium-loaded kidneys regardless
of the previous sodium intake of the perfusors. The lower sodium output in
the sodium-deprived kidneys was the combined result of a decreased glomerular
filtration rate and of an increased fractional reabsorption ; the renal blood flow was
lower in the sodium-deprived kidneys, the filtration fraction was equal. No
relationship was evidenced between the natriuresis and the arterial or venous plasma
renin activity or the release of renin by the transplanted kidney [19]. The existence
of other intrarenal factors modulating filtration and reabsorption is suggested.

8. CONCLUSIONS

   The experiments performed with isolated and transplanted kidneys contribute
to demonstrate several intrarenal functions modulating the excretion of sodium.
- The kidneys are extremely sensitive to acute changes in various indices of blood
dilution ; glomerular filtration increases and fractional reabsorption decreases.

- In the case of 'saline natriuresis', a humoral control of extrarenal origin, depending on intravascular or interstitial expansion, is of lesser quantitative importance than the changes in blood concentration. The evidence of a control by blood volume is however suggested by the renal response to intravascular expansion without dilution.

- The sensitivity of the kidneys to an acute saline load depends on the dietary sodium balance ; this sensitivity is reduced when the sodium intake is low. The differences are due to adjustments of glomerular filtration and of tubular reabsorption ; they can be dissociated from some parameters of the renin-angiotensin system (plasma renin activity and renin release by the kidneys).

- Intrarenal mechanisms adjust glomerular filtration as a response to changes in tubular reabsorption. Some of these mechanisms result in a quantitative equilibrium between the two functions over a wide range of sodium excretion levels ; final sodium excretion depends on a readjustment of this tubulo-glomerular equilibrium.

- The kidneys of sodium-loaded dogs release into the blood a material that potentiate the response to blood dilution. This material seems to be related in some way with renal prostaglandins.

REFERENCES

1. Craig, G.M., Mills, I.H., Osbaldiston, G.W. and Wise, B.L. (1966) J. Physiol. (Lond), 186, 113 p - 114 p.

2. Nizet, A. (1972) Kidney International, 1, 27-37.

3. Nizet, A. (1976) Arch. Intern. Physiol. Biochim., 84, 997-1015.

4. Nizet, A. (1976) Pflügers Arch., 361, 121-126.

5. Lichardus, B. and Nizet, A. (1972). Clin. Science, 42, 701-709.

6. Nizet, A., Tost, H. and Foidart-Willems, J. (1974). Pflügers Arch., 350, 287-298.

7. Nizet, A. (1973). Pflügers Arch., 341, 209-217 .

8. Richet, G., and Hornych, A. (1969). Nephron, 6, 365-378.

9. Nizet, A., Merchie, G. and Robin, M. (1976). Pflügers Arch., 364, 59-64.

10. Nizet, A., Robin, M., Merchie, G. and Godon, J.P. (1978). Contributions to Nephrology, Karger, Basel, vol. 13, pp 21-26

11. Pearce, J.W., Lichardus, B., Sonnenberg, H. and Veress, A.T. (1970). Proc. 4th int. Congr. Nephrol. Stockholm 1969, Karger, Basel, München, New York, vol. 2, pp 80-87

12. Gonick, H.C. and Saldanha, L.F. (1975). J. Clin. Invest. 56, 247–255.

13. Nizet, A. (1979). Pflügers Arch. 378, 223–225.

14. Thurau, K. and Schnermann, J. (1965). Klin. Wochenschr. 43, 410–413.

15. Navar, L.G. (1978) Am. J. Physiol., 234, F 357–F 370.

16. Schnermann, J., Stowe, N., Yarimizu, S, Magnussen, M. and
    Tingwald, G. (1977) Am. J. Physiol., 233, F 217–F 224.

17. Dev, B., Drescher, C. and Schnermann, J. Pflügers Arch. 346, 263–277.

18. Nizet, A. (1979). Pflügers Arch. 217–223.

19. Nizet, A., Deheneffe, J. and Robin, M. Clinical Science (in print).

Hormonal Regulation of Sodium Excretion,
B. Lichardus, R.W. Schrier and J. Ponec, eds.
© 1980 Elsevier/North-Holland Biomedical Press

INFLUENCE OF MEDULLARY HEMODYNAMICS ON THE NATRIURESIS OF DRUG-INDUCED RENAL VASODILATION

N. LAMEIRE, R. VANHOLDER, S. RINGOIR, I. LEUSEN[*] with technical assistance
of M.A. WATERLOOS and V. VANDERBIESEN
University Hospital Ghent, Renal Division of the Department of Medicine and the Laboratory of Normal and Pathological Physiology[*], De Pintelaan, 135, B-9000 Gent, Belgium.

INTRODUCTION

Intrarenal infusion of vasodilators is generally associated with an increase in urinary sodium excretion. However, intrarenal administration of secretin (S) produces a dose-related increase in renal blood flow without a significant rise in urinary sodium excretion (1). Recent experiments in the dog showed that S did not augment the renal papillary plasma flow (PPF), suggesting at least in this animal, that alterations in medullary hemodynamics were of importance in the natriuresis of drug-induced vasodilation (2).

Until now, the effects of S on the relationship between total renal and medullary hemodynamics and sodium excretion have not been studied in the rat. In this study, we have examined this relationship with S, in comparison with acetylcholine (ACh); in addition, renal function and PPF measurements were undertaken with both vasodilators after the administration of a prostaglandin (PG) synthesis inhibitor (meclofenamate).

METHODS

Clearance studies

All studies were performed in male Wistar rats. A tracheostomy was performed, one carotid and one jugular vein were cannulated and the bladder was catheterized. For infusion of the vasodilators, a polyethylene tube (PE_{50}) was threaded through the left iliac artery into the aorta at the level of both renal arteries. An isotonic Ringer solution containing 10 % Inulin and 1.7 % PAH was infused I.V.

At the end, four groups of experimental clearance studies were performed.

Group I, Acetylcholine studies (n=10). ACh (4 μg/kg/min) was infused into the aorta. Fifteen min. later, experimental clearance collections were started.

Group II, Secretin studies (n=14). Same protocol as in group I, but S (Karolinska Institutet, Stockholm, Sweden) was administered in a dose of 75 mU/kg/min.

Group III, Meclofenamate plus acetylcholine (n=8). Meclofenamate (Parke Davis & Co, Detroit, Mich.) (5 mg/kg body weight) was given intravenously over 5 min. Fifteen min. later, the intra-aortic infusion with ACh was started and the experimental clearances were obtained as in group I.

Group IV, Meclofenamate plus secretin (n=7). Fifteen minutes after the administration of meclofenamate, an intra-aortic infusion with S was commenced and the experimental clearances were obtained as in group II.

PPF was determined by a modification of the original method of Lilienfield et al.
(3), as previously described (4). All PPF measurements were performed at a transit
time of 15 sec. PPF was determined in 13 control rats 60 – 90 minutes after the intra-
aortic infusion of isotonic Ringer solution at a rate of 0.02 ml/min (Group I). In 18
rats, PPF was measured 30 to 40 min. after the infusion of either ACh (n=10)
(group II) or S (n=8) (group III). In the groups IV and V, PPF was measured in meclofenamate treated animals (5 mg/kg IV), 30 to 40 min. after infusion with either ACh
(n=8) or S (n=9). In all these PPF studies, abovementioned doses of both vasodilators
were used.

RESULTS

The effects of both vasodilators on kidney function, absolute and fractional sodium
excretion and urinary osmolality are shown in Table 1.

TABLE 1

SUMMARY OF ACETYLCHOLINE AND SECRETIN   RENAL FUNCTION STUDIES

	GFR (ml/min)		PAHCl (ml/min)		$U_{Na}V$ (μEq/min)		FE_{Na} (%)		U_{Osm} (mOsm/kg)	
	C	E	C	E	C	E	C	E	C	E
Acetylcholine (n=10)	1.95	2.30*	5.81	7.92*	0.33	2.10**	0.19	0.65**	1167	730*
SEM	0.11	0.12	0.22	0.52	0.13	0.33	0.05	0.19	121	78
Secretin (n=14)	2.05	2.10	5.98	8.19**	0.46	0.51	0.15	0.17	1145	1078
SEM	0.15	0.12	0.38	0.43	0.12	0.10	0.06	0.04	136	119

* p<0.05
** p<0.01

During ACh infusion, a significant increase in both glomerular filtration rate (GFR)
(p<0.05) and effective renal plasma flow (ERFF) (p<0.01) was noted. Absolute and
fractional excretion of sodium increased and there was a significant fall in urine osmolality.

During S infusion, no significant changes in GFR were observed. However, a
significant increase in PAH clearance was present. Despite this increasing ERPF, no
change in absolute or fractional excretion of sodium was noted under secretin infusion.

TABLE 2

SUMMARY OF ACETYLCHOLINE AND SECRETIN RENAL FUNCTION STUDIES
IN MECLOFENAMATE PRETREATED ANIMALS

		GFR (ml/min)		PAHCl (ml/min)		$U_{Na}V$ (μEq/min)		FE_{Na} (%)		U_{Osm} (mOsm/kg)	
		C	E	C	E	C	E	C	E	C	E
Acetylcholine (n=8)		2.15	2.17	6.15	6.12	0.39	0.77	0.13	0.24	1085	926
	SEM	0.14	0.12	0.19	0.17	0.06	0.06	0.04	0.07	89	92
Secretin (n=7)		2.07	1.98	6.09	7.69**	0.32	0.50	0.12	0.17	1207	1302
	SEM	0.13	0.11	0.27	0.32	0.08	0.06	0.03	0.04	125	133

* $p < 0.05$
** $p < 0.01$

Table 2 summarizes the effects of a pretreatment with meclofenamate on kidney function under ACh and S administration. In ACh treated animals, both the increase in GFR and in ERPF were blocked by pretreatment with meclofenamate. Changes in absolute and fractional excretion of sodium were not significant and no significant fall in urine osmolality occurred.

The experiments in which the effects of meclofenamate on kidney function under S infusion were studied, show changes completely comparable with the results obtained with S alone. There was a significant rise in PAH clearance ($p < 0.01$) while all other parameters remained unchanged.

Despite a comparable increase in ERPF, it is apparent that the increase in absolute and fractional sodium excretion is much greater after ACh compared to S. The effects of ACh on kidney function and sodium excretion were almost completely blocked by pretreatment of the animals with meclofenamate.

The figure shows the PPF measurements obtained for both kidneys in control animals and in the ACh and S infused animals. The mean PPF after S was significantly higher compared to control conditions. The increase in PPF after ACh however was significantly greater. In animals pretreated with meclofenamate, no effect of meclofenamate on PPF after S infusion was noted. In contrast, meclofenamate appears to block substantially the medullary vasodilatation by ACh.

EFFECT OF VASODILATORS ON PPF

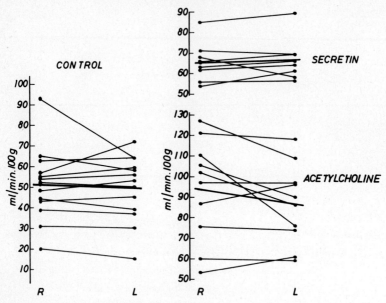

Summary of PPF data. PPF values are shown for control rats as well as rats infused with either ACh or S. Individual data for right (R) and left (L) kidneys are given.

DISCUSSION

These studies in the rat confirm the previously observed results obtained in the dog, showing that S increases the ERPF without a substantial effect on the urinary sodium excretion. In contrast, ACh produces a concomitant renal vasodilation and increase in natriuresis. One of the mechanisms that has been proposed to explain this different behaviour is the failure of S to influence the intrarenal interstitial pressure (5).

The possibility that lack of alteration in PPF might be involved in the natriuretic defect of S was investigated in the present studies and the renal effects of S were compared to the effects of ACh, a vasodilating and natriuretic substance.

An increase in medullary plasma and blood flow has been proposed to influence net sodium reabsorption in the medullary tubular structures in the so-called "medullary wash-out" theory (6, 7). Dissipation of the medullary hypertonicity would decrease passive water loss from descending limbs of Henle's loop, increase volume flow through ascending limbs and reduce absolute solute reabsorption by the ascending limbs. Since compared to ACh, S has only a trivial influence on PPF, it is conceivable that the lack of this hemodynamic effect can explain, at least in part, the absence of its natriuretic effect.

That an increase in medullary blood flow is obtained with ACh has already been suggested by previous microsphere studies in the dog, where a marked redistribution of the renal blood flow towards inner cortical zones was observed (8). However, direct measurements of PPF after ACh infusion were not available. Preliminary studies in this laboratory, using microspheres in the rat did not show redistribution of cortical blood flow with S (unpublished results).

If the minimal papillary vasodilatation observed with S is the reflection of the absence of inner cortical blood flow redistribution, an alternative second hypothesis can be offered to explain the dissociation between renal blood flow and sodium excretion with S. It has been demonstrated that ACh induced vasodilatation causes no redistribution of glomerular filtrate (9). If glomerular filtrate distribution is unchanged while plasma flow is disproportionately increased in juxtamedullary nephrons, the filtration fraction (FF) would be reduced to a greater extent in the deep nephrons. Studies on ACh and bradykinin administration by Stein et al. (10) have indeed shown a greater fall in FF in deep nephrons, presumably leading to a lower oncotic pressure in their postglomerular circulation. Consequently, this would result in a greater fall in sodium reabsorption in the deep nephrons and enhanced sodium excretion. Since S, despite its vasodilatory effect, has no influence on cortical blood flow distribution, a more pronounced change in deep nephron filtration and increased sodium excretion cannot be expected.

In the second part of this study, an attempt was made to further elucidate the mechanism of the renal and medullary vasodilation of ACh, by repeating the experiments after administration of meclofenamate. Previous studies have indicated that administration of renal vasodilating substances as bradykinin was associated with renal PG release (11). It has also been shown that PG inhibition produces a fall in PPF in the rat. In fact, in the present study, the rise in both the effective total renal and the medullary plasma flow with ACh were inhibited to a great extent by meclofenamate. The natriuretic response in these animals was also markedly attenuated in comparison to the natriuresis observed in the intact animals.

In contrast, no effect of the PG inhibitor on either total or medullary plasma flow was observed in the S infused rats. As far as we know, data on the effects of ACh on PG secretion is not available in the literature. However, preliminary studies in our laboratory in which the urinary excretion of PGE_2 and $PGF_{2\alpha}$ were studied after either ACh or S in conscious rats, show that the PG excretion is elevated after administration of ACh but remains unaltered after S. The same results for PGE_2 excretion after S were obtained in the anesthetized dog (2). This does not suggest that PG's are a major determinant of the vasodilatory effects of S.

In summary, the present studies confirm in the rat the dissociation between the renal vasodilation and the natriuresis obtained with S. They further suggest that the absence of a natriuretic response observed with this drug is related to its incapacity to increase substantially the medullary blood flow. Finally, the results are compatible with the view that PG release is of importance in the vasodilating and natriuretic responses obtained with ACh.

ACKNOWLEDGEMENTS

We wish to express our appreciation to Miss C. VAN DEN BERGHE for secretarial assistance. These studies were supported by a grant of the Nationaal Fonds voor Wetenschappelijk Onderzoek.

REFERENCES

1. MARCHAND, G.R. et al. (1972) Proc. Soc. Exptl. Biol. Med.,139, 1356–1358.
2. FADEM, S. et al. (1977) Kid. Int., 12, 557 (abstract).
3. LILIENFIELD, L.S. et al. (1961) Circ. Res., 9, 614–617.
4. LAMEIRE, N.H. et al. (1978) Methods in Pharmacology, Plenum Press/New York, pp. 41–74.
5. MARCHAND, G.R. et al. (1977) Am. J. Physiol., 232, F147–F151.
6. EARLEY, L.E. and FRIEDLER, R.M. (1965) J. Clin. Invest., 44, 1857–1865.
7. EARLEY, L.E. and FRIEDLER, R.M. (1966) J. Clin. Invest., 45, 542–551.
8. STEIN, J.H. et al. (1971) J. Clin. Invest., 50, 1429–1438.
9. STEIN, J.H. et al. (1971) Am. J. Physiol., 220, 227–236.
10. STEIN, J.H. et al. (1972) J. Clin. Invest., 51, 1709–1721.
11. McGIFF, J.C. et al. (1972) Circ. Res.,31, 36–43.

Hormonal Regulation of Sodium Excretion,
B. Lichardus, R.W. Schrier and J. Ponec, eds.
© 1980 Elsevier/North-Holland Biomedical Press

VOLUME AS A DETERMINANT OF THE NATRIURETIC EFFECT OF RENAL PROSTAGLANDIN E
(PGE) IN MAN

MURRAY EPSTEIN AND MEYER D. LIFSCHITZ

Departments of Medicine, University of Miami School of Medicine and the
University of Texas Health Science Center at San Antonio and the Veterans
Administration Medical Centers, Miami, Florida 33125 and San Antonio,
Texas 78284, U.S.A.

INTRODUCTION

Despite extensive study, the role of renal prostaglandins in the maintenance
of external sodium balance remains controversial[1-7]. The contradictory
nature of the available data may relate to a number of factors including
the use of multiple animal species and models, and the use of anesthesia
(a maneuver which has been shown to increase renal prostaglandin synthesis).
Nevertheless, even studies using apparently identical protocols performed in
different laboratories have led to conflicting results and conclusions. A
review of several of these available studies have suggested the possibility
that the volume status of the subject may constitute an important determinant
of the effects of renal PGE on renal sodium handling.

The present study was carried out to examine in a kinetic fashion the
relative contribution of renal prostaglandins to renal sodium handling during
different states of sodium balance. We assessed the natriuretic response to
acute volume expansion in identical subjects during the sodium-replete state
and following dietary sodium restriction, before and after partial inhibition
of prostaglandin synthesis by indomethacin. Since previous studies from
our laboratory have demonstrated that water immersion to the neck (NI)
constitutes a potent "central volume stimulus" without the necessity of

infusing exogenous volume expanders, and thus without altering plasma composition[8-11], the immersion model was used as the means of inducing volume expansion.

METHODS

Eleven normal male subjects between the ages of 22 and 51 years were studied. Nine subjects were studied during the sodium-replete state while eight of the subjects were studied following dietary sodium restriction. The sodium-replete subjects underwent water immersion to the neck on two occasions separated by a 5 to 7-day interval. Prior to the second immersion study, the subjects were pretreated with indomethacin 50 mg per os every 6 hours for the 24-hour period preceding study (NI + Ind). Subsequently, eight of the subjects underwent additional immersion studies following dietary sodium restriction. During the latter studies, the subjects were housed in an environmentally controlled metabolic ward at a constant temperature. Each consumed a diet, the composition of which remained unchanged throughout the study, containing 10 meq of sodium, 100 meq of potassium, and 2500 ml of water per day. Daily 24-hour urine collections were made for the determination of sodium, potassium, and creatinine. After dietary equilibration, each subject underwent an immersion study without indomethacin administration (NI), followed 5-7 days later by a repeat immersion study preceded by 24 hours of indomethacin administration (NI + Ind).

The experimental protocols on the two immersion study days were similar and were carried out as detailed in an earlier publication[11]. In brief, the subject sat in the tank immersed in water to the neck for 4 hours (9:00 am to 1:00 pm), preceded and followed by 1 hour of quiet sitting outside the tank (prestudy and recovery hours, respectively).

Each subject stood briefly to void spontaneously at hourly intervals during the study. To maintain an adequate urine flow, 200 ml of water was administered orally every hour during the study. Sodium, potassium and creatinine were measured in samples of the hourly urine collections, and samples of the prestudy hour urine specimen were frozen promptly for prostaglandin E determinations.

Immersion was carried out in a waterproof tank described in detail in previous communications[11]. Urine PGE was assayed utilizing a hepatic radio-receptor assay. The extraction and assay procedure have been detailed in earlier communications[12]. Data were evaluated statistically by paired or unpaired "t" analysis. Differences with $p<0.05$ or greater were considered significant.

RESULTS

Urinary Prostaglandin Excretion

Urinary PGE determinations were carried out in all subjects to ascertain that indomethacin administration reduced renal prostaglandin excretion, and presumably synthesis. Basal PGE excretion ($U_{PGE}V$) during the prestudy hour of NI was 6.4 ± 1.4 ng/min. During the NI + Ind study, indomethacin pretreatment resulted in a 56% decrement in basal $U_{PGE}V$ as compared to the corresponding values during NI. Similar changes were observed in the subjects studied following dietary sodium restriction: basal UPGEV during the prestudy of NI was 4.7 ± 0.7 ng/min and indomethacin administration resulted in a 78% decrement in basal $U_{PGE}V$ during the prestudy hour of NI + Ind.

Urinary Sodium, Potassium and Fluid Excretion

Sodium-replete Studies. The effects of 4 hours of water immersion on urinary sodium excretion are shown in Figure 1.

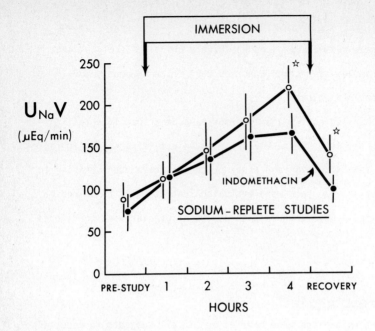

Figure 1. Effect of water immersion on the rate of sodium excretion ($U_{Na}V$) in the subjects studied during sodium-replete state. Immersion without indomethacin pretreatment resulted in a marked natriuresis. The natriuretic response following indomethacin pretreatment was similar although mean $U_{Na}V$ was less during hour 4 of immersion and the recovery hour.

Immersion without indomethacin pretreatment (NI) resulted in a progressive increase in $U_{Na}V$ to levels which were almost 3-fold greater than the prestudy values during the 4th hour of immersion ($p<0.005$). Cessation of immersion (recovery) was associated with a prompt decrement in $U_{Na}V$ although it continued to exceed prestudy levels (p<0.005). When the subjects underwent a repeat immersion following indomethacin pretreatment (NI + Ind), the natriuretic pattern did not differ from that of NI; although mean $U_{Na}V$ was less during hour 4 of immersion and the recovery hour, the cumulative sodium excreted during the 4 hours of NI + Ind did not differ from NI alone (NS).

The kaliuretic response during NI was characterized by an increase in U_KV from 40±8 to levels of 74-79 µeq/min during hrs 2 and 3 of immersion (p<0.05). The kaliuretic response during NI + Ind did not differ from that observed during NI.

NI was associated with a marked diuresis throughout immersion with urine flow (V) increasing to levels of 5.6-5.9 ml/min (Figure 2). The diuretic response during NI + Ind was unaltered compared to NI.

Studies Following Dietary Sodium Restriction

The effects of 4 hours of NI on urinary sodium and potassium excretion are shown in Figure 3 (lower panel). NI resulted in a progressive increase in $U_{Na}V$ from 3±1 to 38±7 µeq/min (p<0.01). Recovery was associated with a decrement in $U_{Na}V$ to 10±3 µeq/min, (p<0.005 for recovery compared to hr 4). When the same eight subjects were restudied during NI + Ind, the natriuretic response was markedly attenuated, with a peak $U_{Na}V$ of 4±1 µeq/min during hr 4 of immersion comprising only one-tenth of peak $U_{Na}V$ during NI. Examination of the individual natriuretic responses of the subjects during NI + Ind disclosed that none of the subjects attained peak $U_{Na}V$'s exceeding 10 µeq/min, with six of the subjects manifesting peak $U_{Na}V$'s of 6 µeq/min. Cumulative sodium excretion during the 4 hours of NI + Ind was significantly less than the amount excreted during NI (p<0.05) mirroring the changes in $U_{Na}V$.

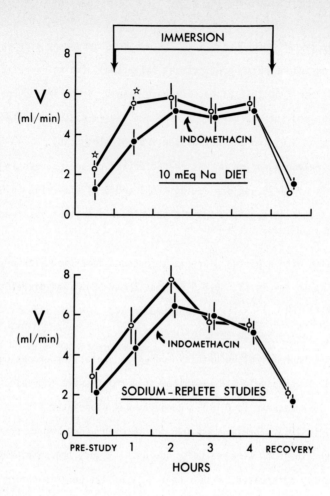

Figure 2. Effects of water immersion on urinary flow rate (V) in both the sodium-replete (lower panel) and sodium-restricted (upper panel) state. Whereas during the sodium-replete studies, indomethacin administration did not modify the diuretic response, in the sodium-restricted group, indomethacin resulted in a decrease in V during the prestudy hour and hr 1 of immersion.

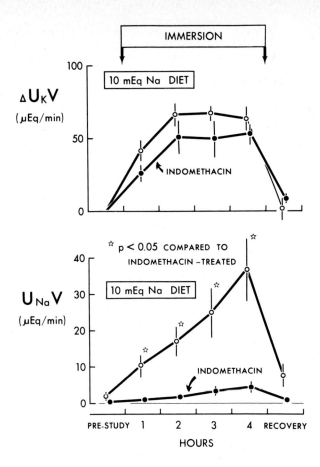

Figure 3. Effects of water immersion on the rate of sodium excretion ($U_{Na}V$) and potassium excretion (U_KV) following dietary sodium restriction. Data for U_KV are expressed in terms of the absolute changes from the prestudy hour (ΔU_KV). Indomethacin pretreatment resulted in a marked attenuation of the natriuretic response to immersion.

U_KV increased during NI from 40±6 to levels of 111-117 µeq/min during the 4-hr immersion period. Recovery was associated with a prompt return of U_KV to prestudy levels. Indomethacin pretreatment resulted in a modest decrease in basal U_KV during the prestudy hour (24 µeq/min during NI + Ind vs. 40 µeq/min during NI). To permit a comparison of the relative kaliuretic responses, the data were expressed as the absolute changes from the prestudy hour. (Figure 3, upper panel). As can be seen, ΔU_KV during NI + Ind did not differ from the response during NI.

NI was associated with a marked diuresis with V more than doubling during hrs 1-4 of immersion compared to the prestudy hour. Despite identical hydration protocols, NI + Ind was associated with a lower mean V during both the prestudy hour and hr 1 of immersion as compared to NI ($p < 0.05$). During the subsequent 4 hrs of immersion, V was similar during NI and NI + Ind. (Figure 2).

DISCUSSION

Attempts to define the effect of prostaglandin release on the natriuresis of extracellular fluid volume expansion (ECVE) by inhibition of prostaglandin synthesis have been marked by contradictory findings, with reports suggesting that inhibition of prostaglandin synthesis may be either antinatriuretic, natriuretic, or fail to affect renal sodium handling[1-7]. Furthermore, only two studies to date have attempted to assess the effect of acute ECVE in *man*[5,13]. Since in both studies, acute ECVE was induced by the administration of an intravenous saline load, a maneuver which presumably alters plasma composition and may thus affect the hormonal system under study.

The present study assessed the effects of acute volume expansion in *man* without resorting to exogenous volume expanders. It was demonstrated that indomethacin pretreatment markedly attenuated the natriuretic response to immersion in sodium-depleted normal subjects. In contrast, when the identical subjects were studied during the sodium-replete state using an identical regimen, indomethacin failed to alter the absolute amount of sodium excreted during the four hours of immersion. The demonstration that synthetase inhibition blunted sodium excretion only in the sodium-depleted state despite comparable suppression of basal urinary PGE is consistent with the formulation that the contribution of renal prostaglandins to sodium homeostasis is magnified under conditions of volume contraction.

Several lines of evidence in man suggest that the present observations regarding the importance of volume as a determinant of the natriuretic response of renal prostaglandins are not isolated findings. Thus, Boyer and Reynold [14] observed that the administration of indomethacin to cirrhotic patients with ascites resulted in significant decrements in p-aminohippurate and creatinine clearances and marked sodium retention. In contrast, these deleterious effects were not observed in compensated cirrhotic patients

202

without ascites. Recently, Zipser et al [15]extended these studies and demonstrated that either indomethacin or ibuprofen resulted in acute renal insufficiency and even more avid renal retention of sodium in their ascitic patients. Of interest, they observed that within their study population, the patients with the most intense secondary hyperaldosteronism and the most avid sodium retention manifested the greatest decrement in GFR following prostaglandin synthetase inhibition.

Such alterations in renal function are not unique to cirrhosis but subtend a wide range of disease states. Thus, Arisz er al [16] studied a large group of nephrotic patients on a restricted sodium intake and observed that indomethacin administration was associated with an immediate decrement in GFR which was completely reversible upon discontinuation of the drug. Recently, Walshe and Venuto [17] extended these observations to congestive heart failure. They observed that the administration of indomethacin to a patient with compensated congestive heart failure resulted in an acute reduction of GFR and marked sodium retention.

Studies in normal man utilizing several different agents which inhibit prostaglandin synthetase have complemented the above studies, lending additional support to the suggestion that the importance of renal prostaglandins in maintaining renal function is accentuated in the setting of volume contraction. Thus, Berg et al [3] observed that the administration of acetylsalicylic acid to normal men ingesting a moderately restricted sodium intake (70 meq Na/day) resulted in a decrease in urine flow and in sodium excretion. The present studies in which renal sodium handling was assessed systematically in identical subjects during different states of sodium balance extends and amplifies these earlier observations.

In summary, we have demonstrated that the administration of indomethacin (and presumably prostaglandin synthetase inhibition) blunted the natriuretic response to immersion-induced central volume expansion only in the sodium-depleted state despite comparable suppression of basal urinary PGE. Bearing in mind the caveat that indomethacin exerts multiple effects in addition to prostaglandin synthetase inhibition, the present findings are consistent with the formulation that renal prostaglandins are critical modulators of renal sodium handling during conditions or disease states characterized by volume contraction.

ACKNOWLEDGEMENTS

These investigations were supported by designated Veterans Administration Research funds and by a grant from the National Aeronautics and Space Administration (NAS 9-15473). The authors are indebted to Ms. Audrey M. Lorenz for her expert preparation of the manuscript.

REFERENCES

1. Dunn, M.J. and Hood, V.L. (1977) Prostaglandins and the kidney. Am. J. Physiol. 233, F169-F184.

2. Donker, A.J.M., Arisz, L., Brentjens, J.R.H., van der Hem, G.K. and Hollemans, H.J.G. (1976) The effect of indomethacin on kidney function and plasma renin activity in man. Nephron 17, 288-296.

3. Berg, K.J. (1977) Acute effects of acetylsalicylic acid on renal function in normal man. Eur. J. Clin. Pharmacol. 11, 117-123.

4. Kirschenbaum, M.A. and Stein, J.H. (1976) The effect of inhibition of prostaglandin synthesis on urinary sodium excretion in the conscious dog. J. Clin. Invest. 57, 517-521.

5. Mountokalakis, T., Karambasis, T., Mayopoulou-Symvoulidou, D., and Merikas, G. (1978) Effect of inhibition of prostaglandin synthesis on the natriuresis induced by saline infusion in man. Clin. Sci. Mol. Med. 54, 47-50.

6. Brater, D.C. (1979) Effect of indomethacin on salt and water homeostasis. Clin. Pharmacol. Ther. 25, 322-330.

7. Work, J., Baehler, R.W., Kotchen, T.A., Talwalkar, R., and Luke, R.G. (1980) Effect of prostaglandin inhibition on sodium chloride reabsorption in the diluting segment of the conscious dog. Kidney Int. 17, 24-30.

8. Epstein, M. (1978) Renal effects of head-out water immersion in man. Implications for an understanding of volume homeostasis. Physiol. Rev. 58, 529-581.

9. Epstein, M., Levinson, R., and Loutzenhiser, R. (1976) Effects of
    water immersion on renal hemodynamics in normal man. J. Appl. Physiol.
    41, 230-233.

10. Begin, R., Epstein, M., Sackner, M.A., Levinson, R., Dougherty, R. and
    Duncan, D. (1976) Effects of water immersion to the neck on pulmonary
    circulation and tissue volume in man. J. Appl. Physiol. 40, 293-299.

11. Epstein, M., Katsikas, J.L. and Duncan, D.C. (1973) Role of mineralo-
    corticoids in the natriuresis of water immersion in man. Circ. Res.
    32, 228-236.

12. Epstein, M., Lifschitz, M.D., Hoffman, D.S., and Stein, J.H. (1979)
    Relationship between renal prostaglandin E and renal sodium handling
    during water immersion in normal man. Circ. Res. 45, 71-80.

13. Papanicolaou, N., Safar, M., Hornych, A., Fontaliran, F., Weiss, Y.,
    Bariety, J. and Milliez, P. (1975) The release of renal prostaglandins
    during saline infusion in normal and hypertensive subjects. Clin.
    Sci. Mol. Med. 49, 459-463.

14. Boyer, T.D, Zia, P. and Reynolds, T.B. (1979) Effect of indomethacin
    and prostaglandin A_1 on renal function and plasma renin activity in
    alcoholic liver disease. Gastroenterology 77, 215-222.

15. Zipser, R.D., Hoefs, J.C., Speckart, P.F., Zia, P.K. and Horton, R.
    (1979) Prostaglandins: Modulators of renal function and pressor
    resistance in chronic liver disease. J. Clin. Endocrinol. & Metab.
    48, 895-900.

16. Arisz, L., Donker, A.J.M., Brentjens, J.R.H. and van der Hem, G.K.
    (1976) The effect of indomethacin on proteinuria and kidney function
    in the nephrotic syndrome. Acta. Med. Scand. 199, 121-125.

17. Walshe, J.J., and Venuto, R.C. (1979) Acute oliguric renal failure
    induced by indomethacin: Possible mechanism. Ann. Intern. Med.
    91, 47-49.

Hormonal Regulation of Sodium Excretion,
B. Lichardus, R.W. Schrier and J. Ponec, eds.
© 1980 Elsevier/North-Holland Biomedical Press

A POSSIBLE ROLE FOR PROSTAGLANDINS IN THE REGULATION OF RENAL SODIUM AND CHLORIDE EXCRETION

RAINER DÜSING and HERBERT J. KRAMER

Medizinische Universitäts-Poliklinik Bonn, Wilhelmstr. 35-37,

5300 Bonn, West Germany

INTRODUCTION

Since the original observation of naturally occurring prostaglandins (PG) in the rabbit renal medulla by Lee and coworkers[1], controversial studies have appeared addressing a possible role of PG in the regulation of renal sodium and chloride excretion[2]. Numerous studies have described an increase in urinary sodium excretion following infusion of exogenous prostaglandins[3,4]. In analogy, dietary depletion of essential fatty acids including the PG-precursor arachidonic acid was shown to impair renal excretion of sodium and potassium suggesting that this effect might be due to endogenous prostaglandin deficiency[5]. A different approach to this question was made possible by the observation that nonsteroidal anti-inflammatory drugs such as aspirin and indomethacin competitively inhibit the prostaglandin synthesizing enzyme system[6].

The adaptation of renal tubular function with its resulting natriuresis following intravenous infusion of isotonic saline may be independent of changes in glomerular filtration rate (GFR) or aldosterone activity[7]. Therefore, other determinants of tubular reabsorption of NaCl such as a natriuretic hormone[8-10], peritubular physical factors [11-13], and changes in intrarenal hemodynamics [14, 15] have been postulated. In the present paper, studies will be described which investigate the extent to which PG may be involved in the natriuresis of acute expansion of the extracellular fluid volume (ECV). Furthermore, possible mechanisms and tubular sites of a PG mediated effect on renal handling of sodium and chloride will be reviewed on the basis of studies performed in this laboratory[16-22].

PROSTAGLANDINS AND RENAL FUNCTION IN ACUTE EXTRACELLULAR VOLUME EXPANSION: STUDIES IN THE RAT

In a first series of studies, a total of 37 conscious female Sprague-Dawley rats were infused with isotonic saline until an increase in body weight of 10% was achieved. Prior to expansion, 21 animals received 10 mg/kg body weight of indomethacin by stomach tube. In addition, six non-expanded rats were also treated with indomethacin in the same manner.

In non-expanded control rats indomethacin had no effect on GFR, renal blood flow or renal excretory function. However, in rats expanded with isotonic saline, indomethacin significantly decreased renal blood flow and urinary excretion of sodium and potassium (figure 1).

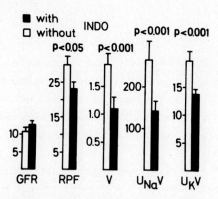

Fig. 1.   Glomerular filtration rate (GFR) (ml min^{-1}kg^{-1}b.wt.), total renal plasma flow (RPF) (ml min^{-1}kg^{-1}b.wt.), urine flow (V) (ml min^{-1}kg^{-1}b.wt.), and urinary excretion of sodium (U$_{Na}$V) and potassium (U$_K$V) (μmol min^{-1}kg^{-1}b.wt.) in acutely salt loaded rats with and without pretreatment with indomethacin (INDO) (n=37)[18].

In this study, determinations of cortical, medullary, and papillary Na-K-ATPase activities revealed no differences between expanded rats without and with concomitant indomethacin administration. However, in contrast to non-expanded rats, in which indomethacin had no effect on total renal blood flow and its intracortical distribution, inhibition of prostaglandin synthesis during ECV-expansion significantly decreased total renal blood flow by 24% which was entirely due to a decrease in outer cortical perfusion[19]. These results suggested that at least one of the mechanisms by which PG may affect renal excretory function might be through changes in intrarenal hemodynamics.

EVALUATION OF PROXIMAL AND DISTAL TUBULAR FUNCTION DURING INHIBITION OF PROSTAGLANDIN SYNTHESIS: STUDIES IN NORMAL MAN

Studies from this laboratory[16-19,22] and other groups of investigators[23,24] have clearly demonstrated that the sodium retention during administration of non-steroidal anti-inflammatory drugs may occur in the absence of changes in glomeru-lar filtration rate. The exact mechanism and the tubular site of a PG mediated effect on renal NaCl excretion, however, remain unclear. Infusion of PGE_2 into the renal artery of the dog had no effect on proximal tubular function despite a marked increase in urinary sodium excretion[4]. Also, micropuncture experiments have largely excluded the proximal tubule from participating in sodium retention during inhibi-tion of PG synthesis[23,25,26]. First evidence pointing to the distal tubule as one site of action of renal PG on tubular NaCl absorption was presented by Ganguli et al.[27]. In their study, rat papillary chloride concentration was significantly increased during inhibition of PG synthesis. Since this increase in inner medullary solute concentra-tion was not dependent on changes in papillary blood flow their results suggested that PG may inhibit electrolyte transport in either the ascending limb of Henle or the collecting duct. Furthermore, in vitro studies have shown that PGE_2 inhibits NaCl transport in isolated segments of rabbit nephrons such as the isolated medullary thick ascending limb of Henle[28] and the cortical and outer medullary collecting tubule[29, 30].

We therefore performed a second series of studies to investigate the effect of prostaglandin synthesis inhibition on proximal and distal tubular function using clearance methods in normal volunteers. Studies were performed during sustained water diuresis and intravenous infusion of hypotonic (0.45%) saline at increasing rates of 0.09, 0.18, and 0.36 ml $min^{-1}kg^{-1}$ b.wt. each for a 45 minute period, respectively. Proximal tubular function was assessed by calculating delivery of proximal tubular fluid to the distal tubules (distal delivery) $[(CH_2O + C_{Cl})/GFR \times 100]$. Distal fractional chloride reabsorption was estimated as $[CH_2O/(CH_2O + C_{Cl})]$ [31].

Furosemide is a potent inhibitor of chloride reabsorption in the ascending limb of Henle[32]. Its action has been suggested to be - at least in part - mediated by PG since some investigators have found an increase in urinary PG excretion during furosemide treatment[21,33-35] and its natriuretic effect may be blunted during concomitant inhibition of PG biosynthesis[21,36-38]. Therefore, proximal and distal tubular function were also investigated during administration of furosemide and during combined treatment with furosemide and indomethacin.

In the absence of changes in GFR, indomethacin significantly decreased mean urinary excretion of chloride, sodium and potassium (figure 2).

208

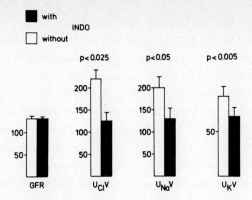

Fig. 2. Glomerular filtration rate (GFR) (ml/min) and urinary excretion of chloride $(U_{Cl}V)$ (µmol/min), sodium $(U_{Na}V)$ (µmol/min), and potassium (U_KV) (µmol/min) in six healthy volunteers during hypotonic saline infusion with and without pretreatment with indomethacin (INDO). Values given represent mean ± SEM over all three clearance periods.

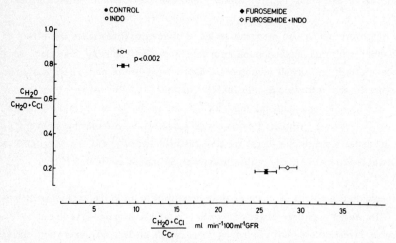

Fig. 3. Distal fractional chloride reabsorption $[CH_2O/(CH_2O + C_{Cl})]$ plotted as function of distal fractional delivery $[(CH_2O + C_{Cl})/GFR \times 100]$. Illustrated are mean ± SEM calulated over all three clearance periods. Note that in the absence of an effect of indomethacin (INDO) on distal delivery, it significantly increased distal fractional chloride reabsorption during hypotonic saline infusion alone but did not affect the changes in proximal and distal tubular function induced by furosemide.

209

This electrolyte retention was not associated with changes in distal delivery suggesting that proximal tubular function was unchanged. However, there was a highly significant increase in distal fractional chloride reabsorption during indomethacin treatment pointing to the diluting segments of the nephron as the tubular site of action of renal prostaglandins.

Various studies in healthy volunteers and in patients with different renal and electrolyte disorders have shown that treatment with drugs which are capable of inhibiting PG synthesis is associated with sodium retention and a subsequent escape from the sodium retaining effect of such treatment[39-42]. It is therefore important to note that in the studies reported in this paper, indomethacin treatment was started shortly before investigations were undertaken.

Furosemide induced an almost twelve-fold increase in urinary NaCl excretion and an approximately three-fold increase in urinary excretion of potassium. These changes in renal excretory function occurred in the absence of changes in GFR but were associated with a marked increase in distal delivery and a highly significant ($p < 0.001$) inhibition of distal fractional chloride reabsorption. Furosemide also increased urinary excretion of PGE_2 from 1.45 ± 0.12 to 2.94 ± 0.34 pmol/min ($p < 0.05$) which was markedly decreased to 0.56 ± 0.13 pmol/min during combined treatment with furosemide and indomethacin. Despite these marked differences in the activity of the intrarenal PG system, none of the furosemide induced changes in renal function was significantly altered during combined treatment with furosemide and indomethacin (figure 3). Our results therefore suggest, that the effect of furosemide on proximal and distal tubular reabsorptive capacity may not be mediated by prostaglandins.

CONCLUSIONS

In the present paper, further evidence is presented that administration of drugs which inhibit PG biosynthesis may promote renal salt retention. Altered renal excretory function is observed in the absence of changes in glomerular filtration rate and proximal tubular function. Results of differential clearance methods point to the diluting segments of the nephron as the site of action of endogenous prostaglandins. Furosemide stimulates intrarenal PG biosynthesis, but its action on proximal as well as distal tubular function appears not to be mediated by the prostaglandin system.

210

REFERENCES

1. Lee, J.B., Crowshaw, K., Takman, B.H., Attrep, K.A., and Gougoutas, J.Z. (1967) Biochem. J. 105, 1251-1260.

2. Düsing, R. and Kramer, H.J. (1978) Renal Prostaglandins, Eden Press, Montreal, pp. 92-107.

3. Gross, J.B. and Bartter, F.C. (1973) Am. J. Physiol. 225, 218-224.

4. Strandhoy, J.W., Ott, C.E., Schneider, E.G., Willis, L.R., Beck, N.P., Davis, B.B., and Knox, F.G. (1974) Am. J. Physiol. 226, 1015-1021.

5. Rosenthal, J., Simone, P.G., and Silbergleit, A. (1974) Prostaglandins 5, 435-440.

6. Vane, J.R. (1971) Nat. New. Biol. 231, 232-235.

7. Rector, F.C., van Giesen, G., Kill, F., and Seldin, D.V. (1964) J. clin. Invest. 43, 341-348.

8. DeWardener, H.E., Mills, J.H., Clapham, W.F., and Hayter, C.J. (1961) Clin.Sci. 21, 249-258.

9. Kramer, H.J. and Krück, F. (1978) Natriuretic Hormone. Springer (Berlin-Heidelberg-New York)

10. Kramer, H.J., Gonick, H.C., and Krück, F. (1972) Klin. Wschr. 50, 893-897.

11. Brenner, B.M., Falchuk, K.H., and Berliner, R.W. (1969) J. clin. Invest. 48, 1519-1531.

12. Windhager, E.E., Lewy, J.E., and Spitzer, A. (1969) Nephron 6, 247-259.

13. Martino, J.A. and Earley, L.E. (1968) J. clin. In vest. 46, 1963-1978.

14. Jamison, R.L. and Lacy, F.P. (1971) Am. J. Physiol. 221, 690-697.

15. Bartoli, E. and Earley, L.E. (1971) J. clin. Invest. 50, 2191-2203.

16. Düsing, R., Opitz, W.D., and Kramer, H.J. (1975) Kidney Int. 8, 473.

17. Düsing, R., Opitz, W.D., and Kramer, H.J. (1977) Nephron 18, 212-219.

18. Düsing, R., Melder, B., and Kramer, H.J. (1976)Prostaglandins 12, 3-10.

19. Düsing, R., Melder, B., and Kramer, H.J. (1977) Circ. Res. 41, 287-291.

20. Kramer, H.J., Prior, W., Stinnesbeck, B., Bäcker, A., Eden, J., and Düsing. R. (1980) Advances in Prostaglandin and Thromboxane Research, Vol. 7. Raven Press, New York, pp. 1021-1026.

21. Kramer, H.J., Düsing., R., Stinnesbeck, B., Prior, W., Bäcker, A., Eden, J., Kipnowski, J., Glänzer, K., and Krück, F. (1980) Clin. Sci. in press.

22. Düsing, R., Nicolas, V., Glänzer, K., Kipnowski, J., and Kramer, H.J. (1980) submitted for publication.

23. Higashihara, E., Stokes, J.B., Kokko, J.P., Campbell, W.B., and DuBose, T.D. (1979) J. Clin. Invest. 64, 1277-1287.

24. Higashihara, E. und Kokko, J.P. (1978) 7th International Congress of Nephrology, Montreal. Q-3.

25. Leyssac, P.P., Christensen, P., Hill, R., and Skinner, S.L. (1975) Acta. Physiol. Scand. 94, 484-496.

26. Foman, R.J. and Kauker, M.L. (1978) Am. J. Physiol. 235, F111-F118.

27. Ganguli, M., Tobian, L., Azar, S., and O'Donnel, M. (1977) Circ. Res. Suppl. 40, 1135-1139.

28 Stokes, J.B., (1979) J. Clin. Invest. 64, 495-502.

29. Stokes, J.B. and Kokko, J.P. (1977) J. Clin. Invest. 49, 1099-1104.

30. Iino, Y. and Imai, M. (1978) Pflügers Arch. Eur. J. Physiol. 373, 125-132.

31. Danovitch, G.M. and Bricker, N.S. (1976) Kidney Int. 10, 229-238.

32. Burg, M.B. (1976) Kidney Int. 9, 189-197.

33. Abe, K., Yasujima, M., Chiba, S., Irokawa, N., Ito, T., and Yoshinaga, K. (1977) Prostaglandins 14, 513-521.

34. Williamson, H.E., Bourland, W.A., Marchand, G.R., Farley, D.B., and van Orden, D.E. (1975) Proc. Soc. exp. Biol. 150, 104-106.

35. Patak, R.V., Fadem, S.Z., Rosenblatt, S.G., Lifschitz, M.D., and Stein, J.H. (1979) Am. J. Physiol. 236, F494-F500.

36. Frölich, J.C., Hollifield, J.W., Dormois, J.C., Frölich, B.L., Seyberth, H., Michelakis, A.M., and Oates, J.A. (1976) Circ. Res. 39, 447-452.

37. Patak, R.V., Mookerjee, B.K., Bentzel, C.J., Hysert, P.E., Babej, M., and Lee, J.B. (1975) Prostaglandins 10, 649-659.

38. Oliw, E., Kover, G., Larsson, C., and Anggard, E. (1978) Eur. J. Pharmacol. 38, 95-100.

39. Gill, J.R., Jr., Frölich, J.C., Bowden, R.E., Taylor, A.A., Keiser, H.R., Seyberth, H.W., Oates, J.A., and Bartter, F.C. (1976) Am. J. Med. 61, 43-51.

212

40.   Berg, K.J. (1977) Eur. J. Clin. Pharmacol. 11, 117-123.

41.   Donker, A.J.M., Arisz, L., Brentjens, J.R.H., van der Hem, G.K., and Hollemanns, H.J.G. (1976) Nephron 17, 228-296.

42.   Güllner, H.-G., Gill, J.R., Jr., Bartter, F.C., and Düsing, R. (1980) Am. J. Med. in press.

Hormonal Regulation of Sodium Excretion,
B. Lichardus, R.W. Schrier and J. Ponec, eds.
© 1980 Elsevier/North-Holland Biomedical Press

THE ROLE OF INTRARENAL PROSTAGLANDIN E IN THE ACTION OF DIURETICS

GEORGES DAGHER* and ADEL BERBARI**

*INSERM U.7, Hôpital Necker, 161 rue de Sèvres, 75015 Paris, France.

**Department of Physiology, American University, Beirut, Lebanon.

INTRODUCTION

The role of PGE in the control of Na handling has given rise to controversial findings. Infusion of PGE in the anaesthetized dog or conscious man result in natriuresis[1-5]. Intrarenal administration of PG in the dog inhibited Na reabsorption in the proximal tubule[3,4,5].

However, the injection of Arachidonic acid, a precursor of PG synthesis did not increase Na excretion in the PG depleted kidney[7]. Moreover, the inhibition of PG synthesis by Meclofenamate caused a natriuresis in the conscious dog[6].

The participation of PG in the natriuretic action of some diuretics has also been studied. Renal venous level of PGE increased in anaesthetized dogs after administration of ethacrinic acid a loop diuretic[8]. Indomethacin reduced the furosemide induced diuresis and natriuresis in rabbits and man[9, 10]. In contrast Willamson and Weber demonstrated that indomethacin did not decrease the response to furosemide or ethacrinic acid in dog and man[11, 12].

In the context of these preliminary findings the role of PGs in the action of diuretics is still controversial and further studies are needed before a definite conclusion can be drawn.

The aim of these experiments was to investigate whether PGE has a modulating effect on the diuretic action of furosemide and hydrochlorothiazide in rats.

MATERIALS AND METHODS

40 females sprague-dawley rats weighing 180-240 gms were maintained on Laboratory chow diet and Tap Water.

A prior pilot experiment on a group of 5 rats to determine time-dose effect of hydrochlorothiazide (HCT), and furosemide showed a maximum diuresis 1 hr after administration by stomach tube of 5 mg/kg HCT or 25 mg/kg furosemide in 1 ml 2.5 % Tween 80 (polysorbate 80).

HCT, Furosemide and indomethacin lactate were disolved in 1 ml 2.5 % Tween 80 and were given by stomach tube. Rats were divided into 5 groups.

Group 1 : Control
          5 rats were given 2.5 % Tween 80 in 1 ml distilled water.
Group 2 : 5 rats were given 5 mg/kg hydrochlorthiazide.
Group 3 : 5 rats were given 25 mg/kg furosemide.
Group 4 and 5 : rats were treated with 3 mg/kg/day of indomethacin lactate
                in 2.5 % Tween 80 for 1 week. On the seventh day :
     Group 4 : 10 rats received 5 mg/kg HCT
     Group 5 : 10 rats received 25 mg/kg furosemide.

After treatment, rats were placed in metabolic cages and allowed free access
to water. Urine was collected for 1 hr after which the animals, anaesthetized-
with Na pentobarbital 30 mg/kg intraperitoneally- were sacrified and Carotid
Blood Collected in Tubes containing 17 mg EDTA/ml H_2O. After centrifugation,
plasma was separated and kept frozen at -20° C for PGE and PRA determination.
The hematocrit was determined by the micromethod technique.

Both kidneys were removed, weighed, cut and homogenized in 1 ml 0.9 % saline
and 0.4 ml of IN HCL.

Renal and plasma PGE levels where determined according to the method of
Orezyk and Behrman. Standard solutions of PGE with concentrations of 20, 35,
50, 75, 100, 200, 400 and 800 pg/ml were prepared for a standard curve. Antiserum to PGE (supplied with PGE kit from Calbiochem-Switzerland) diluted in
phosphosaline buffer (PH = 7.4), ^{3}H-PGE and charcoal were added to standard and
unknown dried samples. The mixtures was centrifuged and supernatant added to
Saclay's scintillation coktail (PPO, POPOP, Naphthalene, Dioxane) and counted*.

Ln of the independent variable (PG conc) was plotted versus the dependent
variable (Radioactivity), and the least square line was drawn using the method
of least squares. The unknown values of PG conc., calculated directly from the
equation of the obtained line, were reported in pg/g tissue/100 gr. body weight
and pg/ml plasma.

PRA was determined using radioimmunoassay technique of HABER and values were
reported in nanograms of AgI released per ml plasma per hr (ng/ml/hr). Urine
vol. was measured and urinary Na and K conc. were determined by flame photome-
try+ and expressed, in ml/hr and meq/hr respectively.

For statistical significance the means $\pm$ SE of different parameters between
groups were compaired using student t-test and were considered significant
when p 0.05.

* Tris-carb scintillation spectrometer, Model 3320, Packard Instrument
  Company, Inc. Illinois.
+ Flame Photometer, Model 143, Instrumentation Laboratory Inc. Massachusetts.

RESULTS

1. Effects of Hydrochlorothiazide

One hour after administration of HCT 5 mg/kg the observed Urine Vol. (1.7 ± 0.32) and urinary Na excretion (190.9 ± 30.5) were significantly higher than the values reported for control group (V = 0.5 ± 0.25, UNa 18.04 ± 8.7) PRA, Plasma PGE, Renal PGE or Hematocrit values of the two groups were not stastically different.

2. Comparison of the effect of HCT in normal and indomethacin treated rats

Rats treated with 3 mg/kg indomethacin for seven days had one hour after administration of HCT a urine volume of 1.1 ± 0.16 and a plasma PGE level of 68.3 ± 9.6 and Renal PGE level of 5.22 ± 0.4.

These values were significantly lower than those reported for HCT treated rats (group II) (V : 1.7 ± 0.3, Plasma PGE : 161 ± 23.5, Renal PGE : 23.16 ± 2.7).

However Urinary Na excretion and Hematocrit ratios were not significantly different.

3. Effets of Furosemide

The urine vol. (1.9 ± 0.24) and the urinary Na excretion (152 ± 32.1) observed one hour after the administration of 25 mg/kg of furosemide were markedly higher than the values reported for control group (V = 0.5 ± 0.25, UNa : 18.04 ± 8.7).

The furosemide induced diuresis was associated with a significantly elevated PRA level of 5.7 ± 3.4 while the control group had a PRA level of 1.8 ± 0.76.

Plasma and renal PGE levels and hematocrit ratio of the two groups were not statistically different.

4. Comparison of the effects of furosemide in normal and indomethacin treated rats

Rats treated with 3 mg/kg indomethacin for seven days had 1 hr after administration of furosemide a urine volume of 3.3 ± 0.3 and a urine Na excretion of 480 ± 111.3. These values were significantly higher than those reported for furosemide only (V. 1.9 ± 0.24 UNa : 152 ± 32.1). In contrast Renal PGE level was markedly lower (6.7 ± 1.46 versus 12.0 ± 2.24).

However Plasma PGE, PRA and hematocrit values were not statistically different.

TABLE 1

Effect of Hydrochlorothiazide (HCT) of Furosemide on Renal PGE, Plasma PGE, Urine Vol. Urinary Na excretion (UNa), Urinary K excretion, Plasma Renin activity and hematocrit in normal and indomethacin treated rats.

	Renal PGE pg/gm tissue/ 100 gm B.W.	Plasma PGE pg/ml	U. Vol. ml/hr	U. Na meq/hr	U. K. meq/hr	PRA ng/ml/hr	hematocrit ratio
Control	16.24 $\pm$ 2.64	203.2 $\pm$ 43.3	0.5 $\pm$ 0.25	18.04 $\pm$ 8.7	4.96 $\pm$ 0.9	1.8 $\pm$ 0.76	42.1
HCT	23.16[a] $\pm$ 2.7	161[c] $\pm$ 23.5	*1.7[d] $\pm$ 0.3	*190.9 $\pm$ 30.5	14.1 $\pm$ 2.7	2.1 $\pm$ 2.3	41.9
HCT + Indomethacin	*5.22[a] $\pm$ 0.4	*68.3[c] $\pm$ 9.6	*1.1[d] $\pm$ 0.16	*146.3 $\pm$ 33.6	*12.3 $\pm$ 1.15	1.2 $\pm$ 0.7	40.5
Furosemide	12.0[b] $\pm$ 2.24	287.9 $\pm$ 165	*1.9[e] $\pm$ 0.24	*152[f] $\pm$ 32.1	*19.6 $\pm$ 1.7	*5.7[g] $\pm$ 3.4	42.8
Furosemide + Indomethacin	*6.7[b] $\pm$ 1.46	*103.5 $\pm$ 17.2	*3.3[e] $\pm$ 0.3	*480[f] $\pm$ 111.3	*28.6 $\pm$ 6.2	3[g] $\pm$ 1.4	39.6

* : Significantly different from the control value $p < 0.05$

a,b,c etc : the 2 values labelled a are significantly different from each other (the same for the other values labelled either b, c, d, etc...) $p < 0.05$

$\pm$ SE : the SE reported to that of the mean within the same group $= SD/\sqrt{n}$

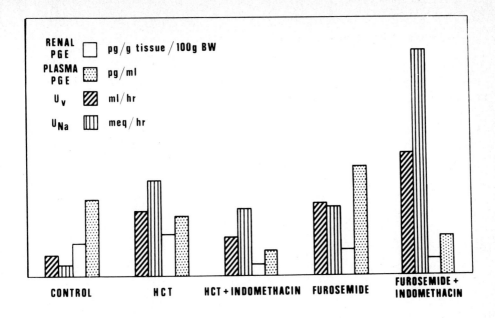

Fig. 1 Summary graph. Comparison of the effect of HCT & Furosemide on Urine
volume (Uv), Urinary Na excretion (U_{na}) Renal and Plasma PGE.

DISCUSSION

The results of the present experiments indicate that :

1. HCT and Furosemide induce a diuresis and natriuresis of similar magnitude
with no change in plasma or renal PGE level indicating that PGE do not mediate
the diuretic action of the two drugs.

2. The diuretic response following hydrochlorothiazide in indomethacin treated
rat was less marked, and is associated with a reduction in Plasma and renal
PGE levels. Na or K excretions were however unchanged.

The reduced diuresis may be due to a reduction in intrarenal PGE level. This
is supported by the observation that indomethacin enhance vasopressin induced
water reabsorption in the toad bladder[14, 15]. In addition, PGE was reported to
inhibit vasopressin induced water reabsorption in toad bladder and collecting
duct[16, 17, 18].

3. Most striking was the potentiation of furosemide induced diuresis and natriu-

resis by indomethacin, associated with a significant depression in Renal PG. This enhanced diuretic and natriuretic response may be due to :

a) decreased synthesis of antinatriuretic PGF 2 by indomethacin PGF 2 when infused to dogs was shown to decrease decreased urine volume and urine Na excretion[19].

b) decreased synthesis of PGE. Several observations have suggested that PGE might be antinatriuretic. An increase in Na excretion was observed after indomethacin infusion into the renal artery of both anaesthetized and conscious dogs [20, 21]. Moreover, PG inhibition with Meclofenamate and Ro 20-572 caused a natriuresis in the conscious dog[13]. Furthermore in vitro studies showed that PGE enhances Na reabsorption in toad bladder and distal tubule[22]. In contrast Oliw E. showed a decrease in furosemide induced diuresis after indomethacin infusion to anaesthetized surgically traumatized rabbits[10]. Williamson reported that indomethacin infusion did not alter the furosemide induced diuresis in anaesthetized dogs[11].

The discrepancies among the above studies are not clear and may be due to the anaesthetized state, the mode of administration of indomethacin or specie differences.

4. Indomethacin treatment inhibited hypereninemia of furosemide treated rats. Similar observations were made Oliw E., Meyer, Patak and Weber on rabbits and man[9, 10, 13, 23].

The lack of response of renin to furosemide in indomethacin treated rats is not clear. The administration of PG was shown to stimulate renin secretion[24, 25]. It could be postulated that a decrease in intrarenal PG concentration might inhibit furosemide induced renin secretion.

The findings of the present experiment suggest that intrarenal PGE plays a role in the mechanism of furosemide diuresis and natriuresis in the rat.

REFERENCES
1. Lee, J.B., Mc Giff, J.C., Kannegiessir, H., Aykent, Y.Y., Mudd, J.G., Frawley, T.F. (1971) Antihypertensive renal effects on Prostaglandin A, in patients with essential hypertension. Ann Intern Med 74, 703.
2. Vander, A.J. (1968) Direct effects of Prostaglandin on Renal function and renin release in anaesthetized dog. Am.J.Physiol. 214, 218.
3. Martinez-Maldonadon, M., Tsaparas, M.N., Eknoyan, G., Suki, W.N. (1972) Renal actions of Prostaglandins : comparison with Acetylcholine and volume expansion. Am.J.Physiol. 222, 1147.

4. Johnston, H.H., Herzog, J.P., Lauler, D.P. (1968) Effects of Prostaglandin E_1 on renal hemodynamics, sodium and water excretion. Am.J.Physiol. 213, 939.

5. Strankhoy, J., Ott, C.E., Schneider, E.G., Willis, L.R., Beck, N.P., Davis, B.B., Knox, F.G. (1974) Effects of Prostaglandins E_1 & E_2 on renal sodium reabsorption and starling forces. Am.J.Physiol. 226, 1015.

6. Kirshenbaum, M.A., Stein, J.H. (1976) The effect of inhibition of Prostaglandin synthesis on Urinary Na excretion in conscious dogs. J.Clin. Invest. 57, 517.

7. Kirschenbaum, M.A., Bay, W.H., Ferris, T.F., Stein, J.H. (1975) The effect of prostaglandin inhibition on the natriuresis of drug induced renal vasolidation (abstract) Clin.Res. 23, 36.

8. Williamson, H., Marchand, G., Bourland, W., Farley, D., Van Orden, D. (1976) Ethacrinic acid induced release of PGE to increase renal blood flow Prostaglandins 11(3), 519.

9. Patak, R., Mookerjec, B., Bentzel, G., Hysert, P., Babej, M., Lee, J. (1975) Antagonism of the effects of furosemide by indomethacin in normal and hypertensive man Prostaglandins 10(4), 649.

10. Oliw, E., Kover, C., Larsson, and Anggard, E. (1976) Reduction by indomethacin of furosemide effects in the rabbit European.J.Pharmcol. 38, 95.

11. Williamson, H., Bourland, W., Marchand, G. (1975) Inhibition of furosemide induced increase in renal blood flow by indomethacin. Proc.Soc.Exp.Biol. Med. 148, 164.

12. Williamson, H., Bourland, W.A., Marchand, G. (1974) Inhibition of ethacrinic acid induce increase in renal blood flow by indomethacin Prostaglandin 8, 297.

13. Weber, P., Scherer, B., Larrson, C. (1977) Increase of free arachidonic acid by furosemide in man as the cause of Prostaglandin and renin release Eur.J.Pharmacol. 41, 329.

14. Albert, W., Handler, J. (1974) Effect of PGE, indomethacin and polyphlorelin phosphate on toad bladder response by ADH. Am.J.Physiol. 226, 1382.

15. Flores, A., Sharp, G. (1972) Endogenous prostaglandins and osmatic water flow in the toad bladder. Am.J.Physiol. 223, 1392.

16. Orloff, J., Handler, J., Bergstrom, S. (1971) Effect of PGE, on the permeability of the toad bladder to vasopression. Nature(Lond.) 205, 397.

17. Flores, J., Witkum, P.A., Beckman, B., Sharp, G. (1975) Stimulation of osmotic water flow in toad bladder by PGE. J.Clin.Invest. 56, 256.

18. Beck, N.P., Kaneko, T., Zor, U., Field, J., Davis, B. (1971) Effect of vasopressin and PGE on the adeny cyclase cyclic 3' 5' adenosine mono-phosphate system of the renal medulla of the rat. J.Clin.Invest. 50.

19. Barac, G. (1969) Action de la prostaglandin PGE sur la diurèse et le dé-bit sanguin rénal chez le chien Soc.Belge Biol. 163, 1233.

20. Satoh, S., Zimmermann, B. (1975) Influence of the renin-angiotensin sys-tem on the effect of prostaglandin synthesis inhibition in the renal vas-culation. Circ.Res. 36(suppl. 1) 89.

21. Gill, J., Alexander, R., Halashka, P., Pisano, J., Keiser, H. (1975) Indo-methacin inhibits distal sodium reabsorption in the dog (abstract) Clin. Res. 23, 431.

22. Owen, T., Ehrhart, J., Haddy, F.J. (1974) Effects of indomethacin on blood flow, ractive hyperemia and autoregulation in the dog kidney. Fed.Proc. 33, 348.

23. Meyer, P., Menard, J., Papanicalan (1968) Mechanism of Renin release fol-lowing furosemide diuresis in Rabbits. Am.J.Physiol. 215, 908.

24. Werning, C., Vetter, W., Weidmann, P., Schwiekert, U., Stiel, D., Sicgen-thaler, W. (1971) Effects of Prostaglandin E, on renin in the dog. Am.J. Physiol. 220, 852.

25. Larsson, C., Weber, P., Angaard, E. (1974) Arachidonic acid increases and indomethacin decreases plasma renin in the rabbit. Eur.J.Pharmcol. 28, 391.

Hormonal Regulation of Sodium Excretion,
B. Lichardus, R.W. Schrier and J. Ponec, eds.
© 1980 Elsevier/North-Holland Biomedical Press

MICROPUNCTURE EXAMINATION OF CHLORIDE TRANSPORT IN RAT CORTICAL AND MEDULLARY NEPHRON SEGMENTS DURING ACUTE VOLUME EXPANSION WITH AND WITHOUT INHIBITORS OF PROSTAGLANDIN SYNTHESIS.

T. DuBose, Jr., E. Higashihara, and J. Kokko. Department of Internal Medicine University of Texas Health Science Center, Dallas, Texas 75235.

INTRODUCTION.

The precise role of the kidney in extracellular fluid volume homeostasis has long been a subject of intense investigation. Most micropuncture and clearance studies have placed emphasis on the segments of the nephron responsible for the regulation of sodium chloride excretion during variations in extracellular fluid volume status. Other studies have attempted to characterize the contribution of various humoral agents, peritubular capillary forces, or sympathetic nerve activity which might affect the regulation of salt excretion. Although it has been widely appreciated that numerous factors may participate in this regulatory process, the demonstration that prostaglandins are saliuretic[1-3] and produced endogenously[4,5] has lead to investigation of the effects of these compounds on segmental sodium chloride reabsorption[6-8]. While the hemodynamic effects of prostaglandins have been well documented, controversy exists with regard to a direct tubular effect of prostaglandins on sodium chloride transport[6,7].

Stokes and Kokko[6], and Stokes[8] have demonstrated a direct effect of PGE_2 on sodium[6] and chloride[8] transport in both the isolated perfused cortical and outer medullary collecting tubule[6] and the medullary thick ascending limb of Henle[8]. In the former study it was demonstrated that PGE_2 significantly reduced the negative transepithelial potential and reversibly inhibited net sodium efflux in the collecting tubule. Similar findings were reported by Iiono and Imai[9]. The findings of these two studies do not agree with the studies of Fine and Trizna[7], in which no effect of PGE_2, $PGF_{2\alpha}$, or PGA_2 on net sodium flux or potential difference was demonstrated in the medullary collecting tubule. Furthermore, these same investigators were unable to demonstrate a direct effect of these compounds on the medullary thick ascending limb[7]. In contrast, Stokes[8] has demonstrated selective inhibition by PGE_2 of chloride transport in the medullary, but not the cortical thick ascending limb. Although several possible explanations for these discrepancies exist, it is likely that the activity of PGE_2 in rabbit serum[7] differs from that in artificial solution[8].

Recently, it has been suggested that the most terminal segments of the nephron may play a major role in modulating the magnitude of the saliuresis of acute isotonic volume expansion. Previous studies from our laboratory[10], and from Stein and associates[11] have provided evidence that the juxtamedullary nephrons contribute a proportionately greater load of sodium chloride than the superficial nephrons to the final urine during volume expansion. Since prostaglandins are present in the renal medulla in large amounts[4,5], and since nonsteroidal anti-inflammatory drugs may promote salt retention[12-14], it has been interesting to speculate that prostaglandins may play a role in the regulation of salt excretion. If, for example, prostaglandins play a role in the saliuresis of acute volume expansion, inhibiting their production should blunt the associated saliuresis. Recent studies in our laboratory were designed to examine this hypothesis.

METHODS AND MATERIALS.

In these studies either meclofenamate or indomethacin was administered to both hydropenic and acutely volume expanded rats. The site of action of these agents was evaluated by micropuncture of both the accessible portions of the superficial cortex and the surgically exposed papilla of the mutant Munich-Wistar rat.

The following experimental groups were examined:
1. Hydropenic controls
2. Hydropenia plus meclofenamate (3mg/kg bolus and 4mg/kg/hr).
3. Volume expansion controls (10% Body weight Ringer's bicarbonate).
4. Volume expansion during inhibition of prostaglandin production (meclofenamate or indomethacin).

The concentration of prostaglandin E_2 and $F_{2\alpha}$ in urine samples obtained from the same volume expanded animals used for micropuncture were measured according to the method of Dray, et al[15].

Results:

Whole Kidney Data. Urine volume was decreased significantly by both meclofenamate and indomethacin during both hydropenia and volume expansion. The glomerular filtration rate, however, was not affected by either meclofenamate or indomethacin. Urinary chloride excretion decreased approximately 50% after either meclofenamate or indomethacin during hydropenia and volume expansion.

Micropuncture data. Single nephron glomerular filtration rates obtained from distal tubular punctures were not altered by meclofenamate or indomethacin.

The segmental micropuncture data are summarized in figures 1-3 and will be reviewed sequentially.

Proximal tubule. The fraction of chloride remaining at the superficial late proximal tubule was not altered by either meclofenamate or indomethacin during acute volume expansion (Fig. 1, 2).

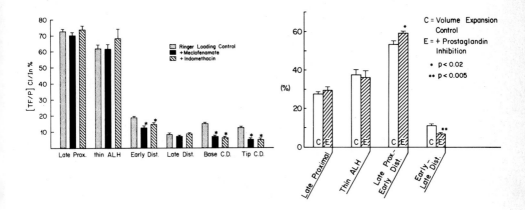

Fig. 1. Fraction of filtered chloride remaining at each micropuncture site during volume expansion before and after prostaglandins inhibitor.

Fig. 2. Fraction of filtered chloride reabsorbed along each nephron segment.

Thin limb of Henle. The fraction of filtered chloride remaining at the thin limb of juxtamedullary nephrons was not affected by meclofenamate during hydropenia although the chloride concentration ratio increased from 2.47 to 4.10 (p < 0.001) Similarly, the fraction of chloride remaining at this site during volume expansion was not changed after meclofenamate or indomethacin (Fig. 1). Thus, meclofenamate and indomethacin did not alter chloride reabsorption up to the thin limb of the juxtamedullary nephron in either hydropenia or volume expansion (Fig's. 1, 2).

Superficial loop of Henle. The fraction of chloride delivered to the early
distal tubule was significantly decreased by both meclofenamate (18.5 vs
12.7%, p < 0.001) and indomethacin (14.4%, p < 0.02) during volume expansion
(Fig. 1). Therefore, the fraction of chloride reabsorbed between the late
proximal tubule and the early distal tubule (short loop of Henle) increased
from 53.1 ± 1.7% to 57.3 ± 1.4% (p < 0.05) after meclofenamate and to 60.2 ±
1.6% (p < 0.02) after indomethacin (Fig. 2).

Distal tubule. The fraction of chloride remaining at the late distal
tubule was not changed significantly by meclofenamate or indomethacin during
hydropenia or volume expansion (Fig. 1). The fraction of chloride reabsorbed
between the early and late distal tubule decreased, however, from 11.0 to 7.0%
after meclofenamate and to 5.5% after indomethacin during volume expansion
(Fig. 2).

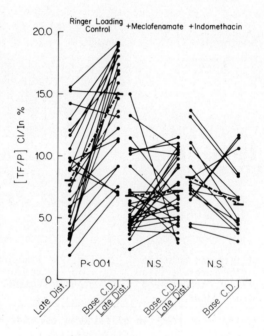

Fig. 3. Comparison of fraction of filtered chloride remaining between the
late distal tubule and base collecting duct during volume expansion and after
either meclofenamate or indomethacin.

Superficial late distal tubule to base collecting duct. The results comparing the fraction of filtered chloride remaining at the late distal tubule

to that fraction remaining at the base of the collecting duct are displayed in
Fig. 3. In the volume expansion "controls" net addition of chloride was observed between the superficial late distal tubule and the base of the collecting duct. There was no significant difference in the fraction of chloride
remaining at either of these two nephron sites during hydropenia or after
administration of meclofenamate. The fraction of chloride remaining at the
base of the collecting duct was significantly reduced by meclofenamate
(15.0 vs 7.2%, p < 0.001) and indomethacin (15.0 vs 6.1%, p < 0.001). Thus,
meclofenamate and indomethacin reversed the pattern of addition of chloride
observed between the late distal tubule and the base of the collecting duct
during volume expansion.

Papillary collecting duct. The fraction of chloride remaining at the tip
of the collecting duct decreased from 1.7 to 1.0% after meclofenamate during
hydropenia. A similar decrease in the fraction of chloride remaining at this
site was observed during volume expansion. Chloride reabsorption between the
base and tip of the collecting duct was noted in every experimental group,
however. The filtered chloride reabsorbed along 1 mm collecting duct during
volume expansion, volume expansion with meclofenamate, and indomethacin was
2.4, 1.9, and 1.0% respectively. Since the magnitude of chloride delivered to
the base collecting duct was less with meclofenamate and indomethacin, and
since the chloride reabsorption across the papillary collecting duct has been
demonstrated to be load dependent[10,16], the percentage of delivered chloride
reabsorbed along the papillary collecting duct was calculated. The data
indicate that both meclofenamate and indomethacin had no effect on chloride
reabsorption in the papillary collecting duct.

Urinary prostaglandins. Urinary excretion of PGE_2 and $F_{2\alpha}$ was suppressed
approximately 95% with both drugs during volume expansion. There was no
significant difference in the urinary prostaglandin excretion observed between
the meclofenamate and indomethacin treated groups.

Papillary tissue chloride concentration. During hydropenia, meclofenamate
administration resulted in a significant increase in chloride concentration
(119 to 215 mEq/kg tissue H_2O). Similarly, during volume expansion, both
meclofenamate and indomethacin administration were associated with a significant increase in papillary tissue chloride concentration (127 ± 15 to 181 ± 9
and 220 ± 13 mEq/kg tissue H_2O, respectively) (p < 0.01, and p < 0.001).
Discussion.

In summary, our study demonstrates that both indomethacin and meclofenamate, when administered in amounts sufficient to reduce urinary excretion of

prostaglandins, reduced urinary chloride excretion in both hydropenic and acutely volume expanded rats without changes in glomerular filtration rate. The failure to demonstrate an effect of either of these agents on proximal chloride reabsorption is in agreement with other studies[17,18]. The increase in chloride reabsorption observed between the late proximal and early distal tubule after indomethacin could be a result of increased reabsorption in either the superficial pars recta, the thin descending limb of Henle, or the thick ascending limb of Henle. Based on the available information relevant to the transport of chloride in these segments[8,19], it is most likely that this increase in reabsorption occurred in the thick ascending limb of Henle.

Since both inhibitors of prostaglandin synthesis increased chloride re-absorption in the superficial loop, most likely as a result of an increase in chloride transport in the thick ascending limb, it is probable that the observed reduction in chloride delivery to the base of the collecting duct was a result of an increase in chloride reabsorption in the medullary thick ascending limb of Henle of the juxtamedullary nephron population. Although prostaglandin inhibition has been associated with a decrease in papillary blood flow[20], it is unlikely that a reduction in papillary blood flow alone can explain the observed decrease in chloride delivery to the base collecting duct. The increase in the concentration of chloride in the papillary interstitium after administration of either meclofenamate or indomethacin as demonstrated in this study and as previously reported by Ganguli, et al[21] could be a result of either a decrease in papillary blood flow (a decreased "washout") or an increase in net NaCl efflux from the medullary portion of the ascending limb of Henle or both. Whatever the mechanism(s), the observed increase in papillary interstitial chloride concentration would create a less favorable, not a more favorable, gradient for passive chloride reabsorption in the thin ascending limb of Henle and could result in this manner in an increase in chloride delivery to the base of the collecting tubule.

The findings indirectly support a role for endogenous prostaglandins in the transport of chloride in the thick ascending limb of Henle and the cortical and outer medullary collecting tubule in vivo and are thus compatible with the observations cited previously in the isolated perfused cortical collecting tubule and thick ascending limb in vitro[6,8]. These studies when considered together strongly suggest that endogenous renal prostaglandins have a direct tubular effect and may play a role in the natriuresis and chloruresis of acute volume expansion by decreasing fractional salt reabsorption in the juxtamedullary nephron. An increase in medullary prostaglandin production in response to volume expansion could then act to inhibit chloride reabsorption in the thick ascending limb of Henle. The demonstration that PGE_2 inhibits chloride transport in the medullary, but not the cortical thick ascending limb[8] is supportive of this hypothesis. The basis for such a functionally heterogeneous response and the mechanism by which this response is elicited remains to be determined.

The observation that the net addition of chloride between the superficial late distal tubule and base of the collecting duct associated with acute volume expansion was blunted by inhibition of endogenous prostaglandin production supports an important role for heterogeneity of nephron function as an important determinant of final urinary sodium chloride excretion.

ACKNOWLEDGEMENTS
This work was supported in part by NIH Research Grants 5R01 AM14677, 5R01 AM25730 and Training Grant 5T32 AM07257.

REFERENCES
1. Strandhoy, J.W., Ott, C.E., Schneider E.G, Willis L.R, Beck N.P., Davis, B.B. and Knox F.G., (1974) Am. J. Physiol. 226, 1015.

2. Martinez-Maldonado, M., Tsaparas N., Eknoyan G., and Suki W.N., (1972) Am. J. Physiol. 222, 1147.

3. Johnston, H.H., Herzog J.P., and Lauler D.P., (1967) Am. J. Physiol. 213, 939.

4. Lee, J.B., Crowshaw K., Takman B.H., Attrep K.A., and Gougoutas J.Z., (1967) Biochem J. 105, 1251.

5. Larsson, C. and Anggard E., (1976) J. Pharm. Pharmacol. 28, 326.

6. Stokes, J.B. and Kokko, J.P., (1977) J. Clin. Invest. 49, 1099.

7. Fine, L.J. and Trizna, W. (1977) Am. J. Physiol. 232, F383.

8. Stokes, J.B., (1979) J. Clin. Invest. 64, 495.

9. Iino, Y. and M. Imai, (1978) Biochem. J. 116, 421.

10. Higashihara, E., DuBose, T.D. Jr., and Kokko, J.P., (1978) Am. J. Physiol. 235, F219.

11. Stein, J.H., Osgood, R.W. and Kunau, R.T., Jr., (1976) J. Clin. Invest. 58, 767.

12. Frolich, J.C., Hollifield, J.W., Dormois, J.C., Frolich B.L., Seyberth, H., Michelakis, A.M. and Oates, J.A. (1976) Circ. Res. 39, 447.

13. Feldman, D., Loose, D.S. and Tan S.Y., Am. J. Physiol. 234, F490.

14. Altsheler, P., Klahr, S. Rosenbaum, R. and Slatopolsky, E. (1978) Am. J. Physiol. 235, F338.

15. Dray, F., Chardonnel, B. and Maclouf, J. (1975) Europ. J. Clin. Invest. 5, 311.

16. DuBose, T.D., Jr., Seldin, D.W. and Kokko, J.P. (1978) Am. J. Physiol. 234, F97.

17. Leyssac, P.P., Christensen, P., Hill, R. and Skinner S.L. (1975) Acta. Physiol. Scand. 94, 484.

18. Foman, R.J., Kauker, M.L. (1978) Am. J. Physiol. 235, F111.

19. Kokko, J.P. (1970) J. Clin. Invest. 49, 1838.

20. Chuang, E.L., Reineck, J., Osgood, R.W., Kunau, R.T., Jr. and Stein, J.H. J. Clin. Invest. 61, 633.

21. Ganguli, M., Tobian, L., Azar, S. and O'Donnel, M., (1977) Circ. Res. Suppl. 40, 1135.

Hormonal Regulation of Sodium Excretion,
B. Lichardus, R.W. Schrier and J. Ponec, eds.
© 1980 Elsevier/North-Holland Biomedical Press

RENAL MINERALOCORTICOID TARGET SITES

DIANA MARVER, MICHAEL J. SCHWARTZ, KEVIN PETTY, AND WILLIAM E. LOMBARD.
University of Texas Health Science Center, Depts. of Internal Medicine and
Biochemistry, Dallas, Texas 75235.

INTRODUCTION

The localization of mineralocorticoid target sites within the kidney remains unclear. Several indirect studies have suggested that both the cortex and outer medulla, but not papilla contain mineralocorticoid-sensitive cells. The data supporting this include the existence of mineralocorticoid-specific receptors in these two renal zones as well as enhanced incorporation of labeled amino acids into total protein in fractions obtained from the renal cortex and outer medulla of adrenalectomized rats following acute aldosterone administration[1-3]. However attempts to further define mineralocorticoid target sites within these broad regions, utilizing microperfusion or micropuncture techniques, have yielded conflicting results. An ultramicro enzyme assay for NaK ATPase activity along isolated nephrons has also been used in an attempt to define aldosterone target sites, but again, some results were discordant with in-vitro microperfusion data. Thus, posited sites have included the proximal convoluted tubule, the cortical thick ascending limb of Henle, the distal convoluted tubule, and the cortical collecting duct within the cortex, as well as an undefined region within the medulla[4-11].

Studies performed in the toad bladder have suggested that the condensing enzyme of the Krebs cycle, citrate synthase, may function as a marker of aldosterone activity. In this tissue, aldosterone increased citrate synthase activity with the same time course as the rise in short circuit current (SCC) and both of these parameters were inhibited by protein and RNA-synthesis inhibitors[12]. Furthermore, the incremental rise in SCC (equivalent to active Na^+ transport) mimicked the incremental rise in enzyme activity. This phenomenon did not appear to be secondary to changes in luminal Na^+ entry, as removal of mucosal Na^+ did not diminish the rise in citrate synthase activity even though it inhibited the rise in SCC. Additionally, vasopressin or a combination of cAMP and theophylline, agents known to stimulate Na^+ transport in this tissue, did not alter citrate synthase levels[13]. Therefore by a number of criteria, this enzyme appeared to be one of the specific proteins induced by aldosterone in the toad bladder.

Studies in the rat supported this proposal. Adrenalectomy reduced citrate synthase activity in the renal cortex and outer medulla, but not in the inner medulla. This reduced activity in adrenalectomized animals could be restored to normal levels by the injection of modest doses of aldosterone, while similar doses of dexamethasone were ineffective[14]. Furthermore, spirolactone blocked the aldosterone-stimulated rise in enzyme activity. Control studies showed that the increase in apparent enzyme activity was the result of a net increase in enzyme molecules, rather than the result of a change in the affinity of either of the substrates, oxaloacetate or acetyl coenzyme A. Therefore when antibodies directed against citrate synthase were used to titrate renal samples, the results confirmed those obtained by enzymatic assay: i.e. that adrenalectomy reduced citrate synthase levels and that this enzyme was elevated again after the acute administration of aldosterone. The inference was that aldosterone, by regulating citrate synthase levels in target cells, increased the flux of substrate through the Krebs cycle. This would result in an enhanced capacity to synthesize ATP, a necessary substrate for active transport.

Based on this information, we have examined the question of the localization of mineralocorticoid target sites along the rabbit nephron by utilizing an ultramicro assay for citrate synthase. Also based on foregoing data, special emphasis was given to sites within the renal cortex and outer medulla.

MATERIALS AND METHODS

New Zealand white female rabbits (1-2 kg) were used throughout the study. Adrenalectomy, where studied, was performed 1-2 weeks prior to sacrifice and during this time animals were maintained on saline drinking water. Adrenalectomized animals were given aldosterone or dexamethasone intravenously, 90 min. prior to sacrifice by decapitation. Spirolactone (SC 26304) was administered intraperitoneally 30 min. before administration of aldosterone.

Macro enzyme assays. Sonicates of renal mitochondrial fractions were prepared and assayed for citrate synthase activity, measuring the rate of product formation at 412 nm (28°C) in the presence of DTNB (5-5'-dithiobis-2-nitrobenzoic acid)[15]. Renal NaK ATPase activity was determined on microsomal fractions[16] of rabbit cortex and outer medulla (37°C) in the presence of 0.1% deoxycholate, 50mM NaCl, 5mM KCl, 3mM ATP and ± 2 mM ouabain. Proteins were assayed by the Lowry method[17].

Ultramicro enzyme assays. Individual nephron segments were dissected free-hand from a coronal slice of rabbit kidney placed in an electrolyte solution designed to simulate an ultrafiltrate of plasma[18]. Segments were identified and dissected as reported previously [19-21]. Following dissection, the iso- lated segments were rapidly rinsed with distilled water to remove excess salt and immediately frozen over dry ice. They were then lyophilized and finally maintained at -80C until ready for assay. On the day of enzymatic assay, the pieces were warmed to room temperature, further divided into 100 μm pieces, weighed on a quartz fiber balance and placed in a nl volume of reagent covered with oil to prevent evaporation[22]. Citrate synthase levels were determined using a method adapted from a procedure developed by Lowry and co-workers for single muscle fibers[23]. The general procedure is outlined in Fig. 1. Using this procedure, we found the assay to be linear with respect to time (0-30 min.), tubule weight (0-40 ng), and moles of citrate entered in step A (3-200 x 10^{-12} moles).

CITRATE SYNTHASE ASSAY

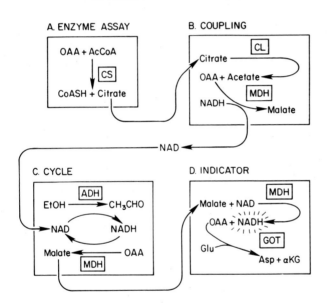

Fig. 1 The ultramicro assay for citrate synthase. Abbreviations used are OAA = oxaloacetate, AcCoA = acetyl coenzyme A, CoASH = coenzyme A, CS = citrate synthase, CL = bacterial citrate lyase, MDH = malate dehydrogenase, ADH = alcohol dehydrogenase, and GOT = glutamate-oxaloacetate transaminase.

RESULTS

Whole tissue studies. The citrate synthase activities for the mitochon- drial sonicates obtained from whole rabbit renal cortex and outer medulla are displayed in Table 1. The previously reported values of Law and Edelman for rat kidney are added for comparison. In the cortex, adrenalectomy produced a 14% and 13% decrease in citrate synthase activity in rabbit and rat, respectively.

TABLE 1
CHANGES IN CITRATE SYNTHASE (CS) AND NaK ATPase ACTIVITIES FOLLOWING ADRENALECTOMY

Tissue	Rat[a]		Rabbit			
	CS Act.[b]	%↓	CS Act.[b]	%↓	NaK ATPase Activity[c]	%↓
RENAL CORTEX						
Normals	0.46 ± 0.01		0.80 ± 0.07		34.0 ± 2.2	
Adx.	0.40 ± 0.01	13%	0.69 ± 0.04	14%	32.0 ± 9.7	6%
OUTER MEDULLA	p <0.001		p = N.S.		p = N.S.	
Normals	0.86 ± 0.02		0.95 ± 0.04		91.3 ± 10.4	
Adx.	0.69 ± 0.03	25%	0.78 ± 0.04	18%	47.9 ± 2.8	48%
LIVER	p <0.001		p<0.02		p <0.001	
Normals	0.16 ± 0.005		0.12 ± 0.005			
Adx.	0.15 ± 0.01		0.12 ± 0.005			
	p = N.S.		p = N.S.			

[a] Rat data from Law/Edelman, 1978[14].
[b] Citrate synthase activities are given in terms of units/mg protein at either 28°C. (rabbits) or room temp. (rats).
[c] NaK ATPase activities are given in terms of μmoles P_i/mg protein/hr (37°C). All values ± SEM. N = 5-8 for rabbits and 9 for rats.

Similarly, citrate synthase activity was reduced in the outer medulla by 18% in rabbit and 25% in rat post adrenalectomy. Enzyme activity of liver mitochondria, on the other hand, did not change in response to surgery in either animal. In comparison, renal cortical NaK ATPase activity in the rabbit was similar in microsomal fractions obtained from both normal and adrenalectomized rabbits, while there was a marked reduction (48%) in this enzyme level in outer medullary samples after adrenalectomy. [Mg ATPase values for these same rabbits were 54.8 ± 2.4 and 49.8 ± 1.1 for cortex, and 138 ± 13.7 and 114 ± 10.0 for outer medullary fractions (normal vs adx)]. A comparison of the NaK ATPase and citrate synthase data in these two zones suggests that there may be a qualitative difference between the effects of adrenalectomy upon these transport-related enzymes. Since some debate exists concerning the factor(s) responsible for modulation of renal NaK ATPase following corticoid with-drawal[24], citrate synthase was used as a preferable marker for possible aldo-sterone-sensitive sites in the rabbit cortex and outer medulla. Figure 2 schematically shows those portions of the rabbit nephron which are localized within the cortex and outer medulla.

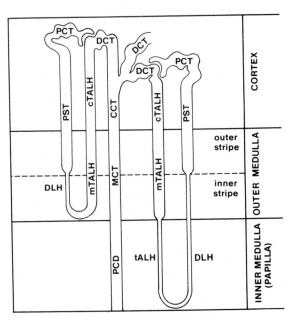

Fig. 2. .A schematic representation of the disposition of superficial and juxtamedullary nephrons within the kidney.

Enzyme analysis in isolated tubule segments. To define those sites in the cortical nephron which have decreased citrate synthase activity in response to adrenalectomy, this enzyme was assayed in tubule segments obtained from both normal and adrenalectomized rabbits. The results are displayed in Figure 3. Those segments assayed in the cortex were: proximal convoluted tubule, proxi-mal straight tubule, cortical thick ascending limb of Henle, distal convoluted tubule and the cortical collecting duct (CCT). Except for the proximal straight tubule, all of these have been postulated targets of aldosterone using a variety of techniques. Among the cortical segments, however, only collecting duct citrate synthase activity was significantly reduced by adrenalectomy. When aldosterone was replaced in physiological quantities,

234

citrate synthase activity in this segment was restored to control levels, while unchanged in the other segments of the cortex. On the other hand, replacement with dexamethasone did not significantly increase citrate synthase activity in the CCT above the adrenalectomized level. Lastly, if spirolactone was given prior to aldosterone administration, the rise in citrate synthase activity was abrogated. It is thus inferred that the sole target of aldosterone induced changes in citrate synthase activity within the renal cortex is the cortical collecting tubule.

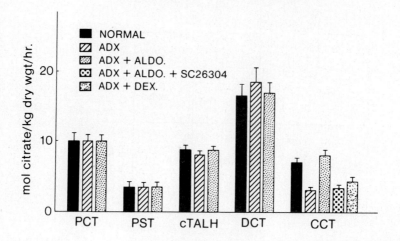

Fig. 3. Citrate synthase activities in various portions of the rabbit cortical nephron. The segments assayed were proximal convoluted tubule (PCT), proximal straight tubule (PST), thick ascending limb of Henle (cTALH), distal convoluted tubule (DCT), and cortical collecting tubule (CCT). Both aldosterone and dexamethasone were given (1 µg/100 gm body wgt) 90 min. prior to sacrifice. Spirolactone SC 26304 (150 µg/100 gm body wgt) was injected 30 min. before aldosterone. Results are ± SEM.

DISCUSSION

It is clear from physiologic measurements that the kidney is capable of responding to aldosterone by altering the transport of Na^+, K^+ and H^+. The site(s) at which these events take place have been difficult to define.

The whole tissue mitochondrial studies demonstrated that there is a 14%

decrease in citrate synthase activity in cortex and 18% decrease in outer medulla in response to adrenalectomy. This supports the concept that citrate synthase is a marker of adrenal hormone action as proposed previously. By examining individual cortical nephron segments it was further demonstrated that the cortical collecting tubule alone appeared to account for this reduced activity. In view of the relatively low proportion of cortical protein contributed by the cortical collecting duct, it is not surprising that there was only a small statistically insignificant reduction in citrate synthase activity of whole cortex after adrenalectomy. The fact that enzyme activity in the CCT was rapidly restored by physiological quantities of aldosterone administered 90 min. before sacrifice is strong evidence that the response of citrate synthase to adrenalectomy is not merely a non-specific response to the physiologic and morphometric developments of the adrenalectomized state. Thus we would conclude from these studies that the nephron segment which responds to aldosterone in the renal cortex, as monitored by citrate synthase, is the cortical collecting tubule. These findings correlate well with physiologic measurements of transepithelial voltage and sodium flux and ADH responsiveness measured in the same segment under varying mineralocorticoid status[7-9,25]. Studies are currently underway to examine the postulated target sites for aldosterone in the outer medulla, as well as the relationship between NaK ATP levels and adrenal steroids within the kidney.

ACKNOWLEDGEMENTS

Spirolactone SC 26304 was kindly supplied by the G.D. Searle Co. The studies noted in this paper were supported by National Institutes of Health grant number AM 21576. D.M. is an Established Investigator of the American Heart Association.

REFERENCES

1. Funder, J.W., Feldman, D. and Edelman, I.S. (1973) Endocrinology, 92, 994.

2. Marver, D. (1980) Endocrinology, 106, 611.

3. Law, P.Y., and Edelman, I.S. (1978) J. Membrane Biol., 41, 15.

4. Wiederholt, M. (1966) Pflugers Arch., 292, 334.

5. Wiederholt, M., Behn, C., Schoormans, W, and Hansen, L. (1972) J. Steroid Biochem., 3, 151.

6. Hierholzer, K., and Stolte, H. (1969) Nephron, 6, 188.

7. Gross, J.B., and Kokko, J.P. (1977) J. Clin. Invest., 59, 82.

8. Schwartz, G.J., and Burg, M.B. (1978) Am. J. Physiology, 235, F576.

9. O'Neil, R.G., and Helman, S.I. (1977) Am. J. Physiology, 233, F544.

10. Schmidt, U., Schmid, J., Schmid, H. and Dubach, U.C. (1975). J. Clin. Invest. 55, 655.

11. Horster, M., Schmid, H., and Schmidt, U. (1980). Pflugers Arch., 384, 203.

12. Kirsten, E., Kirsten, R., Leaf, A. and Sharp, G.W.G. (1968) Pflugers Arch., 300, 213.

13. Kirsten, E., Kirsten, R. and Sharp, G.W.G. (1970) Pflugers Arch., 316, 26.

14. Law, P.Y., and Edelman, I.S. (1978) J. Membrane Biol., 41, 41.

15. Srere, P.A., Brazil, and Gonen, L. (1963) Acta. Chem. Scand., 17, S129.

16. Lo, C.S., August, T.R., Liberman, U.A., and Edelman, I.S. (1976), J. Biol. Chem., 251, 7826.

17. Lowry, O.H., Rosenbrough, N.J., Farr, A.L. and Randall, R.J. (1951) J. Biol. Chem. 193, 265.

18. Stokes, J.B. and Kokko, J.P. (1977) J. Clin. Invest., 59, 1099.

19. Jacobson, H.R. and Kokko, J.P. (1976) J. Clin. Invest. 57, 818.

20. Kawamura, S., Imai, M., Seldin, D.W. and Kokko, J.P. (1975) J. Clin. Invest., 55, 1269.

21. Stokes, J.B. (1979) J. Clin. Invest. 64, 495.

22. Lowry, O.H. and Passonneau, J.V. (1972) A Flexible System of Enzymatic Analysis, Academic Press, New York, pp. 43-60 and 223-260.

23. Lowry, C.V., Kimmey, J.S., Felder, S., Chi, M. M-Y, Kaiser, K.K., Passonneau, P.N., Kirk, K.A. and Lowry, O.H. (1978) J. Biol. Chem., 253, 8269.

24. Marver, D., (1980) Vitamins and Hormones, Vol. 37, Academic Press N.Y., In press.

25. Schwartz, M.J. and Kokko, J.P. (1980) J. Clin. Invest., 65, In press.

KALLIKREIN-KININ SYSTEM

Hormonal Regulation of Sodium Excretion,
B. Lichardus, R.W. Schrier and J. Ponec, eds.
© 1980 Elsevier/North-Holland Biomedical Press

THE REGULATION OF URINARY KININ EXCRETION

GARY L. ROBERTSON AND MARY L. CONDER
University of Chicago, Pritzker School of Medicine, and the V. A. Hospital,
Indianapolis, Indiana

INTRODUCTION

After many years of comparative neglect, the kallikrein kinin system is receiving increased attention from a variety of basic and clinical scientists. This upsurge of investigative interest was spawned by advances in methods for measuring various components of the system and a growing awareness of its potential importance in the regulation of many vital biologic processes. Of particular concern to students of fluid and electrolyte homeostasis is that part of the kallikrein-kinin system located in the kidney. Though still quite sketchy, our knowledge about the actions of this system raises a number of intriguing questions about its role in the control of important variables such as salt and water excretion or blood pressure[1]. Most of this information is based upon measurements of urinary kallikrein, a protease that cleaves a peptide precursor (kininogen) to generate the biologically active kinins[2]. However, serious questions have arisen about the accuracy with which some of these assays reflect intrinsic kinin levels[3]. Recently, radioimmunoassays have been developed which provide simple and sensitive methods for measuring the kinins directly. These new methods and the altered perspective on the role of kinins in renal function which they are providing are the subject of this review.

CHEMISTRY

In man and other mammals, the kinins occur in three forms which differ only by the addition of one or two amino acid residues on the N-terminus of the molecule (Figure 1). Bradykinin (BK), the shortest peptide, is the principal kinin of plasma. Lysyl-bradykinin (1-BK or kallidin) is found chiefly in urine which also contains variable amounts of BK[4]. Metlysylbradykinin (ml-BK) has also been found in urine, but it appears to be an artifact formed by the action of uropepsin when strong acids are added as a preservative[4]. Besides kinins, urine also contains kallikrein[2], kininogen[5], and kininases[6]. Consequently, it is prudent to treat samples in such a way as to prevent the formation and/or

```
         1   2   3   4   5   6   7   8   9
   H-Arg-Pro-Pro-Gly-Phe-Ser-Pro-Phe-Arg-OH
                 Bradykinin
```

```
   H-Lys-Arg-Pro-Pro-Gly-Phe-Ser-Pro-Phe-Arg-OH
                  Kallidin
```

```
   H-Met-Lys-Arg-Pro-Pro-Gly-Phe-Ser-Pro-Phe-Arg-OH
               Metlysylbradykinin
```

```
   Arg-Pro-Pro-Gly-Phe-Ser-Pro-Tyr-Arg-OH
               Tyr-8-Bradykinin
```

Fig. 1. Primary structure of mammalian kinins and a kinin analogue which can be iodinated and used as tracer in radioimmunoassay.

degradation of kinins during storage and/or processing.   The combination of immediate acidification and refrigeration or extraction is usually satisfactory, although some workers also add inhibitors of kallikrein uropepsin and/or kininase. In urine and other protein poor fluids, kinins may also be lost by adsorption on the wall of the collection vessel. This adsorption is greatest at neutral and alkaline pH and, in the case of glass, incompletely prevented by presence of carrier proteins (Conder, M. L., Alexander, R., and Robertson, G. L., unpublished observations). Therefore, samples should always be collected, processed and assayed entirely in plastic and kept at pH 4 whenever carrier proteins are absent.

ASSAY

   For many years, the only methods available for measuring kinins were bioassays. These methods were cumbersome, insensitive, and of dubious specificity. Recently, several laboratories have succeeded in developing radioimmunoassays which are much simpler to perform and several orders of magnitude more sensitive[7-16]. These advances were made possible by the introduction of methods

for enhancing bradykinin antigenicity by coupling it to larger molecules[7] and
for preparing a radioiodinated tracer by substituting tyrosine for phenylalanine
in the 8 (or 5) position of the molecule (Figure 1)[9]. These techniques as well
as improved methods for purifying ^{125}I-tyr-BK by Sephadex chromatography
(Figures 2 and 3) have made it possible to develop radioimmunoassays capable of

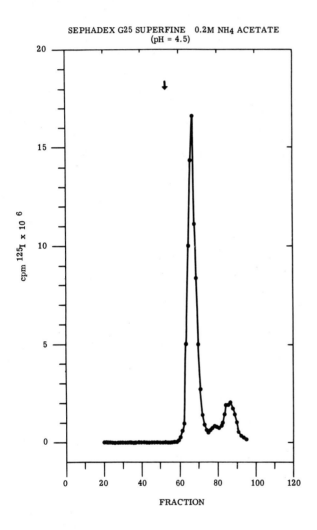

SEPHADEX G25 SUPERFINE   0.2M NH4 ACETATE
(pH = 4.5)

cpm ^{125}I x 10^6

FRACTION

Fig. 2. Sephadex G-25
elution profile of
^{125}I-tyr-8-BK prepared
and purified as pre-
viously described (9).
Note that the gel fil-
tration in Walpole's
acetate, pH = 4.5, with
0.5 mg/ml crystalline
lysozyme separates the
^{125}I-tyr-8-BK (tall
peak) from residual
radioactive contami-
nants (low trailing
peak) as well as un-
reacted ^{125}I-tyr-8-BK
(vertical arrow).

detecting as little as 2 pg of BK and other kinins (Figure 4.) Many of these
assays also react slightly with kininogen which, therefore, must be eliminated
prior to assay. The simplest and most widely used approach is to selectively
precipitate the kininogen by extraction with an organic solvent such as ace-

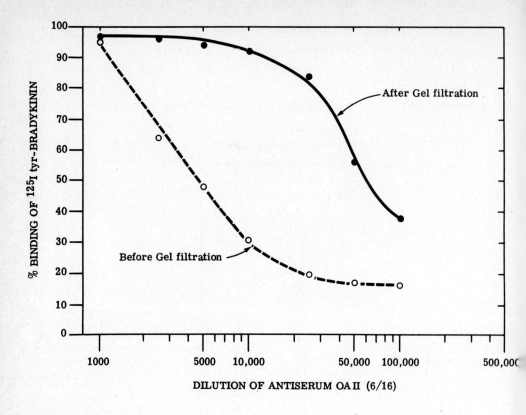

Fig. 3. Effect of Sephadex chromatography on proportion of ^{125}I-tyr-8-BK bound by serial dilutions of one BK-antiserum. Note that chromatograpjic purification of the tracer permits the use of more dilute antiserum, thereby providing greater assay sensitivity.

tone[16] or ethanol[16]. Alternatively, kinins and kininogens may be separated by more elaborate methods such as gel filtration or ion exchange chromatography[3, 4, 5]. All these methods have the added advantage of eliminating kininases, thereby removing another potential immunoassay artifact caused by tracer "damage". As noted above, immediate elimination of kininogen and kininases also removes the possibility of artifacts due to production and/or degradation of kinins in the sample before and during the assay procedures.

These techniques have been successfully applied to measure basal and/or kallikrein-generated kinins in urine[12-16]. All of these assays cross-react equally well with BK, 1-BK and ml-BK and thus reflect total urinary kinins. However, they vary considerably in their susceptibility to kininogen and/or other nonkinin constituents of urine. One assay has been used without extrac-

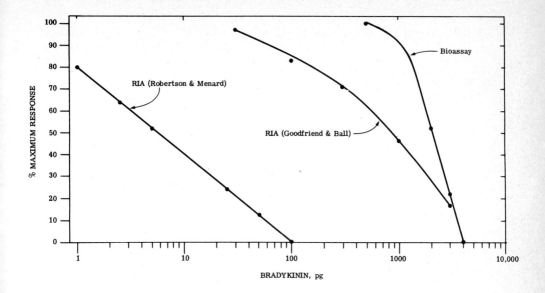

Fig. 4. Relative sensitivities of a typical bioassay and two immunoassays. Note the improvement achieved with the first immunoassay (9) and even greater sensitivities possible with current methods (Robertson, G. and Menard, J., unpublished observations).

tion because Sephadex chromatography of raw urine revealed no immunoreactivity distinguishable from BK^{12}. On the other hand, using a different assay[16] and a more highly resolving chromatographic system[4], we consistently find significant amounts of nonkinin immunoactivity in unextracted urine (Table 1). Extraction with acetone completely eliminates the nonkinin immunoactivity but leaves unchanged the other 2 peaks which cochromatograph with standard BK and $1-BK^{16}$. This acetone soluble activity also cross-reacts in parallel with standard BK and is rapidly and completely destroyed by incubation with kininase[16]. Hence, combining acetone extraction with our radioimmunoassay appears to provide an accurate measure of total intact endogenous urinary kinins.

These observations make it clear that careful characterization of urine immunoactivity seen by each assay system is a prerequisite for meaningful study of urinary kinins. Chromatographic systems capable of resolving ml-BK from the other two kinins are especially useful in this regard because absence of the former also reassures that results are not being distorted by artifacts due to the action of uropepsin.

244

TABLE 1

Elution profile of immunorcactivity from unextracted urines during gradient-
elution ion-exchange chromatography on CM Sephadex C25 (4). Varying amounts
of immunoactivity consistently are recovered in the void volume widely separated from that which elutes in positions identical to standard BK (Peak 1) or
l-BK (Peak 3). No activity is ever detectable in the elution position of
standard ml-BK (Peak 2).

Urine	Void	Peak 1 (BK)	Peak 2 (ml-BK) ng/ml	Peak 3 (1-BK)
1.	12.1	0.2	< 0.1	7.1
2.	1.6	19.7	"	1.8
3.	31.0	< 0.1	"	41.8
4.	16.6	"	"	8.0
5.	1.0	1.9	"	3.8
6.	1.3	< 0.1	"	2.7
7.	7.1	"	"	6.3
8.	0.9	10.5	"	0.3
9.	0.1	0.1	"	< 0.1
10.	3.0	< 0.1	"	1.9
11.	1.9	0.4	"	6.5
12.	0.2	2.3	"	< 0.1
13.	0.1	1.3	"	0.4
Mean	5.9	2.8	< 0.1	6.2
± SE	2.5	1.6	0	3.1

ORIGINS

Urinary kinins appear to originate in the distal and/or collecting tubules
of the nephron[17]. Normally, none are derived by glomerular filtration since
direct infusion of BK into the renal artery does not increase urinary kinins[18].
Moreover, BK injected into the proximal tubule is promptly destroyed while that
injected into the distal tubule is recovered intact[19]. This is probably due to
the high level of kininase activity in the brush border of the proximal convoluted tubules[20] since urine and plasma kinins do change in parallel if kininase
inhibitor is infused simultaneously with BK in the renal artery[18].

The kinins that arise in the distal nephron probably are formed *de novo* in
the kidney. Kallikrein is present in renal tissue[21], particularly in the distal
tubules[22] and its substrate, low molecular kininogen, is also present in
urine[5]. *De novo* renal origin of urinary kinins also is attested by the preponderance of 1-BK (Table 1). Unlike plasma kallikrein which cleaves kininogen
in such a way as to release only BK, the renal kallikrein produces l-BK which
is subsequently converted to BK in urine by a ubiquitous amino-peptidase. The
fact that urinary kallikreins and kinins both originate in the distal nephron[17]

further supports this concept. However, stop flow studies also have shown that urinary kinins arise in two locations, the largest and more distal of which is not associated with significant increase in urinary kallikrein[17]. This partial dissociation suggests that the rate of *de novo* formation may not be the only or even the major determinant of urinary kinins, a possibility also suggested by recent studies of factors that influence the rate of excretion of the two substances.

REGULATION

In healthy adults on a normal diet, the rate of excretion of urinary kinins averages from 11 to 38 µg/day[4, 12, 15] or about 25 µg per mg of creatinine[16]. Allowing for individual and genetic variation as well as differences in the standards and methods of collection, extraction and assay used in the various laboratories, the reported values agree reasonably well. When related to creatinine[4, 16], the rate of kinin excretion is similar in men and women and does not appear to be influenced by posture or activity[16]. It is also un-affected by changes in sodium and potassium intake or the administration of mineralocorticoids, all of which cause pronounced changes in kallikrein ex-cretion. However, we found recently that the rate of kinin excretion is signi-ficantly depressed by water loading[16]: From a mean basal value around 25 µg/mg creatinine, kinin excretion falls in parallel with plasma and urinary osmola-lity, reaching a nadir averaging about 3 µg/mg creatinine at the height of the water diuresis. As the water load is excreted and plasma and urine osmolality return to basal values, the rate of kinin excretion also returns to normal. Interestingly, water loading does not depress urinary kallikreins[24], suggesting that some other factor such as an increase in kininase activity might be re-sponsible for the fall in kinins.

In patients with familial neurogenic diabetes insipidus, we also found that kinin excretion is low before treatment but rises to normal along with urine osmolality following injection of aqueous Pitressin[16]. These observations and the changes produced by water loading suggest that the rate of kinin excretion may be regulated in part by changes in plasma vasopressin. However, alternative possibilities must be considered because Pitressin may be contaminated with other pituitary hormones, like oxytocin or β-endorphin, which also can respond to changes in hydration. Moreover, we recently observed a patient with severe neurogenic diabetes insipidus in whom prolonged fluid deprivation increased the rate of kinin excretion to normal without raising either plasma vasopressin or or urine osmolality (Robertson, G. L., and Conder, M. L., unpublished observations). This finding clearly indicates that total kinin excretion also may be significantly influenced by one or more factors which lack antidiuretic action yet can respond to modest changes in the tonicity and/or volume of body fluids. Aldosterone stimulation of renal kallikrein cannot be excluded because the lack of kinin effect observed previously[23] might have been due to relatively large and possibly offsetting contributions from adjacent sites sensitive to vasopressin or other stimuli (*vide infra*).

Essential hypertension appears to be one condition associated with parallel reductions in urinary kallikrein and kinins[12, 25]. The cause of this depression is unknown. Renal damage *per se* might be responsible for the decrease in urinary kinins since the latter are also low in patients with renal transplants and chronic glomerulonephritis[12].

FUNCTION

The effect of urinary kinins on renal function in man continues to elude precise definition. The major obstacle is that the kinins are administered experimentally via the renal artery and, therefore, may not duplicate either the levels or the site of action of those formed in the distal and collecting tubules or urine. Nevertheless, there is a large and varied body of circumstantial evidence that renal kinins increase water and electrolyte excretion as well as blood flow in the kidney[26]. These actions may be mediated at least in part by renal prostaglandins since the latter not only are stimulated by kinins[27] but can also mimic many of the renal effects of kinins[28]. Of particular interest in this regard is the ability of both prostaglandin E and kinin to inhibit vasopressin-induced hydroosmotic permeability in toad bladders[29, 30]. When coupled with the probable effect of vasopressin on urinary kinins[16], these observations suggest the operation of a local or short loop feedback system which serves to attenuate the antidiuretic effects of vasopressin.

Fig. 5. Hypothetical Scheme of Kinin Regulation and Action in Collecting Tubule

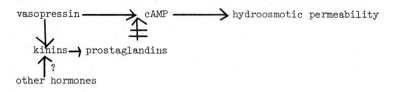

This scheme obviously cannot account for the putative naturetic effect of urinary kinins. However, the latter can be accommodated by postulating the second site of kinin formation and action that is proximal to the collecting tubule, responds to aldosterone instead of vasopressin and inhibits sodium readsorption rather than water permeability. Such duality of urinary kinin regulation and action in the nephron is consistent with the stop flow data showing two sites of formation, only one of which was associated with kallikrein formation[17] and the apparent dissociation of urinary kallikrein and kinin changes during water loading (*vide supra*) and mineralocorticoid administration[23]. This hypothesis lends itself to several predictions that can easily be tested. If verified, it would have significant implications for further studies of the renal-kallikrein-kinin system in normal and disordered states of salt and water balance.

REFERENCES

1. Margolius, H.S. (1978) J. Lab. Clin. Med., 91, 717-720.

2. Margolius, H.S., Horwitz, D., Pisano, J.J., and Keiser, H.R. (1976) Proceedings of the Federation of American Societies for Experimental Biology, 35, 203-206.

3. Levinsky, N.G., ole-MoiYoi, O., Austen, K.F., and Spragg, J. (1979) Biochem. Pharmacol., 28, 2491-2495.

4. Hial, V., Keiser, H.R., and Pisano, J.J. (1976) Biochem. Pharmacol., 25, 2499-2503.

5. Pisano, J.J., Yates, K., and Pierce, J.V. (1978) Agents and Actions, 8, 153.

6. Erdös, E.G., Sloane, E.M., and Wohler, I.M. (1964) Biochem. Pharmacol., 13, 893-905.

7. Talamo, R.C., Haber, E., and Austen, K.F. (1968) J.Immunol., 101, 333-341.

8. Talamo, R.C., Haber, E., and Austen, K.F. (1969) J. Lab. Clin. Med. 74, 816.

9. Goodfriend, T.L. and Ball, D.L. (1969) J. Lab. Clin. Med. 73, 501-511.

10. Mashford, M.L., and Roberts, M.L. (1972) Biochem. Pharmacol. 21, 2727-2735.

11. Hulthen, U.L., and Borge, T. (1976) Scand. J. Lab. Invest. 36, 833-839.

12. Shimamoto, K., Ando, T., Nakao, T., Tanaka, S., Sakuma, M., and Miyahara, M. (1978) J. Lab. Clin. Med. 91, 721-728.

13. Carretero, O.A., Oza, N.B., Piwonska, A., Ocholik, T., and Scicli, A.G. (1976) Biochem. Pharmacol. 25, 2265-2270.

14. Stocker, M. and Hornung, J. (1978) Klin. Wochenschr. 56 (Suppl. 1), 127-129.

15. Vinci, J.M., Gill, J.R., Jr., Bowden, R.E., Pisano, J.J., Izzo, J.L., Jr., Radfar, N., Taylor, A.A., Zusman, R.M., Bartter, F.C., and Keiser, H.R. (1978) J. Clin. Invest. 61, 1671-1682

16. Robertson, G.L. and Conder, M.L. (1980) Clin. Res. 28, 454A.

17. Scicli, A.G., Gandolfi, R., and Carretero, O.A. (1978) Am. J. Physiol. 234, F36-40.

18. Nasjletti, A., Colina-Chourio, J., and McGill, J.C. (1975) Circ. Res. 37, 59-65.

19. Carone, F.A., Pullman, T.N., Oparil, S., Nakamura, S. (1976) Am. J. Physiol. 230, 1420-1424.

20. Ward, P.E., Gedney, C.D., Dowben, R.M., Erdös̈t, E.G. (1975) Biochem. J. 151, 755-758.

21. Pisano, J.J. (1975) Proteases and Biological Control, Cold Spring Harbor Conference on Cell Proliferation 2, 199-222.

22. Orstavik, T.B., Nostad, K., Brandtzaeg, P., and Pierce, J.V. (1976) J. Histochem. Cytochem. 24, 1037-1039.

23. Vinci, J.M., Zusman, R.M., Izzo, J.L., Jr., Bowden, R.E., Horwitz, D., Pisano, J.J., and Keiser, H.R. (1979) Circ. Res. 44, 228-237.

24. Croxatto, H.R., Huidobro, F., Rojas, M., Roblero, J., Albertini, R. (1975) Advan. Exp. Med. Biol. 70, 361-373.

25. Margolius, H.S., Horwitz, D., Pisano, J.J., Keiser, H.R. (1974) Circ. Res. 35, 820-825.

26. Levinsky, N.G. (1979) Circ. Res. 44, 442-451.

27. Nasjletti, A., and Colina-Chourio, J. (1976) Proceedings of the Federation of American Societies for Experimental Biology 35, 189-193.

28. Dunn, M.J., and Hood, V.L. (1977) Am. J. Physiol. 233, F169-184.

29. Lipson, L.C., and Sharp, G.W.G. (1971) Am. J. Physiol. 220, 1046-1052.

30. Furtado, M.R.F. (1971) J. Membr. Biol. 4, 165-178.

Hormonal Regulation of Sodium Excretion,
B. Lichardus, R.W. Schrier and J. Ponec, eds.
© 1980 Elsevier/North-Holland Biomedical Press

PARTIAL RESTORATION OF NATRIURESIS BY VASOPRESSIN DURING RAISED KALLIKREIN
EXCRETION PRODUCED BY WATER LOADING IN DOGS: RELATIONSHIP TO THE NATRIURETIC
HORMONAL CASCADE

IVOR H. MILLS and PAMELA A. NEWPORT
Department of Medicine, University of Cambridge, Cambridge, CB2 2QQ, England

Volume expansion by infusion of saline operates by two factors in increasing
sodium excretion; one is the effect of dilution of the blood and the other is
the effect of volume expansion[1,2]. The dilution factor has been shown to
operate in entirely isolated perfused kidneys[3,4]. This indicates that an intrarenal mechanism can respond to dilution of the perfusing blood by increasing
sodium excretion, when no other tissues are in the circuit to alter the
constituents of the blood.

The afferent pathway which is stimulated by volume expansion could be the
atrial receptors with their pathway up the vagus, receptors in the heart with
their pathway to the spinal cord via the first four sympathetic rami, or
arterial baroceptors whose afferents arise from the aortic arch or carotid
arteries.

Gauer and Henry[5] first indicated that stretch of the atria increased urine
flow which they thought was by decrease in ADH secretion. Subsequently they
proved their supposition[6]. Goetz and his colleagues carried out extensive
experiments on the role of the atria in the regulation of salt and water
excretion. They reviewed the subject[7] and came to the conclusion that
alteration of the pressure on the atria from fluid in a pericardial atrial pouch
they constructed, could not be relied upon to produce alteration in stimuli
arising from the atria alone. Usually a change in arterial baroceptor
stimulation also occurred.

Linden and his colleagues have shown that stretch of the atria by a balloon
in the appendix increased urine flow. The effect was abolished by cutting the
vagi. When one kidney was perfused via plastic tubes it also responded to
atrial stretch by increased urine flow[8]. However, their conclusion that the
renal response is due to an alteration in a circulating substance is only
valid if one includes the other normal and still innervated kidney as a possible
source of the active substance which affects the isolated, perfused kidney.
They have now shown that atrial stretch increases the levels of a plasma
component which can inhibit the secretion by the Malpighian tubules of the

blood-sucking Hemipteran Rhodnius[9].

Apart from the implications of Goetz and his colleagues[7] that arterial baroceptors probably play a part in the response of the kidney to changes in blood volume, more direct evidence arises from the studies of Keeler[10]. Stimulation of carotid baroceptors by stretch led to natriuresis and increased urine flow in rats loaded with ADH. When the upper six thoracic sympathetic rami were destroyed bilaterally in dogs and hypertension produced by a Page-type kidney, the blood volume was always 20% above control values[11]. This may indicate that these nervous pathways play some role in volume regulation.

During volume expansion with dextran, Schad and Seller[12] showed clearly a decrease in the nerve traffic down the renal nerves. Further evidence on this has now been presented by Linden et al[13]. On the contrary, it has been shown by Bello-Reuss et al[14] and by Zambraski et al[15] that stimulation of the renal nerves can decrease sodium excretion without change in glomerular filtration rate. If one intact and innervated kidney is present during volume expansion, it can be the source of an active circulating substance affecting a denervated kidney. So far, no volume expansion studies have been carried out when the animal had only denervated kidneys. Marin-Grez et al[16] showed that the free bradykinin in the plasma of dogs rises during saline infusion into the stomach, but only if the kidneys are intact. This suggests that volume expansion released renal kallikrein into the circulation to increase the bradykinin levels. Clearly, this is an example of an active circulating substance responding to volume expansion but arising from the kidney itself.

The same argument applies to the cross-circulation between rats carried out by Pearce and his colleagues[17]. Rats treated with DOCA were cross-circulated with rats on a low salt diet. The latter did not have a natriuresis with blood volume expansion before the cross-circulation but did afterwards. The DOCA animals transferred an active substance to the salt deprived rats but there is no evidence as to the source of the substance and it could have been the kidneys of the DOCA treated animals.

Lichardus and his colleagues produced evidence that the posterior pituitary was the source of an active substance which enabled a rat to respond to volume expansion by natriuresis[18]. Physiological doses of ADH did not restore the response to volume expansion but Lichardus has now stated that the amounts of ADH in the posterior pituitary are enough to enable the hypophysectomised rats to respond normally to volume expansion (Personal communication).

It has been pointed out[19] that unilateral natriuresis can be effected in a variety of ways and particularly by wrapping one kidney in latex during volume expansion. This manoeuvre does not prevent the increase in C_{PAH} and C_{IN} during rapid saline infusion but it markedly decreases the sodium excretion and the excretion of kallikrein from the wrapped kidney[20]. This indicates that it is unlikely that volume expansion releases into the circulation a natriuretic substance which can act directly on the renal tubules. It could, however, act via a mechanism sensitive to changes in intra-renal vascular pressure (such as substance P[21]).

Intra-renal natriuretic mechanisms

Dopamine. Volume expansion with saline was shown by Alexander et al[22] and by Faucheux et al[23] to increase dopamine excretion in the urine. The latter workers showed that the rise in dopamine excretion could not be explained by increased clearance from the plasma. Baines and Chan[24] have shown that a denervated kidney can excrete radio-active dopamine from labelled dopa injected under the capsule. Most of the labelled dopamine appeared in the urine of the injected kidney.

Ball and Lee[25] demonstrated that the dopa decarboxylase inhibitor carbidopa decreased sodium excretion in normal subjects. They have since shown that changing sodium intake in normal subjects produces a corresponding change in dopamine excretion.

Dopamine is well known to be natriuretic[26]. When given intra-arterially to dogs the natriuresis was correlated with the rise in kallikrein excretion in the urine. This stimulation could be blocked by haloperidol but not with α and β-adrenergic inhibitors[27].

It appears, therefore, that changes in oral or intravenous sodium intake change renal dopamine excretion; that this may not require the renal nerves to be intact and that the natriuretic action of dopamine is associated with renal kallikrein release. How the increased sodium status is communicated to the kidney is unknown.

Renal kallikrein/kinin system

Renal kallikrein resembles glandular-type kallikreins and is closely similar to urinary kallikrein[28]. It enters the urine at a point in the tubule corresponding to the distal tubule[29] and has been shown by immuno-fluorescence to be in the tubule cells beyond the macula densa[30]. Besides entering the urine it also is released into the renal lymph, at a rate which correlates with its release into the urine during volume expansion[31].

A relationship between kallikrein excretion and sodium excretion was first suggested by Marin-Grez and Carretero[32] in rats and by Adetuyibi and Mills[33] in man. The relationship in rats on a free sodium intake was confirmed by Mills et al[20] and was shown in rabbits on a free sodium intake by Mills and Ward[34]. The latter workers showed that the relationship of sodium intake and kallikrein excretion depends upon a volume mechanism because altering sodium intake with constant water intake does not change kallikrein excretion.

The relation between kallikrein and sodium excretion is a complex one when one considers the sodium depletion end of the salt intake spectrum. Sodium depletion in man increases kallikrein excretion[35,36] as it does also in the rat[37,38]. It has been suggested by Mills[39] that at the lowest end of the sodium scale kallikrein is stimulated by the renin/angiotensin system: as sodium intake rises the kallikrein excretion falls and then rises again when kallikrein excretion is related to sodium excretion.

Kallikrein excretion is directly related to renal artery pressure[40]. When angiotensin is initially infused into the renal artery, the kallikrein excretion falls as the renal artery is constricted. Angiotensin stimulates the release of prostaglandin E (PGE) from the kidney[41]. Prostaglandin E_1 infused into the renal artery stimulates release of kallikrein[42]. It is probably this mechanism which leads to tachyphyllaxis of the renal vessels to angiotensin. If the dose of angiotensin is high enough to produce hypertension, the direct pressure effect stimulates the release of more kallikrein and natriuresis occurs[43]. If a constriction on the renal artery prevents the hypertension affecting the infused renal artery, the kallikrein excretion remains low, the renal vasculature does not develop tachyphyllaxis and sodium excretion falls[44].

If indomethacin is superimposed on arterial infusion of angiotensin at 5 μg per minute, it suppresses the natriuresis and the kallikrein excretion[45]. Similarly if noradrenaline is infused at 2 μg per minute into the same renal artery as the angiotensin at 5 μg per minute, vasoconstriction occurs and decreased sodium and kallikrein excretion[46].

Very small doses of noradrenaline (10 ng per minute) infused into the renal artery increase kallikrein excretion and produce a natriuresis[47]. Both effects are blocked by indomethacin, indicating that the effect is due to the PGE, which noradrenaline releases[41], causing release of kallikrein.

Margolius and his colleagues[48] have suggested that aldosterone directly stimulates kallikrein release from the kidney. Mills[49] has discussed in detail why this is unlikely to be true, although chronic administration of sodium-retaining steroids increases kallikrein excretion as the "escape" phase develops[33]. More recently we have shown that infusion of aldosterone into the

renal artery of the dog does not stimulate kallikrein release in acute
experiments (Mills and Newport, unpublished observations).

In summary, kallikrein release into the urine is stimulated by volume
expansion with saline and this mechanism probably involves stimulation of renal
dopamine release. Kallikrein excretion rises with increase in renal artery
pressure and falls with decrease in pressure. All renal artery vasodilators
tested increase kallikrein release[21,50] and presumably act via this pressure
mechanism. Angiotensin in natriuretic doses acts partly via release of PGE
which stimulates kallikrein release, and partly by a direct pressure effect
once hypertension develops.

Natriuretic hormones

The kallikrein/kinin system in the kidney appears to be directly involved in
the natriuretic mechanism. However, it is stimulated under two conditions when
natriuresis does not occur. One is in sodium depletion[35] and the other is in
glomerulo-nephritis, in rats[51].

However, the administration of antibodies to bradykinin markedly decreases
the natriuresis of volume expansion[52] and administration of aprotinin
(Trasylol), which inhibits renal kallikrein, to volume expanded rats sharply
decreased the sodium excretion[53]. These facts indicate that the renal
kallikrein/kinin system is part of the natriuretic chain of hormones.

Godon has shown that renal tubular fragments from a salt loaded rat in
tissue culture produce a large molecular weight natriuretic substance which in
assay rats increases the fraction of filtered sodium which is excreted[54]. This
substance is not produced by kidneys of salt-depleted animals nor rats with
glomerulo-nephritis. The molecular weight of the active substance is about
40,000 daltons.

de Wardener and his colleagues have shown that two active natriuretic
fractions occur in human urine[55]. The large molecular weight one has a delayed
and prolonged action: the small molecular weight one has an immediate and
shorter lived action in the assay water-loaded rat. It seems likely that the
larger molecular weight substance leads to the formation of the smaller.

Gonick and Saldanha[56] isolated a small molecular weight substance from
kidneys of saline loaded rats after boiling the kidneys. The material inhibits
Na/K ATPase.

The natriuretic hormonal cascade is shown in figure 1. Inhibiting factors
are shown on the left and stimulating factors on the right. The main
biological inhibiting factor is noradrenaline or renal nerve stimulation.

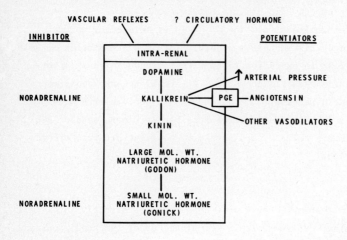

RESPONSE TO VOLUME EXPANSION WITH SALINE

Fig. 1.   The natriuretic hormonal cascade

TABLE 1

CHANGES PRODUCED BY I.V. INFUSION OF 2.5% GLUCOSE — PLASMA

| | Control | \multicolumn{5}{c}{Duration of infusion} | | | | |
		10	30	50	70	90
Plasma						
n	12	5	5	5	5	5
Osmolality	300	− 5	− 10	− 13	− 14	− 11
(m-osmole/kg)	± 3	± 2	± 4	± 4	± 5	± 4
P		n.s.	n.s.	< 0.05	< 0.05	< 0.05
Sodium	143.1	− 0.6	− 4.3	− 3.5	− 4.3	− 3.2
(m-equiv/l)	± 0.7	± 0.8	± 0.9	± 1.4	± 1.9	± 1.3
P		n.s.	< 0.01	n.s.	n.s.	n.s.
P.C.V.(%)	45.9	− 1.9	− 2.6	− 2.3	− 1.8	− 0.9
	± 1.2	± 0.4	± 0.7	± 0.7	± 0.9	± 0.7
P		< 0.01	< 0.02	< 0.05	n.s.	n.s.

Values are means ± S.E.
P.C.V., packed cell volume
(After Mills and Newport, 1979)[57]

255

Volume expansion with 2.5% glucose

In dogs under pentobarbitone anaesthesia with ureters catheterised and inulin and PAH infused for clearance purposes, 2.5% glucose was infused intravenously at 0.35 ml/kg/minute. At this rate glycosuria rarely was detected.

The changes in plasma osmolality, sodium concentration and packed cell volume are shown in Table 1[57]. The osmolality fell significantly below control values by 50 minutes of infusion and remained significantly lower. On the other hand the sodium concentration was significantly below control values only in the samples taken at 30 minutes of infusion.

The packed cell volume had fallen by the end of 10 minutes of infusion and at the end of 70 minutes was no longer different from control values.

The effects on urine flow and sodium and kallikrein excretion are shown in Table 2[57]. Though urine flow rose significantly by 20-40 minutes of infusion, the sodium excretion fell and was significantly below control values after 40 minutes.

Kallikrein excretion rose steadily and reached a plateau from 60 to 100 minutes of infusion. The rise in kallikrein excretion, therefore, occurs with volume expansion with either saline or 2.5% glucose. It would appear to be a response to the volume expansion rather than the nature of the infused solution. Since kallikrein, when infused intravenously, markedly increased vascular permeability[58], it is probable that the response of the renal kallikrein represents a mechanism to maintain a dynamic equilibrium in the circulation. This would fit in with the response of the packed cell volume and sodium concentration in the plasma which were not significantly different from control values when the kallikrein excretion was at a plateau in the last 40 minutes of infusion.

The depression of the natriuretic response must presumably act at a point beyond the kallikrein/kinin system in the natriuretic chain in the kidney. To test if this was affected by suppression of plasma vasopressin, we infused vasopressin into one renal artery in a further series of experiments, at doses between 0.5 and 50 μ units per minute, once the urine flow had reached its plateau.

The results are shown in Table 3[59]. Although this dose of vasopressin had no effect on inulin clearance, urine flow or urinary osmolality, it increased sodium excretion significantly. This was not associated with any further change in kallikrein excretion.

The sodium excretion was still very far short of that seen with volume expansion with saline, when comparable rises in kallikrein excretion occur.

TABLE 2

CHANGES PRODUCED BY I.V. INFUSION OF 2.5% GLUCOSE - URINE

	Control	Infusion periods				
		1,2	3,4	5,6	7,8	9,10
n	18	12	12	12	12	12
Flow	0.54	0.15	0.71	2.26	3.85	4.78
(ml/min)	± 0.07	± 0.10	± 0.29	± 0.52	± 0.53	± 0.56
P		n.s.	< 0.05	< 0.005	< 0.001	< 0.001
Sodium	93.3	8.4	- 3.0	- 38.7	- 42.7	- 40.3
(μ-equiv/min)	± 9.4	± 11.1	± 15.7	± 13.4	± 13.3	± 13.7
P		n.s.	n.s.	< 0.02	< 0.01	< 0.02
Kallikrein	36.5	7.0	31.2	77.7	162.6	176.3
(m-EU/min)	± 4.4	± 4.7	± 11.4	± 14.1	± 19.6	± 22.3
P		n.s.	< 0.02	< 0.001	< 0.001	< 0.001
Osmolality	941	- 78	-259	-666	-824	-856
(m-osmole/kg)	± 86	± 33	± 66	±108	±108	±106
P		< 0.05	< 0.005	< 0.005	< 0.005	< 0.005
C_{IN}	64.4	0	4.0	1.9	- 4.4	- 4.2
(ml/min)	± 5.5	± 2.4	± 1.8	± 3.4	± 4.1	± 4.7
P		n.s.	< 0.05	n.s.	n.s.	n.s.
C_{PAH}	170	5	32	22	- 10	- 25
(ml/min)	± 14	± 12	± 13	± 13	± 10	± 11
P		n.s.	< 0.05	n.s.	n.s.	< 0.05

Values are means ± S.E.

m-EU, milli-esterase unit

C_{IN}, inulin clearance

C_{PAH}, para-amino-hippurate clearance

(After Mills and Newport, 1979)[57]

Presumably one or other or both the renal natriuretic hormones, which follow the kallikrein/kinin system in the cascade is (are) affected by the sustained hypoosmolality of the plasma or the depressed plasma sodium concentrations between 20 and 40 minutes of the infusion of 2.5% glucose. Whether the lack of vasopressin acts directly on a factor in the cascade or in some other way is not clear.

TABLE 3

RENAL EXCRETION BEFORE AND DURING 2.5% GLUCOSE LOADING AND DURING VASOPRESSIN
INFUSION INTO LEFT RENAL ARTERY

	Control n = 24	Water loaded Before ADH n = 27	During ADH n = 22	P
Urine flow (ml/min)	0.64 ± 0.12	5.62 ± 0.6	5.59 ± 0.56	n.s.
Na (μ-equiv/min)	88.7 ± 11.0	72.5 ± 4.5	94.3 ± 6.4	< 0.01
Kallikrein (m-EU/min)	46.1 ± 9.5	190.9 ± 15.7	195.6 ± 17.6	n.s.
Osmolality (m-osmole/kg)	989 ± 99	100 ± 10	111 ± 15	n.s.
C_{IN} (ml/min)	46.1 ± 3.2	47.4 ± 2.8	47.6 ± 2.8	n.s.

P values measured by Student's t test comparing means of observations before and
during ADH infusion.
Na, urinary sodium excretion.
kallikrein, excretion in urine.
C_{IN}, inulin clearance.
(After Mills and Newport, in press)[59]

ACKNOWLEDGEMENT

   This work was supported by the Medical Research Council.

REFERENCES

1. Bahlmann, J., McDonald, S.J., Dunningham, J.G. and de Wardener, H.E. (1967) Clin. Sci., 32, 395-402.

2. Bahlmann, J., McDonald, S.J., Ventom, M.G. and de Wardener, H.E. (1967) Clin. Sci., 32, 403-413.

3. Mills, I.H., Osbaldiston, G.W., Craig, G.M. and Wise, B.L. (1966) Abstracts, III International Congress of Nephrology, Washington, p. 244.

4. Nizet, A., Cuypers, Y., Deetjen, P. and Kramer, K. (1967) Pflügers Archiv., 296, 179-195.

5. Gauer, O.H. and Henry, J.P. (1963) Physiol. Rev., 43, 423-481.

6. Henry, J.P., Gupta, P.D., Meehan, J.P., Sinclair, R. and Share, L. (1968) Can. J. Physiol. Pharmacol., 46, 287-295.

7. Goetz, K.L., Bond, G.C. and Bloxham, D.D. (1975) Physiol. Rev., 55, 157-205.

8. Kappagoda, C.T., Linden, R.J. and Snow, H.M. (1973) J. Physiol., 235, 493-502.

9. Kappagoda, C.T., Knapp, M.F., Linden, R.J., Pearson, M.J. and Whitaker, E.M. (1979) J. Physiol., 291, 381-391.

258

10. Keeler, R. (1975) Can. J. Physiol. Pharmacol., 53, 1193-1197.

11. Chessar, J.R., Ferrario, C.M. and McCubbin, J.W. (1972) Can. J. Physiol. Pharmacol., 50, 1108-1111.

12. Schad, H. and Seller, H. (1976) Pflügers Archiv., 363, 155-159.

13. Linden, R.J., Mary, D.A.S.G. and Weatherill, D. (1980) J. Physiol. 300, 31-40.

14. Bello-Reuss, E., Trevino, D.L. and Gottschalk, C.W. (1976) J. clin. Invest., 57, 1104-1107.

15. Zambraski, E.J., DiBona, G.F. and Kaloyanides, G.J. (1976) Proc. Soc. Exper. Biol. Med., 151, 543-546.

16. Marin-Grez, M., Cottone, P. and Carretero, O.A. (1972) Am. J. Physiol., 223, 794-796.

17. Pearce, J.W., Sonnenberg, H., Veress, A.T. and Ackermann, V. (1969) Can. J. Physiol. Pharmacol., 47, 377-386.

18. Lichardus, B. and Ponec, J. (1975) Curr. Probl. Clin. Biochem., 4, 234-236.

19. Mills, I.H. (1970) Regulation of Body Fluid Volumes by the Kidney, S. Karger, Basel, pp. 165-181.

20. Mills, I.H., Ward, P.E., Macfarlane, N.A.A. and Obika, L.F.O. (1978) Natriuretic Hormone, Springer-Verlag, Berlin, pp. 77-87.

21. Mills, I.H., Macfarlane, N.A.A., Ward, P.E. and Obika, L.F.O. (1976) Fed. Proc., 35, 181-188.

22. Alexander, R.W., Gill, J.R. Jr., Yamabe, H., Lovenberg, W. and Keiser, H.R. (1974) J. clin. Invest., 54, 194-200.

23. Faucheux, B., Buu, N.T. and Küchel, O. (1977) Am. J. Physiol., 232(2), F123-F127.

24. Baines, A.D. and Chan, W. (1980) Life Sciences, 26, 253-259.

25. Ball, S.G. and Lee, M.R. (1977) Br. J. clin. Pharmac., 4, 115-119.

26. Goldberg, L.I., McDonald, R.H. Jr. and Zimmerman, A.M. (1963) New Engl. J. Med., 269, 1060-1064.

27. Mills, I.H. and Obika, L.F.O. (1976) J. Physiol., 263, 150-151P.

28. Nustad, K. (1970) Br. J. Pharmac., 39, 73-86.

29. Scicli, A.G., Carretero, O.A., Hampton, A., Cortes, P. and Oza, N.B. (1976) Am. J. Physiol., 230, 533-536.

30. Ørstavik, T.B., Nustad, K. and Brandtzaeg, P. (1980) Enzymatic Release of Vasoactive Peptides, Raven Press, New York, pp. 137-149.

31. de Bono, E. and Mills, I.H. (1974) J. Physiol. 241, 127-128P.

32. Marin-Grez, M. and Carretero, O.A. (1971) Physiologist, Wash., 14, 189.

33. Adetuyibi, A. and Mills, I.H. (1972) Lancet, 2, 203-207.

34. Mills, I.H. and Ward, P.E. (1975) J. Physiol., 246, 695-707.

35. Margolius, H.S., Horwitz, D., Geller, R.G., Alexander, R.W., Gill, J.R., Jr., Pisano, J.J. and Keiser, H.R. (1974) Circulation Res., 35, 812-819.

36. Levy, S.B., Frigon, R.P. and Stone, R.A. (1978) Clin. Sci. Mol. Med., 54, 39-45.

37. Geller, R.G., Margolius, H.S., Pisano, J.L. and Keiser, H.R. (1972) Circulation Res., XXXI, 857-861.

38. Johnston, C.I., Matthews, P.G. and Dax, E. (1976) Clin. Sci. Mol. Med., 51, 283s-286s.

39. Mills, I.H. (1979) Nephron, 23, 61-71.

40. Bevan, D.R., Macfarlane, N.A.A. and Mills, I.H. (1974) J. Physiol., 241, 34-35P.

41. McGiff, J.C., Crowshaw, K., Terragno, N.A. and Lonigro, A.J. (1970) Nature (Lond), 227, 1255-1257.

42. Mills, I.H. and Obika, L.F.O. (1977) J. Physiol., 273, 459-474.

43. Macfarlane, N.A.A., Adetuyibi, A. and Mills, I.H. (1974) J. Endocr., 61, lxxii.

44. Mills, I.H. and Newport, P.A. (1978) J. Physiol., 284, 153-155P.

45. Mills, I.H., Obika, L.F.O. and Newport, P.A. (1978) Contr. Nephrol., 12, 132-144.

46. Mills, I.H. and Newport, P.A. (1979) J. Physiol., 289, 70-72P.

47. Mills, I.H. and Obika, L.F.O. (1977) J. Physiol., 267, 21-22P.

48. Margolius, H.S., Chao, J. and Kaizu, T. (1976) Clin. Sci. Mol. Med., 51, 279s-282s.

49. Mills, I.H. (1979) Bradykinin, Kallidin and Kallikrein. Supplement to Handbook of Experimental Pharmacology, Vol. XXV, Springer-Verlag, Berlin, pp. 549-567.

50. Mills, I.H. and Obika, L.F.O. (1979) J. Physiol., 292, 37-38P.

51. Godon, J.P. and Damas, J. (1974) Archs int. Physiol. Biochim., 82, 273-277.

52. Marin-Grez, M. (1974) Pflügers Arch., 350, 231-239.

53. Kramer, H.J., Moch, T., von Sicherer, L. and Düsing, R. (1979) Clin. Sci. 56, 547-553.

54. Godon, J.P. (1978) Natriuretic Hormone, Springer-Verlag, Berlin, pp. 88-100.

55. Clarkson, E.M., Raw, S.M. and de Wardener, H.E. (1976) Kidney Internat., 10, 381-394.

56. Gonick, H.C. and Saldanha, L.F. (1975) J. clin. Invest., 56, 247-255.

57. Mills, I.H. and Newport, P.A. (1979) J. Physiol., 295, 102-103P.

58. Macfarlane, N.A.A., Mills, I.H. and Wraight, E.P. (1973) J. Physiol., 231, 45-47P.

59. Mills, I.H. and Newport, P.A. (1980) J. Physiol., in press.

Hormonal Regulation of Sodium Excretion,
B. Lichardus, R.W. Schrier and J. Ponec, eds.
© 1980 Elsevier/North-Holland Biomedical Press

THE KALLIKREIN-KININ AND RENIN-ANGIOTENSIN SYSTEMS : RELATIONSHIPS IN
NORMAL AND SODIUM DEPLETED RATS.

P.G. MATTHEWS, M. YASUJIMA, and C.I. JOHNSTON
Monash University, Department of Medicine, Prince Henry's Hospital,
St. Kilda Road, Melbourne, 3004 (Australia)

INTRODUCTION

The kallikrein-kinin system (KKS) and renin-angiotnesin system (RAS) are
two peptide-generating enzymo systems that participate in blood pressure
regulation and sodium homeostasis[1,2]. In these roles, investigation of KKS
has lagged behind that of RAS. Over the past decade considerable evidence
which implicates the activity of the KKS as one of the regulatory mechanisms
in cardiovascular events has been accumulated[3,4].

The behaviour of each system is expressed by the action of small, potent
and predominantly vasoactive peptide hormones which are generated from independent α_2 globulin substrates by the specific enzymes[1,5]. Both of these enzymes
have been located in high concentration in the renal parenchyma[5,6]. The
actions of the systems is mediated, at least in smooth muscle cells by independent plasma membrane-located hormone receptors[7]. Both agonist peptide
products can significantly modify renal function and blood pressure. The
differences in the two systems are evidenced by the facts that angiotensin II
(AII) is the most potent endogenous vasoconstrictor substance elaborated by
the body, whereas bradykinin (BK) is an extremely potent vasodilator.
Angiotensin converting-enzyme (CE) has been identified as kininase II (KII)
and is ubiquitous in its distribution. CE/KII plays an important but
opposite role in the expression of activity of both systems. In the RAS
it can be considered a permissive or potentiating enzyme since it promotes
the formation of AII. In the KKS, its acts to degrade the agonist product[8].

Since the advent of a new class of drugs, designed to inhibit specifically
CE/KII[9,10], increasing interest in the relationship between these two systems
which have several opposing functional effects, has been stimulated. It is
now possible to examine the role of CE/KII more selectively and because
of the high therapeutic index of the compounds, in more biologically complex
situations[4,11]. The present study examines the relationship of the RAS
to the KKS after a known provocative stimuls to both systems viz. sodium
depletion[1,2]. It examines the dependence of this relationship on CE/KII
activity. Sequential events in the pathways of activity of both systems

have been studied.

MATERIAL AND METHOD

Animals

Male Sprague-Dawley rats (200-250g) were maintained in metabolic cages on normal and low sodium diets for five to seven days after an initial four day period of acclimitization to this environment. When necessary for peptide receptor studies on uterine smooth muscle and when examining the peptide dose responses in the vasculature, female rats of similar age were used. These animals were treated with 500 μg kg^{-1} of diethylstilboestrol daily for two days prior to study.

Assay techniques

Kallikrein. 24 hour urinary kallikrein excretion was assayed on samples from measured 24 hour urine collections by the method of Johnston et al.[12]. The enzyme kinetic assay used as substrate, natural kininogens from dog plasma. The generated kinin was measured by radioimmunoassay.

Renin. Plasma renin activity (PRA) was measured by an enzyme kinetic technique using an incubation of diluted rat venous plasma which had been prepared at 4°C in the presence of angiotensinase inhibitors[13]. Generated angiotensin was measured by radioimmunoassay[14].

Bradykinin. Blood BK was measured by the method of Mashford and Roberts[15] on rat venous blood collected directly into ethanol. The ethanolic extract was washed, evaporated to dryness and assayed by radio-immunoassay[16].

Angiotensin I. Blood angiotensin I (AI) levels were measured on the same ethanolic extract of blood prepared for bradykinin estimation and measured by radioimmunoassay[14]. The extract showed immunologic identity with native hormone. Recovery of added AI through the extraction procedure was 96±5%. The extraction of increasing volumes of blood resulted in proportionate increases in measured AI.

Angiotensin II. Plasma AII values were determined on extracts of venous plasma collected for PRA by a modification of the method of Boyd et al.[17].

Bradykinin receptors. BK receptors have been studied on a plasma membrane enriched subcellular fraction of rat uterine smooth muscle, using a simplification of the method of Kidwai et al.[18]. The subcellular preparation was incubated at 29°C and pH 6.8 with radiolabelled-BK in the absence and presence of an excess of non-radiolabelled BK. The difference was considered to be "specific" receptor binding. The receptors have been assayed by Scatchard analysis of concentration-dependent binding sites performed under equilibrium conditions, from which the apparent equilibrium dissociation (K_D) constant and number of binding sites (N_S) were determined.

Angiotensin receptors. All receptors have been assayed by the technique of Rouzaire-Dubois et al.[19], using radiolabelled angiotensin binding to a microsomal preparation of rat myometrium.

Vasodepressor dose-response effects of bradykinin. These effects were examined in rats, anaesthetised with Inactin[R] (150 mg kg^{-1}), in which had been placed a central venous canula for BK administration and a further canula in the right common carotid artery for blood pressure measurement.

Vasopressor dose-response effects of angiotensin II. The effect of AII on blood pressure in the rat was studied in animals prepared as for BK dose-response. In addition, these animals had undergone vagotomy and ganglion blockade with intraperitoneal pentolinium.

Drugs

Bradykinin and analogues. These were obtained from the Protein Research Foundation, Peninsula Laboratories and Sandoz (Australia).

Angiotensin I. Ile^5-angiotensin I was obtained from MRC, Mill Hill.

Angiotenesin II. Ile^5-angiotensin II was obtained from MRC, Mill Hill. Asp-βamide-val^5-angiotensin II (Hypertensin, Ciba) was used in dose-response curves.

Captopril (SQ 14225). Captopril was a gift of Dr. Z.P. Horowitz, Squibb Institute of Medical Research, Princeton. Captopril was administered by gavage, 8th hourly when 24 hour urine collections were being made. Captopril was given by gavage at a dose of 30 mg kg^{-1} in experiments relating to circulating hormones, by gavage at a dose of 30 mg kg^{-1} in experiments requiring 24 hour urine collection and by intravenous infusion (using osmotic minipumps) at a dose of 100 μg kg^{-1}h^{-1} in experiments assaying receptors and measuring dose-response curves.

RESULTS

The low sodium diet has a profound effect on renal sodium excretion which diminished from 0.69 ± 0.04 mmole d^{-1} to 0.02 ± 0.004 mmole d^{-1}. The changes in renin, kallikrein and circulating peptides after six days on a low sodium diet are shown in Table I. PRA was increased by three to four times. This was accompanied by marked increases in circulating AI and AII levels. The 24h kallikrein excretion was doubled on this diet. Circulating BK on the other hand did not change significantly.

The consequences of the sodium restricted regimen on peptide receptors are seen in Table 2. Binding affinities for either peptide-receptor

TABLE I

EFFECTS OF SODIUM DEPLETION ON HORMONES

Hormone	Normal Diet	Low Sodium Diet	n
Plasma Renin Activity ng AI ml^{-1} h^{-1}	4.15±0.07	14.31±1.69[a]	17
Angiotensin I pg ml^{-1}	129±14	224±28[a]	17
Angiotensin II pg ml^{-1}	125±13	274±26[a]	10
24h Kallikrein excretion mg BK d^{-2}	40.6±2.2	81.8±6.7[a]	58
Bradykinin ng ml^{-1}	2.01±0.20	1.80±0.16	17

[a] $p < 0.05$

interaction were not significantly altered by the dietary modification.
However, the number of specific receptors was significantly increased for
each agonist hormone, to 2.5 times control for AII and about 1.5 times
control levels for BK. The vascular responses to both AII and BK measured
by intermittent intravenous injection into the superior vena cava showed
that the effective dose for half-maximal response (ED_{50}) for AII in rats
after seven days on the sodium deficient regimen did not differ from control rats : 98±10 pmole kg^{-1} for control (n=5) and 98±24 pmole kg^{-1} for
the sodium depleted rats (n=4). Similarly, the ED_{50} values for BK dose-
responses (performed in different rats) did not vary with dietary regimen :
6.0±1.7 nmole kg^{-1} in controls (n=13) and 7.1±2.0 nmole kg^{-1} (n=9).

The effect of CE/KII inhibition on the components of the RAS and KKS
reported above, has been compared in rats already subjected to sodium
depletion and those of a control group. The results are presented as
percentage changes of each parameter from a paired, pre-treatment determination (except in the case of receptor and dose-response studies where
between animal comparisons have been made). 24h renal sodium excretion
was not altered by CE/KII inhibition in normal rats. Although there was
an apparent increase of 44% in sodium excretion in rats on the low sodium
diet, this was not statistically significant, probably because of the
variability in measuring very low urinary sodium concentrations which
these animals generate.

Circulating renin and AI were markedly increased in normal rats after

TABLE 2

PEPTIDE RECEPTOR CHANGES IN DIETARY SODIUM VARIATION

Hormone	Parameter	Normal Diet	Low Sodium Diet
Angiotensin II (n=3)	K_D ($\times 10^9$M)	10.1±1.5	8.4±0.5
	N_s	100	250±42[a]
Bradykinin (n-5)	K_D ($\times 10^9$M)	0.7+0.03	0.7±0.05
	N_s	100	168±3[a]

a p <0.05

TABLE 3

EFFECT OF CONVERTING ENZYME/KININASE II INHIBITION (PERCENTAGE CHANGE FROM CONTROLS)

	Normal Diet	Sodium Depleted Diet
24h sodium excretion	+ 6 (10)	+ 44 (10)
Plasma renin activity	+ 3492 (17)[b]	+ 892 (10)[b]
Blood angiotensin I	+ 997 (17)[b]	+ 446 (10)[b]
Plasma angiotensin II	- 25 (10)[b]	- 53 (10)[b]
24h kallikrein excretion	0 (10)	- 30 (10)[b]
Blood bradykinin	+ 52 (17)[b]	- 19 (9)[b]
Bradykinin receptor[c]: K_D	- 1 (10)	-[d]
Bradykinin receptor : N_s	- 24 (10)[b]	-
Bradykinin ED_{50}	- 97 (6)[b]	-

a Figures in parenthesis = number of paired observations
b p<0.05 or less
c Receptor and dose-response results are between group observations
d not performed

CE/KII inhibition. This same marked increase still occurred in the sodium deficient animals. AII was decreased significantly after CE/KII inhibition and to a relatively greater degree in rats already sodium-restricted. Kallikrein excretion was not influenced by sodium depletion but decreased by 30 per cent when rats were sodium depleted prior to CE/KII inhibition. BK, on the other hand, rose significantly to 150 per cent of control values in rats on normal diets but decreased significantly in rats that were sodium restricted before inhibition.

The affinity of the BK receptor did not change after CE/KII inhibition in normal rats, but the number of sites diminished to three-quarters of those of control rats. The dose of BK for half-maximal response in the dose-response curve was reduced nearly two orders of magnitude by treatment with captopril.

DISCUSSION

The stimulus of sodium depletion in the normal animal is known to result in increases in circulating renin and AII[20]. Less frequently reported, has been the parallel rise in AI[21]. Sodium depletion in the rat has been shown to increase the number of AII receptors in the adrenal and myometrium[22], an often-used model of vascular smooth muscle. Sodium depletion, in our hands has not resulted in a decreased pressor sensitivity to exogenous AII, as evidenced by the lack of change of ED_{50}. This difference from the findings of others may be related to the nature of the preparation and the extent of the examination of the dose-response curve[23]. Our preparation favoured response reflecting more selectively the myotropic action of AII on resistance vessels. Lack of change of receptor affinity was consistent with the unchanged ED_{50}. The increase in receptor number was not explained, but known not to be due to differences in preparation.

The increased urinary kallikrein excretion after sodium depletion and failure of circulating bradykinin levels to change significantly confirmed earlier observations[12,24]. The findings supported suggestions that kallikrein excretion may be a function of aldosterone levels[24]. The BK receptor was not modified in affinity but increased in number. The former finding, similar to the AII receptor, was consistent with the lack of difference of ED_{50} for the vasodepressor effect of exogenous BK.

High dose captopril was used to maximize the inhibition of CE/KII. Pharmacokinetic studies on captopril are not yet available, but it has been shown that hormonal effects of this competitive inhibitor are markedly dose dependent[25]. The RAS is much more sensitive to captopril, perhaps because AI has a lower affinity for CE/KII than BK[26]. CE/KII inhibition significantly reduced the formation of AII, and relatively more so in sodium depletion, consistent with evidence of reduced CE/KII activity in sodium depletion[27]. Proximal to the block, AI and BK both rose significantly

in normals, as predicted should their generation or non-CE/KII degradation
not be impaired. However, with salt depletion, circulating BK levels fell
despite evidence of enzyme blockade. This finding would not be consistent
with easily inhibited, already reduced CE/KII activity, unless other mechanisms such as decreased generation or increased non-CE/KII clearance
played a role. Decreased kallikrein activity during captopril therapy
in sodium depletion would support the former and may be related to these
lower levels. Plasma renin, on the other hand rose remarkably with CE/KII
inhibition in both states probably for several reasons which have been
considered elsewhere[25]. BK receptors after CE/KII inhibition in normal
rats showed no change in affinity but a significant fall in number. This
enzyme inhibition is probably the main reason for the marked reduction in
ED_{50} in these rats. Acute intravenous captopril shifts the BK dose-
response curve almost equivalently to the left and to a similar order of
magnitude as intra-arterial BK (not shown).

The reason for the loss of parallelism of activation of components of
the RAS and the kallikrein system during the stimulus of sodium depletion
was not positively identified in this study. However, it is possible
that a reduction in aldosterone secretion could have led to reduced kallikrein activity (and possibly the variable increase in sodium excretion)
in sodium depleted animals. The relationship between reduced renal/urinary
kallikrein activity and reduced circulating BK was not resolved but suggests that activity of kallikrein in the kidney might influence circulating
BK in some situations.

ACKNOWLEDGEMENTS

Assistance of Monique Straw and Kathy Sowards is acknowledged. PGM is
a Research Fellow of NH&MRC. Project was supported by LIMRF and NHF.
Judy Murphy typed the manuscript.

REFERENCES

1. Erdös, E.D.(ed.) (1979) Handb. Exp. Pharm. 25, Suppl. Springer-Verlag,
   Berlin.

2. Page, I.H. and Bumpus, F.M. (1974) Handb. Exp. Pharm. 37, Springer-
   Verlag, Berlin.

3. Margolius, H.S. and Buse, J.B. (1979) Hormonal Function and the Kidney,
   Churchill Livingstone, New York, pp.115-145.

4. Thurston, H. and Swales, J.D. (1978) Circ. Res. 42, 588-592.

5. Smeby, R.R. and Bumpus, F.M. (1968) Renin, Year Book Medical Publishers,
   Chicago, pp. 14-61.

6. Orstavik, T.B. and Nustad, K. and Brandtzaeg, P. (1979) Clin. Sci.,

57, 239s-241s.

7. Yasujima, M., Johnston, C.I. and Matthews, P.G. (1979) Proc. Aust. Soc. Med. Res. 12, 68.

8. Erdös, E.G. (1979) Handb. Exp. Pharm. 25, Suppl. Springer-Verlag, Berlin, pp. 427-487.

9. Greene, L.J., Camargo, A.C.M., Krieger, E.M., Stewart, J.M. and Ferreira, S.H. (1972) Circ. Res. 20, II-62-II-71.

10. Ondetti, M.A., Rubin, B. and Cushman, D.W. (1977) Science, 196, 441-444.

11. Matthews, P.G., McGrath, B.P. and Johnston, C.I. (1979) Clin. Sci. 57, 135s-138s.

12. Johnston, C.I., Matthews, P.G. and Dax, E. (1976) Systemic Effects of Anti-hypertensive Agents, Stratton Intercontinental Medical Book Corporation, New York, pp. 323-336.

13. Johnston, C.I., Matthews, P.G., Davis, J.M. and Morgan, T. (1975) Pflugers Arch., 356, 277-286.

14. Johnston, C.I., Mendelsohn, F.A.O. and Casley, D. (1969) Proc. Aust. Soc. Med. Res., 2, 271-272.

15. Mashford, M.L. and Roberts, M.L. (1972) Biochem. Pharmacol., 21, 2727-2735.

16. Matthews, P.G. and Johnston, C.I. (1979) Adv. Exptl. Med. Biol., 120B, 447-457.

17. Boyd, G.W., Landon, J. and Peart, W.S. (1967) Lancet, 2, 1002-1005.

18. Kidwai, A.M., Radcliffe, M.A. and Daniel, E.E. (1971) Biochim. Biophys. Acta. 233, 538-549.

19. Rouzaire-Dubois, B., Devynck, M-A., Chevillotte, E. and Meyer, P. (1978) FEBS. Lett. 55, 168-172.

20. Gocke, D.J., Gerten, J., Sherwood, L.M. and Laragh, J.H. (1969) Circ. Res., 24 & 25, I-131-I-148.

21. Waite, M.A. (1937) Clin. Sci. mol. Med. 45, 51-64.

22. Devynck, M-A., Pernollet, M-G., Matthews, P.G., MacDonald, G.J., Raisman, R.S. and Meyer, P. (1979) J. Cardiovasc. Pharmacol. 1, 163-179.

23. Campbell, W.B., Schmitz, J.M. and Itskovitz, H.D. (1979) Clin. Sci. 56, 325-333.

24. Margolius, H.S., Horowitz, D., Geller, R.G., Alexander, R.N., Gill, J.R., Pisano, J.J. and Keiser, H.R. (1974) Circ. Res. 35, 812-819.

25. Matthews, P.G. and Johnston, C.I. (1979) Med. J. Aust. Specl. Suupl. 2, xii-xv.

26. Dorer, F.E., Kahn, J.R., Lentz, K.E., Levine, M. and Skeggs, L.T. (1974) Circ. Res., 34, 824-827.

27. Merrill, J.E., Peach, M.J. and Gilmore, J.P. (1973) Am. J. Physiol. 224, 1104-1108.

Hormonal Regulation of Sodium Excretion,
B. Lichardus, R.W. Schrier and J. Ponec, eds.
© 1980 Elsevier/North-Holland Biomedical Press

URINARY KALLIKREIN ACTIVITY AND ALDOSTERONE EXCRETION RATE IN
YOUNG HYPERTENSIVES AND IN PATIENTS AFTER RENAL TRANSPLANTATION

HELENA BULTASOVÁ, PŘEMYSL PINSKER, JARMILA STŘÍBRNÁ, VOJTĚCH
MARTÍNEK
Institute for Clinical and Experimental Medicine, Vídeňská 800,
14622 Praha 4 - Krč and Postgraduate Medical and Pharmaceutical
Institute, Ruská 85, 10005 Praha 10 - Vinohrady (Czechoslovakia)

INTRODUCTION

The systems renin-angiotensin-aldosterone and kallikrein-kinin-
prostaglandins participate in the regulation of blood pressure not
only by their powerful vasoactive effects, but also through their
influence on salt and water excretion. A decreased kallikrein excretion was observed in essential hypertensive[1,2] and renal transplant patients[3,4]. Moreover, patients with essential hypertension
showed evidence of a decreased prostaglandin E excretion[5,6].

The aim of this study was to evaluate the participation of altered vasodepressor mechanisms in the initiation and development
of essential hypertension and hypertension after renal transplantation.

SUBJECTS AND METHODS

Ten young men (aged 16-25 years) with borderline hypertension
and 10 .age-matched normotensive volunteers participated in the
first part of the study. Informed consent was obtained in each
case. Four of the hypertensives had a positive family history of
essential hypertension. Thus far, none of them has been treated
with antihypertensives and diuretics. All subjects were hospita-
lized and allowed a diet containing 135 mmol sodium and 90 mmol
potassium daily. After a balance period of three days recumbent
blood samples were obtained at 0800 h following a 10 h bed rest.
The subjects were then ambulatory for the next two hours, when
additional blood samples were taken. Four-hour urine samples were
collected for studying circadian periodicity, and during infusions of saline at a rate of 500 ml h^{-1} for 4 h, angiotensin II
(Hypertensin, Ciba-Geigy) at a rate of 3 ng $kg^{-1}min^{-1}$ and 15 ng

$kg^{-1}min^{-1}$ respectively for two consecutive 60 min periods, and β^{1-24}-ACTH (Synacthen, Ciba-Geigy) at a rate of 2 µg h^{-1} for 4 h, applied on the third day of dexamethasone administration (0.5 mg 4 x daily). Urine was collected also for 24 h during the control period and again after 2 and 6 weeks of a β-adrenolytic drug therapy with metipranolol (Trimepranol, Spofa). In the plasma, renin activity (PRA), aldosterone and prostaglandin E (PGE) concentrations were measured, in the urine, kallikrein activity, PGE, aldosterone, sodium and potassium excretion rates were determined.

Urinary kallikrein activity and aldosterone excretion rate were measured also in 21 renal allograft recipients, 1-26 months after transplantation. All but two patients were hypertensive. In the control period, the patients were on free salt and water intake (110-200 mmol sodium daily), in the period of mild salt restriction (10 patients) they were allowed about 60-70 mmol sodium daily. The urine was collected before and after 4-5 days of salt restriction. In 17 patients kallikrein excretion was also measured after an acute water load (12 ml kg^{-1}).

Kallikrein activity was determined by the radiochemical method of Margolius[7], PGE, PRA and aldosterone by radioimmunoassay. The data were analysed by the Student´s t-test. Linear dependencies were examined by regression analysis. Data are given as mean values $\pm$ SEM.

RESULTS AND DISCUSSION

The young men with borderline hypertension had significantly higher values for PRA than age-matched control subjects (supine 3.373 ± 0.540 vs 1.529 ± 0.126; upright 6.737 ± 0.771 vs 3.791 ± 0.264 nmol AI $l^{-1}h^{-1}$, $p < 0.01$). On the contrary, there were no significant differences in plasma and urinary aldosterone, although some of the recumbent plasma values lay above the upper limit. In the young hypertensives urinary kallikrein activity was in the same range as in controls or slightly increased (21.0 ± 3.2 vs 16.3 ± 1.8 EU d^{-1}), but as a group the difference was not significant. Urinary kallikrein activity correlated significantly with aldosterone excretion in both groups ($r = 0.7329$, $p < 0.001$). This correlation persisted during the administration of metipranolol, which produced a similar decrease both in kallikrein activity and aldosterone excretion. However, the relationship between the two parameters disappeared in the 4-hour urine samples collected during the infusion of saline, angiotensin II and ACTH, which led to the expected changes in aldosterone excretion but to variable responses in urinary kallikrein activity. This finding may reflect a delayed response of kallikrein to the changes of mineralocorticoid activity. The blunted circadian periodicity of kallikrein in regard to aldosterone excretion seems to support this possibility (Fig. 1). However, other factors influencing urinary kallikrein activity may be involved. The circadian periodicity of potassium excretion correlated positively with the rhythmicity of aldosterone and kallikrein excretion, while sodium excretion behaved in an opposite manner, especially during the 24 h bed rest (Fig. 2).

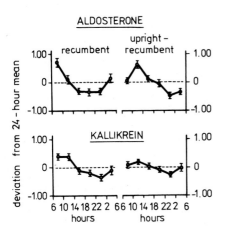

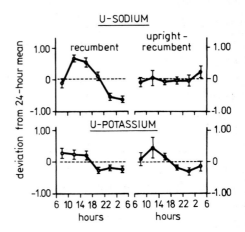

Fig. 1. Circadian rhythms of aldosterone and kallikrein excretion.

Fig. 2. Circadian rhythms of sodium and potassium excretion.

In borderline hypertensive subjects, the plasma and urinary PGE did not significantly differ from controls (plasma 2.118 ± 0.282 vs 2.248 ± 0.101 nmol l^{-1}; urine 2.738 ± 0.647 vs 1.975 ± 0.228 nmol d^{-1}). Decreased values for plasma and urinary PGE occurred only in one patient, the only one with normal PRA. Another patient had elevated PGE excretion, combined with increased urinary kallikrein activity. After all stimuli the changes in PGE excretion parallelled the changes in urine flow (Fig. 3).

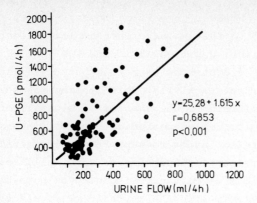

Fig. 3. Correlation between PGE excretion and urine flow in 4-hour samples.

There was no correlation between the excretion of PGE and sodium. A positive correlation appeared only after the two parameters were correlated in each patient separately (r ranged between 0.7057 and 0.9075, p between < 0.05 and < 0.001). The infusion of angiotensin II elicited a moderate increase in plasma PGE concentration, but urinary PGE decreased in accordance with changes in urine flow and sodium excretion. As expected, saline infusion augmented urine flow, sodium output and PGE excretion.

The normal values for urinary kallikrein and PGE in young men with borderline hypertension disprove a potential primary role of a defective synthesis of these compounds in the initiation of essential hypertension. However, it cannot be ruled out that in some of our patients a normal production of kallikrein and PGE failed to sufficiently counterbalance the increased activity of the renin-angiotensin system.

Renal allograft recipients showed a significantly lower urinary kallikrein activity than controls (5.35 ± 1.25 vs 17.4 ± 2.2 EU d^{-1}, p<0.01). Long-term treatment with diuretics led only to a slight increase in kallikrein excretion (6.60 ± 1.38 EU d^{-1}, NS). Most of the low values were found in the first post-transplantation month. Reexamination at later periods showed changes in kallikrein excretion related to the functional capacity of the graft. The urinary kallikrein activity did not significantly correlate with aldosterone excretion rate. However, many of the values found during the phase of stable renal function were within the 95% confidence limits determined in controls (Fig. 4).

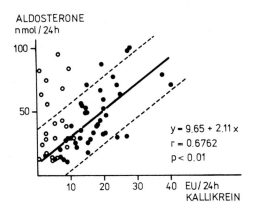

Fig. 4. Correlation between urinary aldosterone and kallikrein activity (see text). Solid circles = controls, empty circles = transplant patients.

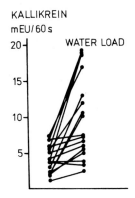

Fig. 5. Effect of acute water load on urinary kallikrein activity in allograft recipients.

Dietary sodium restriction elevated significantly PRA (from 1.98 $\pm$ 0.65 to 4.98 $\pm$ 0.78 nmol AI $l^{-1}h^{-1}$, $p < 0.05$), aldosterone excretion rate (from 25.8 $\pm$ 6.6 to 77.3 $\pm$ 27.2 nmol d^{-1}, $p < 0.05$) and urinary kallikrein activity (from 3.98 $\pm$ 1.13 to 10.79 $\pm$ 2.87 EU d^{-1}, $p < 0.05$). However, the limited number of normotensives in the group of transplant patients did not permit to determine whether the increment of urinary kallikrein activity after sodium deprivation is greater in normotensive than in hypertensive patients, as reported by Margolius[8] in nontransplant subjects. With two exceptions, acute water load elevated kallikrein excretion (Fig. 5).

Judging by our results in renal allograft recipients, 1) urinary kallikrein activity is decreased but related to aldosterone excretion rate in the phase of stabilized renal function, 2) the graft preserves its ability to respond to various stimuli with an increase in kallikrein excretion.

REFERENCES

1. Werle, E. and Korsten, H. (1938) Z. Ges. Exp. Med., 103, 153.
2. Margolius, H.S. et al. (1971) Lancet, 2, 1065-1065.
3. Werle, E. et al. (1968) Klin. Wochenschr., 46, 1315-1317.
4. Carretero, O.A. and Scicli, A.G. (1978) Klin. Wochenschr., 56 (Suppl. 1), 113-125.
5. Tan, S.Y. et al. (1978) Prostaglandins Med., 1, 76-85.
6. Abe, K. et al. (1978) Clin. Sci. Mol. Med., 55 (Suppl. 4), 363s-366s.
7. Margolius, H.S. et al. (1974) Circ. Res., 35, 812-819.
8. Margolius, H.S. et al. (1974) Circ. Res., 320-325.

Hormonal Regulation of Sodium Excretion,
B. Lichardus, R.W. Schrier and J. Ponec, eds.
© 1980 Elsevier/North-Holland Biomedical Press

URINARY KALLIKREIN EXCRETION IN ALLOGRAFT PATIENTS: ACUTE
EFFECT OF FUROSEMIDE AND BETA ADRENERGIC BLOCKADE

J. STŘÍBRNÁ, H. BULTASOVÁ, Z. ROTNÁGLOVÁ, V. MARTÍNEK
Institute for Clinical and Experimental Medicine, Vídeňská 800,
146 22 Praha 4, ČSSR

INTRODUCTION

There is evidence that renal kallikrein (KE) - kinin system
modulates the tubular transport of water and sodium (Na), but
its function as a natriuretic factor is uncertain. Volume expansion with water load[1], infusion of isotonic saline[2] or 2.5%
glucose[3] induces increased KE excretion. Increase in natriuresis
depends on fluid load composition.

Diuretics administration produces increased urinary flow, Na
and KE excretion. KE activation is evidently not mediated by
aldosterone or renal haemodynamic. Increased tubular urine flow
seems to be nonspecific stimulus of KE excretion[4]. Concurrent
administration of a beta adrenergic blocker is reported to enhance the effect of thiazides on KE excretion. On the other
hand some authors observed no changes[5] or a decrease after beta
adrenergic blockade.

Recipients with renal allograft show a decreased KE excretion.
Their response to various stimuli has not yet been studied.
We examined a group of allograft recipients under conditions
of volume expansion with oral water load. Further, we evaluated
the acute effect of furosemide (F) and beta adrenergic blocker
Trimepranol (T) on KE, Na, K and aldosterone excretion, on
plasma renin activity (PRA), and renal haemodynamics.

MATERIAL AND METHODS

A group of 18 allograft recipients, 9 men and 9 women, aged
between 23 to 52 years (mean 34) were investigated 0.5 to 28
months after transplantation. All received immunosuppressive
therapy. All but two patients were hypertensive. Six of them
were on methyldopa medication.

Table 1

Exptl. condition		$C_{in}/1.73m^2$ ml/s	$C_{PAH}/1.73m^2$ ml/s	FF %	V/C_{in} %	U_{Na}/U_K	$U_{KE}V$ mEU/60s	$U_{aldo}V$ pmol/60s	PRA nmol/l/h
Water load	$\bar{x}$	0.69	3.55	19.7	8.27	3.38	9.48	73.1	3.37
n 23-21	s	0.28	1.21	5.9	6.46	2.23	6.44	65.5	1.92
Furosemide	$\bar{x}$	0.67	3.71	18.7	6.32	3.00	8.83	55.6	2.58
Control n 10-8	s	0.24	1.17	5.7	4.34	2.24	3.52	59.5	1.33
F_{40}	$\bar{x}$	0.84	4.50	18.6	25.20	11.20	21.05	188.7	3.61
	s	0.25	1.27	4.5	8.85	4.72	14.48	309.3	0.85
F_{80}	$\bar{x}$	0.71	3.57	18.7	25.90	10.50	19.39	102.5	3.34
	s	0.27	1.49	3.7	6.69	4.39	13.49	91.7	1.95
C: F_{40}	P	0.1%	5%	n.s.	0.1%	0.1%	1%	5%	5%
C: F_{80}	P	n.s.	n.s.	n.s.	0.1%	0.1%	1%	5%	5%
Trimepranol	$\bar{x}$	0.66	3.28	20.0	9.78	2.84	10.64	98.6	4.34
Control n 10-9	s	0.29	1.12	6.4	8.11	1.45	7.78	73.1	1.83
T_{40}	$\bar{x}$	0.61	2.96	21.6	9.99	2.73	10.23	54.8	-
	s	0.22	0.88	8.3	7.94	1.66	7.83	33.0	
T_{80}	$\bar{x}$	0.55	2.86	19.3	8.72	2.17	8.17	51.5	2.94
	s	0.21	0.87	6.9	6.74	1.60	7.96	32.4	1.24
C: T_{40}	P	n.s.	n.s.	n.s.	n.s.	n.s.	n.s.	n.s.	-
C: T_{80}	P	n.s.	n.s.	n.s.	n.s.	1%	n.s.	5%	1%

F_{40}, T_{40}, F_{80}, T_{80}: urine collection from 0 to 40 (80) min after drug administration

Fluid and saline intake was free, but maintained at a constant level for at least 5 days before examination. The examination started in the morning by oral water load administration of 0.2 1/10 kg in the course of 30 min. followed by tests of inulin + PAH clearance. The urine was collected in three 40-min. intervals. After each collection the patient received 0.15-0.2 l of fluid. At the end of the first, i.e. control period, 20 mg and 40 mg i.v. F and oral T, respectively, were administered in 10 examinations each. Peripheral blood samples were collected at the end of control period and 30 and 90 minutes after drug administration. The patients were examined in the sitting position.

Concentrations of inulin, PAH, Na, and K were determined in the blood and urine. Aldosterone and PRA were determined by radioimunoassay. Urinary KE was estimated by Margolius[7] modification of the radiochemical method.

Clearance values, filtration fraction (FF) and mean arterial pressure were calculated in the usual manner. Some value changes (Δ) were calculated as the difference, expressed in % of the control value. Statistical evaluation was done by the Student t-test.

RESULTS

Water load

Mean values are given in table 1. Increased KE excretion correlated with FF values (fig.1). This finding agrees with theopinion that pressures at and beyond vas afferens may be involved in the regulation of KE production[2]. The rate of KE excretion correlated with V/C_{in} value (fig.2). The value indicates the rate of decreased tubular water reabsorption, reflected in urine flow. No relationship of urinary KE to C_{Na}/C_{in}, U_{Na}/U_K value, or to $U_{aldo}V$ was observed.

Furosemide

Mean values from the control and the 2 subsequent periods after F administration are given in table 1. KE excretion correlated with V/C_{in} (fig.3) as well as with C_{Na}/C_{in} values (r:0.579, P: 0.1%). We found no relationship between KE excretion and pa-

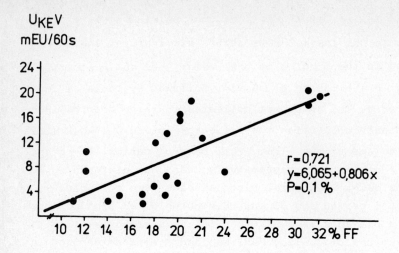

Fig.1. Water load. Correlation between kallikrein excretion ($U_{KE}V$) and filtration fraction (FF).

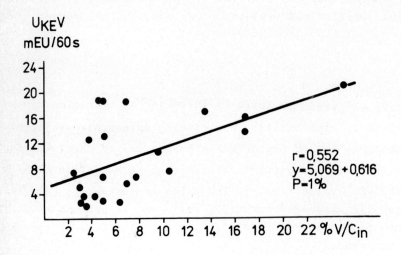

Fig.2. Water load. Correlation between kallikrein excretion ($U_{KE}V$) and excretion fraction of water (V/C_{in}).

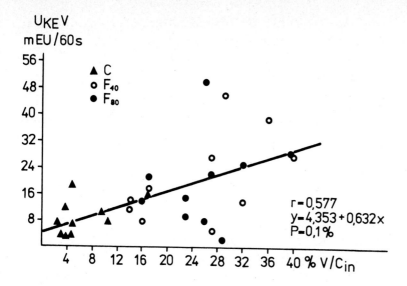

Fig.3. Correlation between kallikrein excretion ($U_{KE}V$) and excretion fraction of water (V/C_{in}). C: control period, F_{40}: 0-40 min, F_{80}: 40-80 min, after furosemide (F) administration.

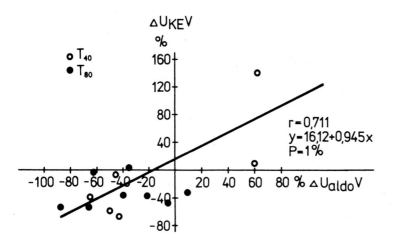

Fig.4. Correlation between the change (Δ) in kallikrein excretion ($U_{KE}V$) and aldosterone excretion ($U_{aldo}V$) after beta adrenergic blocker Trimepranol (T) administration. T_{40}: 0-40 min, T_{80}: 40-80 min after administration.

rameters of renal haemodynamic or between PRA and $U_{aldo}V$. A positive correlation between KE excretion and V/C_{in} after acute water load or F administration may be due to a wash-out effect or stimulated KE secretion. After F the rate of decrease in tubular water reabsorption is determined by inhibition of Na reabsorption. Under this condition the interaction of KE and Na cannot be clearly defined.

Trimepranol

Mean values from the control and the 2 subsequent intervals after beta adrenergic blockade with T are given in tab.1. Between 40-80 min. after T administration, a significant decrease in C_{Na}/C_{in}, U_{Na}/U_K, $U_{aldo}V$ and PRA was observed. At that time KE excretion decreased insignificantly. There was also a positive correlation between Δ PRA and $\Delta U_{aldo}V$ (r: 0.772, P: 5%) and between $\Delta U_{aldo}V$ and $\Delta U_{KE}V$ (fig.4). This finding may reflect the onset of the action of suppressed renin-angiotensin-aldosterone system activity on KE excretion. Presumably evaluation of the effect of beta adrenergic blockade on KE excretion could be influenced by the duration of its action. The decreased C_{Na}/C_{in}, U_{Na}/U_K values resp., were not related to changes in KE excretion.

REFERENCES
1. Croxatto, H.R. et al. (1976) Clin.Sci.Mol.Med.,51, 259-261.
2. Mills, I.H. et al. (1976) Fed.Proc., 35, 181-188.
3. Mills, I.H. and Newport, P.A. (1979) J.Physiol., 295,102-1039 .
4. Nielsen, C.K. et al. (1976) Acta pharmacol.Toxicol., 39, 500-511.
5. Carretero, O.A. and Scicli, A.G. (1978) Klin.Wschr., 50, Suppl.I., 113-125
6. Pinsker, P. et al. - unpubl. data .
7. Margolius, H.S. et al. (1974) Circ.Res., 35, 812-919.

NATRIURETIC HORMONE

Hormonal Regulation of Sodium Excretion,
B. Lichardus, R.W. Schrier and J. Ponec, eds.
© 1980 Elsevier/North-Holland Biomedical Press

EFFECT OF INCREASED EXCRETORY RENAL MASS ON KIDNEY FUNCTION

GEORGE KÖVÉR and HILDA TOST
Institute of Physiology, Semmelweis University Medical School,
Budapest, Hungary.

INTRODUCTION

Acute or progressive reduction of renal mass has been shown
to induce adaptive changes in the remaining nephrons, so that
the overall salt and water balance is well maintained. The mechanisms by which water and electrolyte excretion from the remnant kidney is enhanced shortly after renal mass reduction remain unknown.

It is not clear yet, how the joint function of the two kidneys is regulated, wether the presence and excreting capacity of
one kidney has any influence on the function of the other kidney.

Our present study was designed to examine the acute increase
of nephron mass by acutely connecting a pair of isolated kidneys
into the circulation of an anesthetized dog, and examining the
effect of such a maneuver both on the function of the perfusor's
kidneys in situ, and isolated kidneys. We performed further studies on the in situ kidneys /without increasing the renal mass/
in narcotised dogs where the volume expansion was similar as in
the perfusor dogs. We compared renal function parameters observed in the animals with "two kidneys" and with "four kidneys".

MATERIALS AND METHODS

Studies were performed on mongrel dogs of either sex, weighing between 10-30 kg, anesthetized intravenously with Nembutal
/25 mg/kg/. The animals were deprived of food 24 hours before
the experiment.

Cannulation of the femoral arteries and veins on both sides
were performed in all animals. From a low midline incision the
bladder was exposed and the ureters were catheterized suprave-
sically.

The animals were given 10 ml/kg body weight Ringer solution
i.v. within 4-5 minutes. Each animal then received intravenously

paraamino-hyppuric acid /PAH/ and inulin, dissolved in 40 ml
Ringer solution. The sustaining infusion of inulin and PAH in
Ringer solution, calculated to maintain plasma inulin 30 mg/100
ml, and PAH 2 mg/100 ml, was infused at a rate of 0.25 ml/kg/min.

In the "two kidneys" group, the left kidney was exposed by
flank incision and the renal vein was connected to the left external jugular vein with siliconized rubber tube. A T-extension
of the tube permitted the direct measurement of renal venous
outflow.

In the perfusor dogs /prepared to receive the isolated kid-
neys/ from a midline incision the left carotid artery and the
right external jugular vein were exposed on the neck and were
cannulated using glass tubes.

Femoral arterial blood pressure was continuously registered
with a recorder connected to a strain-gauge. Before connecting
the anastomoses the animals were given 0.1 ml/kg of Heparin intravenously.

An equilibration period of 10 min was then allowed and three
timed /20 min/ urine samples /1, 2, 3/ and midpoint blood samples were obtained. The blood was immediately centrifuged, the
supernatant plasma removed and the red cells were dissolved in
Ringer solution and reinfused.

After the third period a pair of isolated kidneys removed
from another dog was transplanted to the perfusor's neck.

For the preparation of the isolated kidneys the method of
Brull[1] was used.

After connecting the isolated kidneys to the perfusor's circulation, urine from the perfusor's kidney in situ was collected in a 20-minute period /4/.

Following the 4th period the function of the isolated kidneys was investigated together with the parameters of the in
situ kidney in two 20 minute periods /5, 6/.

Studying the function of the in situ and isolated kidneys
the blood flow /$RBF_{dir.}$/ was estimated directly in the middle
of each period from the blood flowing out of the renal veins
using, a graduated cylinder and a stopwatch /the $RBF_{dir.}$ was
not measured in the perfusor's kidney/.

PAH concentration in blood and urine was estimated by the

method of Smith et al[2], inulin concentration by that of Little[3].

Renal clearances $/C_{PAH}$, $C_{inulin}/$ and extractions were calculated by the usual formulas. All data were referred to 100 g
kidney tissue weight with the exception of the total renal vascular resistance, this was calculated per kg kidney tissue.

RESULTS

The changes observed in 30 perfusor dogs kidneys in situ,
represented in the function of time can be seen in Fig. 1, where
the individual points mean the averages for the experimental periods.

Mean arterial blood pressure was not affected by the transplantation, at the same time a small decrease could be observed
in C_{PAH}, glomerular filtration rate $/C_{inulin}/$. The transplantation caused a significant decrease in both urine output and sodium excretion, while urinary osm. activity remained constant.

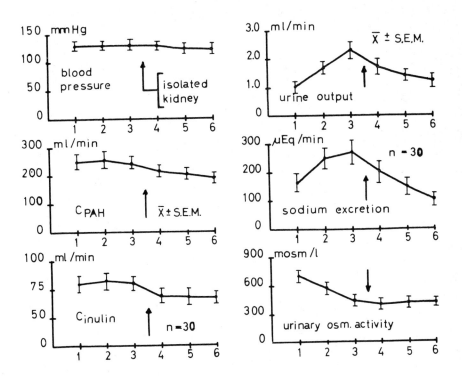

Fig. 1. The renal parameters in the perfusor's kidneys in situ.

TABLE 1

COMPARISON OF THE RENAL PARAMETERS

$$\bar{x} \pm S.E.M.$$

	in situ kidneys		transplanted kidneys		perfusor's kidneys in situ	
n	31	31	30	30	30	30
No of the periods	5	6	5	6	5	6
blood pressure mmHg	125± 3	125± 3	122± 3	122± 4	122± 3	122± 4
RBF dir. ml/min	486±18	489±20	467±18	480±20	-	-
R_{kidney}/kg RPF ml/min	1.62±0.07	1.63±0.08	1.66±0.08	1.59±0.08	-	-
	301±12	303±14	270±11	274±12	-	-
C_{PAH} ml/min	263±18	238±12	205±10	200±12	204±11	180±10
E_{PAH}	0.79±0.02	0.80±0.02	0.74±0.02	0.75±0.02	-	-
C_{PAH}/E_{PAH} ml/min	330± 9	296±10	266±10	266± 8	-	-
C_{inulin} ml/min	73± 4	71± 4	72± 4	72± 4	70± 4	68± 5
E_{inulin}	0.28±0.02	0.22±0.02	0.31±0.02	0.27±0.02	-	-
$C_{in.}/E_{in.}$ ml/min	270± 5	321± 5	245± 7	267± 5	-	-
urine output ml/min	2.65±0.32	2.59±0.31	1.14±0.23	1.23±0.26	1.44±0.21	1.18±0.17
$U_{Na} \cdot V$ /µEq/min	350±45	331±42	120±33	128±33	148±30	100±20
urine osm. conc. mosm/l	427±22	423±23	482±18	442±18	438±21	439±25
hematocrit %	38± 1	38± 1	42± 1	43± 1	42± 1	43± 1
plasma protein conc. g/100 ml	5.42±0.14	4.84±0.14	5.50±0.15	5.50±0.15	5.40±0.14	5.40±0.14

In Table 1 the parameters of the in situ kidneys /without increase of the renal mass/, the isolated kidneys and the perfusor's kidney in situ in two periods, during the steady state /5. 6. periods/, are shown.

The hemodynamic studies were performed in the in situ and isolated kidneys, the $RBF_{dir.}$, $R_{kidney/kg}$, were the same in the two experimental series. As can be observed no significant difference in glomerular filtrations rate, was apparent when the in situ and isolated kidneys were compared. Altough the C_{inulin} was the same in both groups the urine output and the sodium excretion were significantly less in the transplanted kidneys.

There were no significant differences between result obtained in the perfusor's kidney in situ and transplanted kidneys.

DISCUSSION

In the narcotized animals, there is a progressive escape of infused fluid and sodium. The time of stabilization in our experiments is about 60 minutes. There is no further increase of sodium excretion and urine output despite of continued fluid infusion.

Connection of a pair of isolated kidneys into the perfusor's circulation caused sodium excretion and urine output to fell to half of the control values. At the same time the amount of sodium and water excreted by the four kidneys was exactly the same as the amount excreted by the two in situ kidneys during the control periods /5. 6. periods/.

This phenomenon suggests that there is a very precise mechanism regulating sodium and water excretion, and capable of modifying the secreting capacity of the kidney in a few minutes.

The current knowledge regarding sodium excretion indicates the existence of multiple control mechanisms. Among there are the rate of glomerular filtration, the intrarenal distribution of blood flow, hematocrit, physical and hormonal factors, and the adrenergic nervous system /Nizet[4], Lichardus and Nizet[5], Kövér et al.[6]/.

In the conditions described here, the arterial blood pressure, renal blood flow, total vascular resistance, plasma protein concentration, glomerular filtration rate were not significantly different in the in situ and isolated kidneys and certainly in

the perfusor's kidney in situ /we didn't measure the RBF in this
kidney/. This indicating that the decrease of the urine output
and sodium excretion observed in the perfusor's kidney in situ
and transplanted kidney were independent of the previous factors.
Therefore, the differences obtained in the function of the kidney in situ following the connection of the isolated kidney into
the circulation, could only be related either to a decreased
natriuretic or to an increased antinatriuretic stimuli present
in the blood.

The short time rules out a possible role of mineralocorticoids
or vasopressin in this effect.

The results can be commented on as follows:
a./ The kidneys transplanted to the neck release a substance
into the blood /that is not renin/ increasing the tubular sodium
and water reabsorption.
b./ The increase of sodium and water excretion following the saline load might be due, among other causes, to the presence of
natriuretic factor/s/ of extrarenal origin. When four kidneys
are connected to the perfusor's circulation the natriuretic material could be eliminated by the kidneys more rapidly, its
plasma concentration drops, displaying in this way an anti-nat-
riuretic effect. This last point finds some support in our recent experiments.

The production-rate and intrarenal elimination of the natriuretic factor may determine its plasma concentration and so its
natriuretic effect realised in the kidney /Kövér and Tost[7]/.

REFERENCES
1. Brull, L. /1931/ C.R. Soc. Biol. /Paris/, 107, 248-251.
2. Smith, H.W., Finkelstein, N., Aliminosa, L., Crawford, B.,
   Graber, M. /1945/ J. clin. Invest. 24, 388-404.
3. Little, J.M. /1949/ J. biol. Chem. 180, 747-754.
4. Nizet, A. /1972/ Kidney Int. 1, 27-37.
5. Lichardus, B. and Nizet, A. /1972/ Clin. Sci. 42, 701-709.
6. Kövér, G., Bartha, J., Tost Hilda /1976/ Int. Urol. Nephrol.
   8, 237-245.
7. Kövér, G. and Tost Hilda /1978/ Acta physiol. Acad. Sci.
   hung. 51, 41-50.

Hormonal Regulation of Sodium Excretion,
B. Lichardus, R.W. Schrier and J. Ponec, eds.
© 1980 Elsevier/North-Holland Biomedical Press

SENSITIVITY OF PREPUBERTAL RATS TO THE HYPERTENSOGENIC EFFECT
OF SALT - A LACK OF NATRIURETIC FACTOR?

JIŘÍ KŘEČEK, HELENA DLOUHÁ, JELENA A. LAVROVA, JOSEF ZICHA
Institute of Physiology, Czechoslovak Academy of Sciences,
Prague and Sechenov Institute of Evolutionary Physiology and
Biochemistry, Academy of Sciences of USSR, Leningrad

Salt hypertension is one of the most extensively studied
forms of experimental hypertension. Skelton and Guillebeau[1]
first demonstrated that young rats are more susceptible than
adults to the hypertensogenic influence of adrenal regeneration
combined with increased salt intake. Prepuberty was identified
as critical period for hypertension produced by unilateral nephrectomy and 0.6% NaCl solution drinking in Brattleboro rats
with hereditary diabetes insipidus[2]. Hypertension was produced
by nephrectomy performed even in adulthood under the condition
that saline consumption began from prepuberty[3]. Hypertension
was elicited in rats of a sensitive substrain even by mere
high salt diet[4] consumed from youth.

Drinking of hypertonic saline was reported to produce hypertension in rats as well but results obtained by different authors were quite controversial[5,6,7], probably due to the high
mortality of animals used in experiments and to differences
in salt concentration in hypertonic solutions used. In order
to elucidate this confusion an experiment was undertaken in
which rats were offered to drink hypertonic salt solutions
of different concentration either from youth or only in adulthood and the blood pressure (BP) was estimated for several
weeks. Saline consumption began at the age of 4 weeks in the
"young" group, at the age of 12 weeks in the "adult" one.
Each of these groups consisted of 4 subgroups: 1. control
group (rats drinking water), 2. rats drinking 225meq/l NaCl
solution, 3. rats drinking 300meq/l NaCl solution, 4. rats
drinking 375meq/l NaCl solution. Each group was formed by 10
Wistar female rats. BP was measured in unanaesthetized animals
by the tail-cuff method for 17 weeks. While no sustained hyper-

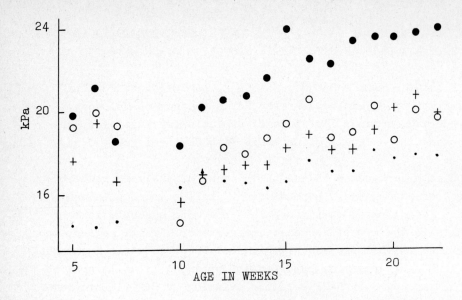

Fig. 1. Blood pressure in rats drinking water • or 225 meq/1 +, 300 meq/1● and 375 meq/1O NaCl solution from the age of 4 weeks

tension was observed in rats drinking salt solutions only in adulthood, increased BP and even hypertension was found in those drinking NaCl solutions from the 4th week (Figure 1). A sustained hypertension appeared only in rats drinking fluid containing 300 meq/l NaCl. No mortality was observed in groups 1 and 2, 2 rats died at the age of 10 weeks in the group 3 and only 4 rats survived the age of 13 weeks in the group 4.

The attention was, thereafter, focused to the effects of the 300 meq/l NaCl solution (hypertonic saline). In order to establish whether hypertension observed in rats drinking hypertonic saline from 4th week of life could be explained by higher saline consumption in youth in comparison with adulthood, fluid intake was estimated. Daily measurements of hypertonic saline were done in rats both drinking saline from the 4th and 12th week of life. An automatic drinkometer was used[8]. Regression lines shown in Figure 2 were calculated from 800 single measurements in each group. It is evident that rats consuming hypertonic saline from youth had higher salt intake at the onset of

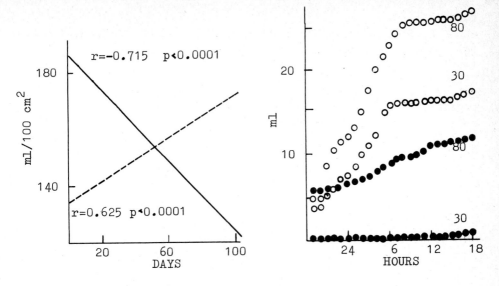

Fig. 2. Hypertonic saline intake in rats drinking it from the
4th (full line) or 12th (inter-
rupted line) week of age. Ordinate: fluid intake related to
the body surface. Abscissa: time from the onset of drinking

Fig. 3. Water o and hypertonic saline ● intake in rats
offered a free choice between these fluids for 24 h.
30 — rats drinking hypertonic saline from 30th day of
age, 80 — from 80th day.

experiment and that the opposite was true for rats drinking saline only in adulthood.

High saline consumption in young rats could be caused either
by thirst or by appetite for salt. The next experiment was designed to make clear which of these mechanisms is more involved.
Again, rats drinking saline from the 5th week of age were compared with those drinking it from the 12th week of age. After 5
days of hypertonic saline drinking rats were offered a free choice to drink water or hypertonic saline. Fluids consumption was
measured each 15 minutes for 24 hours. Figure 3 shows that young
rats drank eagerly water and almost completely refused to drink
hypertonic saline. Adult rats drank water but they consumed hypertonic saline as well. From the distinct preference of water
it could be concluded that young rats are forced to consume
hypertonic saline, representing the only drinking fluid, by thirst.

Sodium concentration in the blood plasma is an important
contributing factor in the regulation of the water intake[9].

TABLE 1

BLOOD PLASMA Na$^+$ CONCENTRATION IN RATS DRINKING HYPERTONIC SALINE EITHER FROM YOUTH OR FROM ADULTHOOD

Day of the experiment	Water to drink from the 4th week	Hypertonic saline from the 4th week	12th week
6	136.4±0.69 (7)	159.3±0.57^a (8)	131.6±0.56^b (7)
11	130.7±1.46 (7)	158.6±0.27^a (9)	136.2±0.96^b (6)
25	130.1±0.55 (5)	160.0±2.21^a (5)	136.6±0.69^b (6)
150	140.3±0.96 (6)	152.5±3.65^a (6)	

In parentheses: number of animals
a Significantly different from Water to drink (p < 0.01)
b Significantly different from the 4th week (p < 0.01)

Blood plasma Na$^+$ concentration was, therefore, determined in rats drinking hypertonic saline either from the 4th or from the 12th week of age. Determinations were performed 6, 11, 25 and in the younger group 150 days after the onset of saline drinking. Table 1 shows that the intake of hypertonic saline caused a well expressed hypernatremia persisting till the adulthood if taken in from the 4th week of age, whereas no change in plasmatic Na$^+$ concentration was observed in rats consuming hypertonic saline only from adulthood. It was assumed that young rats submitted to high salt intake retained more sodium than adults. Bengele and Solomon[10] reported that, in comparison with the natriuretic ability of adult rats, prepubertal rats have a limited capacity to excrete sodium after blood volume or extracellular fluid volume expansion. Recently, this low natriuretic capacity was ascribed to the absence of an blood-born natriuretic factor in young rats. In order to verify this assumption, the experiments of Solomon et al.[11] were repeated.

Wistar rats aged 25-30 days anaesthetized by Inactin were infused through jugular vein for 80 min. with the Ringer solution (0.5ml/h) and after this control period the blood volume expansion was carried out by the infusion of heparinized blood

TABLE 2

URINE VOLUME AND Na^+ EXCRETION IN YOUNG RATS DURING 80 MIN. BEFO-
RE AND AFTER BLOOD VOLUME EXPANSION WITH THE BLOOD FROM EITHER
YOUNG OR ADULT RATS

Treatment	Urine volume ml/100g of body weight	Na excretion μeq/100g of body weight
Before expansion	0.64±0.079 (26)	23.32± 2.918 (26)
Expansion with the blood of young rats	2.79±0.345[a] (17)	219.20±36.648[a] (17)
Expansion with the blood of adult rats	4.10±0.532[ab] (9)	363.06±57.396[ab] (9)

In parentheses: Number of animals
[a] Significantly different from Before expansion ($p < 0.01$)
[b] Significantly different from the blood of young rats ($p < 0.05$)

(2.3ml/100g of body weight, duration of the infusion - 20 min.).
The infused blood was withdrawn either from adult or from 25 - 30
days-old rats. Urine was collected for 80 min. from the outset
of the blood infusion in four 20-min. samples. As shown in Table
2 a polyuria accompanied by intensive Na^+ excretion was elicited
by the infusion of blood taken out from both the young and adult
rats but this response was more expressed if the blood of adult
rats was infused. Thus, the low natriuretic activity of the blood
of young rats was confirmed.

If the lack of natriuretic factor in young rats is responsible
for the sodium retention in their body, the high plasma Na^+ concentration produced by drinking hypertonic saline can be decreased by the infusion of the blood obtained from adult saline
drinking rats. The experiment was, therefore, carried out in
the course of which 30-day-old rats drinking hypertonic saline
from the 25th day of age were infused by the blood taken out
either from 30-day-old or from adult rats drinking hypertonic
saline for 5 days as well. The experimental procedure was as
described in the preceding paragraph. In addition, plasma Na^+
concentration was determined at the onset of the control infusion period and 80 min. after the onset of the blood infusion.

TABLE 3

PLASMA Na$^+$ CONCENTRATION IN YOUNG RATS DRINKING SALINE FROM THE 4th WEEK OF AGE AND INFUSED WITH THE BLOOD FROM YOUNG AND ADULT RATS DRINKING HYPERTONIC SALINE

	Blood plasma Na$^+$ concentration meq/l
Before expansion	159.8$\pm$1.2716 (35)
After expansion with the blood of young rats	159.1$\pm$1.4131 (19)
After expansion with the blood of adult rats	153.9$\pm$2.1281[a] (16)

In parentheses: number of animals
[a] Significantly different from Before expansion (p < 0.02) and from young rats (p < 0.05)

No change of hypernatremia was observed in recipient rats after the infusion of the blood from hypertonic saline drinking young rats, whereas a significant decrease appeared after the infusion of the blood from adult rats (Table 3). However, this drop of

TABLE 4

URINE VOLUME AND Na$^+$ EXCRETION IN YOUNG RATS DRINKING SALINE FROM THE 4th WEEK OF AGE BEFORE AND AFTER EXPANSION WITH THE BLOOD FROM EITHER YOUNG OR ADULT RATS DRINKING HYPERTONIC SALINE

Treatment	Urine volume ml/100g of body weight	Na$^+$ excretion μeq/100g of body weight
Before expansion	0.33$\pm$0.049 (37)	79.46$\pm$13.778 (36)
Expansion with the blood of young rats	2.84$\pm$0.361[a] (20)	412.80$\pm$55.478[a] (20)
Expansion with the blood of adult rats	2.83$\pm$0.328[a] (16)	462.16$\pm$54.132[a] (16)

Legend see Table 2

plasma Na$^+$ concentration was not accompanied by increased Na$^+$ excretion in rats infused with the blood from adult rats in com-

parison with those infused with blood from young rats (Table 4).
If data from Table 4 are confronted with those presented on
Table 2 it may be remarked in recipients which drank hypertonic saline increased Na^+ excretion after infusion of the blood
from young donors and a decrease of urine volume after infusion of the blood from saline drinking adult donors. These con-

TABLE 5
URINARY Na^+ CONCENTRATION IN 20 MIN. SAMPLING PERIODS BEFORE
AND AFTER INFUSION OF THE BLOOD FROM EITHER YOUNG OR ADULT RATS
DRINKING HYPERTONIC SALINE (IN meq/l)

20 min. sampling periods	Before infusion	After the onset of infusion of the blood from young	of the blood from adult rats
I	$317.4^{\pm}19.62$ (32)	$147.0^{\pm}13.82$ (19)	$200.2^{\pm}14.32^{a}$ (16)
II	$280.8^{\pm}16.00$ (28)	$141.5^{\pm}7.73$ (21)	$164.5^{\pm}10.45$ (17)
III	$215.8^{\pm}13.29$ (30)	$135.1^{\pm} 9.84$ (21)	$160.4^{\pm}11.65$ (17)
IV	$162.6^{\pm}13.13$ (31)	$149.4^{\pm}12.30$ (20)	$153.9^{\pm}13.17$ (15)

In parentheses: number of animals
[a] Significantly different from young ($p < 0.02$)

troversial findings were made clear as soon as the urinary Na^+
concentrations were taken into consideration. Sodium concentrations in urine sampled in the course of single 20 min. collecting periods are presented on Table 5. In accordance with the
high salt intake of the recipient young rat,the urinary Na^+
concentration was very high in the I. sampling period. It declined gradually to isotonic values which were attained at the onset of the blood infusion. Isotonic sodium concentration was
kept even after the infusion of the blood from young rats with
high salt intake but it was significantly increased by the
infusion of blood obtained from the adult hypertonic saline
drinking rats. However, urinary Na^+ concentration dropped
down immediately after the interruption of the infusion of the

blood. Hence, a natriuretic activity is contained in the blood of adult rats drinking hypertonic saline, which is capable to reduce hypernatremia produced in young rats by increased salt intake. This decrease of blood plasma Na^+ concentration is achieved by a short time increase of the urinary Na^+ concentration of the recipient rat to hypertonic values. This activity is apparently promptly cleared out of the blood of the recipient because the urinary Na^+ concentration goes down immediately after the interruption of the infusion of the adult blood. This activity is absent in the blood of prepubertal rats.

TABLE 6

URINARY Na^+ CONCENTRATION IN 20 MIN. SAMPLING PERIODS BEFORE AND AFTER INFUSION OF THE BLOOD FROM EITHER YOUNG OR ADULT RATS DRINKING WATER (IN meq/l)

20 min. sampling periods	Before infusion	After the onset of infusion of the blood from young	of the blood from adult rats
I	69.5±9.23 (20)	51.9±10.06 (14)	86.3±11.06[a,b] (8)
II	52.9±9.08 (23)	71.1±8.27[b] (14)	78.7±5.68[b] (9)
III	34.3±6.08 (23)	66.2±6.45[b] (15)	88.5±9.86[b] (8)
IV	35.4±6.26 (24)	82.7±8.12[b] (15)	97.4±5.38[b] (8)

In parentheses: number of animals
[a] Significantly different from young ($p < 0.05$)
[b] Significantly different from Before infusion IV ($p < 0.01$)

On the Table 6 analogous data are presented as on the Table 5 for rats drinking water. Although the urinary Na^+ concentration is lower in all sampling periods than in rats submitted to the hypertonic saline drinking, the transient difference between rats receiving blood from young and adult rats resp. is evident. The difference in natriuretic properties of blood between prepubertal and adult rats is, therefore, independent on the salt intake.

Recently, a sodium retaining activity was found in the

blood of Sprague-Dawley rats sensitive to the hypertensogenic
influence of high salt intake[12]. In present paper, on the other
hand, the absence of a natriuretic factor was documented in
Wistar rats limited to the age period of prepuberty. Prepuberty
is a developmental period of increased sensitivity of rats toward the hypertensogenic effect of salt. A conclusion might be
drawn that a lack of natriuretic activity in young rats drinking
hypertonic saline bring about the retention of sodium in the
body and resulting increase of blood plasma Na^+ concentration.
Intensive thirst is raised as a consequence of hypernatremia.
The rat is forced to drink the only available drinking fluid,
i.e. hypertonic saline. A "circulus vitiosus" is switched on
keeping hypernatremia. The resulting disbalance of the sodium
distribution inside of blood vessels compartments might contribute to increase the sensitivity of these vessels towards vasoactive substances and the BP might be increased.

REFERENCES

1. Skelton, F. R. and Guillebeau, J. (1956) Endocrinology 59, 201 - 214
2. Dlouhá, H. et al. (1977) Pflügers Arch. 369, 177 - 182
3. Dlouhá, H. et al. (1979) Clin. Sci. 57, 273 - 275
4. Dahl, L. K. et al. (1968) Circ. Res. 22, 11 - 18
5. Sapirstein, L. A. et al. (1950) Proc. Soc. Exp. Biol. Med. 73, 82 - 85
6. Haigh, A. S. and Weller, J. M. (1962) Am. J. Physiol. 202, 1144 - 1146
7. Jelínek, J. et al. (1966) Physiol. Bohemoslov. 15, 137 - 147
8. Krpata V. and Křeček J. (1975) Physiol. Bohemoslov. 24, 449
9. Andersson, B. and Westbye O. (1970) Nature (Lond.) 228, 75 - 76
10. Bengele A. H. and Solomon, S. (1974) Am. J. Physiol. 227, 364 - 368
11. Solomon, S. et al. (1979) Biol. Neonate 35, 113 - 120
12. Tobian, L. et al. (1979) Hypertension 1, 316 - 324

Hormonal Regulation of Sodium Excretion,
B. Lichardus, R.W. Schrier and J. Ponec, eds.
© 1980 Elsevier/North-Holland Biomedical Press

RENAL SODIUM EXCRETION IN ACUTELY HYPOPHYSECTOMIZED RATS WITH
EXPANDED EXTRACELLULAR FLUID VOLUME

PÁL BENCSÁTH, GÁBOR SZÉNÁSI, JOZEF PONEC[+], LAJOS TAKÁCS,
BRANISLAV LICHARDUS[+]
Res. Group Clin. Immunol., Nephrol., Endocrinol., MTA-SOTE EKSz,
2nd Dept. Med., Semmelweis Univ. Med. School, Szentkirályi u. 46,
1088 Budapest (Hungary) and Inst. Exp. Endocrinol., Ctr. Physiol.
Sci., Slovak Acad. Sci., Vlárska 3, 809 36 Bratislava-Kramáre,
(Czechoslovakia)

INTRODUCTION

Hypophysectomy performed 120 min prior to a sudden increase of
extracellular fluid volume (ECFV) by blood transfusion or by saline infusion (acute hypophysectomy; a.h.) dissociated, in anesthetized rats, their renal reaction to such a stimulation of the body
fluid volume regulatory mechanisms: the animals enhanced urine output by augmenting mainly the excretion of osmotically free water
but they failed adequately to increase the renal sodium output[1,2,3].
Similar results were obtained also in a.h. dogs[4]. A continuous infusion of antidiuretic doses of vasopressin to a.h. rats cut off
the excretion of free water but did not restore a homeostatically
effective natriuresis[2,5,6,7,8]. A search for other factors possibly
involved in the renal regulation of ECFV revealed that a.h. prevented concomitantly also the increase of cardiac output, as well as
the increase of renal cortical blood flow during the ECFV expansion with saline. As a rule glomerular filtration rate and renal
perfusion pressure were not affected. Thus the failure to increase
renal blood flow was due to a failure to decrease renal vascular
resistance. Consequently in comparison to normal rats which react
by decreasing renal vascular resistance and by increasing renal
blood flow, the hydrostatic pressure in the peritubular capillaries of a.h. rats should be lower and the oncotic pressure higher[1,9,10,11]. This resetting of Starling forces (physical factors)
by means of acute hypophysectomy could facilitate the capillary
uptake of reabsorbate and thereby indirectly increase tubular

reabsorption, thus contributing to the impaired ability of a.h. rats to react to ECFV expansion by adequate natriuresis. Therefore it is probable that extrarenal hormonal factor(s) by regulating renal hemodynamics regulate the operation of physical factors which play a role in the mechanism of renal sodium execution[1,3,9,10]. Such humoral factor(s) may or may not necessarily be identical with a more specific "natriuretic hormone" which is supposed to affect directly tubular sodium transport. In any case humoral factors probably play a primary role in the complex mechanism of renal regulation of ECFV[1,2,3,9].

The aim of the present work was to obtain more direct evidence for the above theory on an interaction between humoral and physical factors in the renal regulation of ECFV by measuring the hydrostatic pressure in peritubular capillaries of sham-operated and a.h. rats. The fractional and absolute reabsorption of water and sodium was also measured by means of micropuncture.

MATERIAL AND METHODS

Eighteen rats were used for direct measurement of hydrostatic pressure in the peritubular capillaries by a servo-nulling device and a further 18 rats were used for micropuncture studies of tubular sodium and water reabsorption (10 sham operated and 8 a.h. rats were in each group). Late proximal and early distal collections were made based on prior intravenous injection of Lissamine green. The rats were of CFY strain, Inst. for Lab Animals, Gödölö, Hungary, weighing 210-300 g. The rats fasted for 14-16 h before the experiment started but tap water was available ad libitum. All experiments were performed in Inactin anesthesia. Pituitaries were removed by a parapharyngeal approach. Sham operation was completed by drilling a hole in the sphenoid bone. Canulas were inserted in the jugular vein, femoral artery and in both ureters of each animal. The left kidneys were exposed and prepared for micropuncture of peritubular capillaries, late proximal, and early distal tubules.

After completing the surgical preparation an equilibration time of an hour was allowed. All studies were then performed during a 20 min urine collection period which followed a 40 min period in which all rats were infused with a volume of isotonic saline corresponding to 6% of their body weight (2/3 of the volume was given in the first half of the period and 1/3 in the second half). GFR was measured as clearance of ^{3}H-Inulin. The experimental procedure as well as the experimental and laboratory micromethods used were described in more detail elsewhere[3,5,6,12].

RESULTS

The results are summarized in the tables.

TABLE 1

EFFECT OF ACUTE HYPOPHYSECTOMY ON HYDROSTATIC PRESSURE IN THE PERITUBULAR CAPILLARIES OF RATS WITH EXPANDED ECFV

Parameters	CONTROL n=10	HYPOX n=8
BP torr	101 ± 3.8	97 ± 3.7
Peritub.capillary torr	13 ± 0.5 (n=21)	10 ± 0.3[a] (n=23)
$U_{Na}V$ /umol/min/g	7.7 ± 0.93	0.1 ± 0.02[b]

All values of the parameters studied are means ± S.E.M. Standard abbrevations are used in all tables. Significance of differences between the respective parameters was evaluated by the Student t-test (a=P< 0.01; b=P< 0.001).

The stricking difference in renal sodium excretion between the control and a.h. rats was accompanied by a difference in the peritubular capillary hydrostatic pressure: higher pressure being accompanied by a much more pronounced natriuresis. Even if the present data do not prove a causal relationship between the two parameters, the basic assumption was confirmed i.e. the hydrostatic pressure in the peritubular capillaries of a.h. rats was found to be lower than in normal rats.

TABLE 2

EFFECT OF ACUTE HYPOPHYSECTOMY ON SOME PARAMETERS OF RENAL
FUNCTION DURING ECFV EXPANSION (CLEARENCE DATA)

Parameters	CONTROL n=10			HYPOX n=8		
BP torr	105.4	$\pm$	1.95	108.9	$\pm$	3.55
GFR ml/min/g	1.738	$\pm$	0.096	0.973	$\pm$	0.086^{b}
V $_{/}$ul/min/g	15.08	$\pm$	2.39	26.78	$\pm$	2.97^{a}
U_{osm} mmol/kg H_2O	1137	$\pm$	115	123.4	$\pm$	8.9^{b}
C_{osm} /ul/min/g	41.09	$\pm$	3.54	10.27	$\pm$	0.85^{b}
C_{H_2O} /ul/min/g	-28.53	$\pm$	2.77	+16.48	$\pm$	2.4^{a}
U_{Na} mmol/l	276.3	$\pm$	18.1	12.03	$\pm$	3.36^{b}
$U_{Na}V$ /umol/min/g	3.554	$\pm$	0.512	0.272	$\pm$	0.078^{b}
U_K mmol/l	131.6	$\pm$	16.6	5.87	$\pm$	0.64^{b}
U_KV /umol/min/g	1.431	$\pm$	0.096	0.141	$\pm$	0.017^{b}
FE_{Na} %	1.654	$\pm$	0.219	0.214	$\pm$	0.07^{b}
SNGFR nl/min (late proximal)	41.7	$\pm$	1.94	29.9	$\pm$	1.19^{b}

n=29, resp. 28

The clearance data of the function of the left and right kidney
were not significantly different, therefore only data from the
left kidneys which were used for micropuncture are presented as
means $\pm$ S.E.M.

The data in TABLE 2 are comparable to those already published
in part[1,3]. The failure of a.h. rats to react by natriuresis to
ECFV expansion is again well documented. However in these experiments GFR was lower in a.h. rats than in controls by about 50%.
As a rule, in several previous series of experiments in which the
micropuncture technique was not used, the differences in GFR between the controls and a.h. rats were not significant (in preparation). Some of this difference in the present experiments might
have been caused by a more extensive surgery. On the other hand,
differences in SNGFR were not so pronounced (about 25%). This dis-
crepancy in the values for GFR and SNGFR may be caused by a re-

distribution of glomerular filtration rate in a.h. rats.

TABLE 3

PARAMETERS OF FRACTIONAL AND ABSOLUTE TUBULAR REABSORPTION IN SHAM OPERATED AND ACUTELY HYPOPHYSECTOMIZED RATS WITH EXPANDED ECFV

Parameters	CONTROL n=10	HYPOX n=8
End proximal collections (n=29)		
FR %	32.24 ± 1.52	48.88 ± 1.17^{b}
AR_{H_2O} nl/min	12.96 ± 0.41	14.22 ± 0.43
AR_{Na} nmol/min	2.13 ± 0.09	2.12 ± 0.09
Beginning distal collections (n=28, resp.26)		
FR %	75.56 ± 0.30	79.20 ± 0.37^{b}
FR_{Na} %	83.30 ± 0.57	88.40 ± 0.61^{b}
AR_{Na} nmol/min	2.71 ± 0.08	1.79 ± 0.07^{b}
Urine		
FR %	99.12 ± 0.12	97.04 ± 0.31^{b}
FR_{Na} %	87.33 ± 0.90	95.00 ± 0.74^{b}
AR_{Na} nmol/min	0.32 ± 0.03	0.24 ± 0.02^{a}

Abbrevations used: FR = fractional reabsorption; AR = absolute reabsorption. Data are presented as means $\pm$ S.E.M.

In proximal tubule absolute reabsorption of fluid is the same even though filtered load is reduced in a.h. rats. This means that proximal transport capacity in this group is increased, in agreement with the experimentally determined reduction of peritubular hydrostatic pressure. By the time fluid reaches the early

distal collection site the differences in fractional reabsorption
of salt and water are less than at the end of the proximal tubule,
indicating the load-dependency of loop transport[13]. As expected,
in the collecting duct water reabsorption is less in a.h. rats.
However, the relative increase in fractional sodium reabsorption
seen in both proximal and distal collections persists and may even
be enhanced. Therefore it is conceivable that a factor which operates against tubular sodium reabsorption in normal rats may be
lacking in a.h. rats. Data on direct measurements of hydrostatic
pressure support the suggestion that the missing factor may be of
a humoral nature, linked to the function of the pituitary and participating in the regulation of renal hemodynamics and consequently in the operation of physical and hemodynamic factors controlling capillary uptake of reabsorbate at least at the level of the
proximal tubule. As for the experimental model used – acute hypo-
physectomy-it seems to be advantageous for revealing the interaction between the operation of hormonal, hemodynamic and physical factors in the mechanism of natriuresis evoked by a sudden
increase of ECFV.

ACKNOWLEDGEMENTS

The authors express their gratitude to Mrs. B. Asztalos for
her technical assistance and to Prof. Harald Sonnenberg for a help-
ful criticism of the presented data.

REFERENCES

1. Lichardus, B., Ponec, J. (1978) In: Natriuretic Hormone
   (eds. H.J. Kramer, F. Krück), Springer, Berlin, pp. 6-15.

2. Ponec, J., Lichardus, B. (1977) Experientia, 33, 685.

3. Lichardus, B. (1978) Mechanizmy rýchlej renálnej regulácie
   objemu extracelulárnej tekutiny, VEDA SAV, Bratislava,
   pp. 115-131.

4. Szalay, L., Bencsáth, P., Takács, L., Ponec, J., Lichardus, B.
   (1975) Experientia, 31, 1298.

5. Lichardus, B., Ponec, J. (1972) Experientia, 28, 471.

6. Lichardus, B., Ponec, J. (1972) Experientia, 28, 1443.

7. Lichardus, B., Ponec, J. (1973) Endokrinologie, 61, 403.

8. Lichardus, B., Ponec, J., Albrecht, I. (1973) In: Endocrinology (ed. R.O. Scow) Excerpta Medica, Amsterdam, pp. 729-732.

9. Lichardus, B., Ponec, J., Turek, R. (1975) 2nd Int. Congr. Pathophysiol., Praha 1975, Abstracta No 230.

10. Lichardus, B., Ponec, J., Turek, R. (1976) Experientia, 32, 884.

11. Reineck, H.J., Stein, J.H. (1978) In: Sodium and Water Homeostasis (eds. B.M. Brenner, J.H. Stein) Churchill Livingstone, New York, pp. 24-50.

12. Bello-Reus, E., Colinders, R.E., Pastoriza-Munoz, E., Mueller, R.A., Gottschalk, C.W.(1975) J. Clin. Invest., 56, 208.

13. Morgan, T., Berliner, R.W. (1969) Amer. J. Physiol., 217, 992.

Hormonal Regulation of Sodium Excretion,
B. Lichardus, R.W. Schrier and J. Ponec, eds.
© 1980 Elsevier/North-Holland Biomedical Press

SOME CHEMICAL PROPERTIES OF THE NATRIURETIC FACTOR

YURI I. IVANOV
Department of Pharmacology, Chernovtsy Medical Institute,
Teatralnaya pl. 2, 274000, Chernovtsy, USSR

It is well known that the expansion of extracellular fluid
volume by intravenous infusion of saline produces an increased
excretion of sodium by the kidney. The investigation of volume
natriuresis showed that the increased sodium excretion was caused
neither by a change of the glomerular filtration rate nor by the
decreased aldosterone secretion nor by other well-known regulators of the kidney function. That is why, it was suggested that
the volume natriuresis was due to increased synthesis of a humoral natriuretic factor. Lately many investigators[1,2,3] have made
an attempt to isolate this factor, to find out its source, and
reveal its chemical composition. It was supposed that the source
of this factor was the brain[1], the kidney[4], but in 1973 we suggested that the natriuretic hormone was synthesized or activated in
the liver, because our experiments had shown that the level of a
natriuretic activity before and after an expansion of the extracellular space was the highest in the blood plasma flowing out of
the liver. In contrast it was significantly lower in the blood
plasma flowing to the brain and kidney and flowing out of them[5].
In rats experimental dystrophy of the liver decreased the content
of the natriuretic factor in blood plasma and the expansion of
extracellular space did not produce any natriuretic effect as
compared to control rats. After pharmacological stimulation of
the liver the volume expansion led to a significant increase of
the excretion of sodium by the kidney, and to the increase of the
content of the natriuretic factor in blood plasma as compared to
control rats[6].

But further investigations on the physiological role of the
natriuretic factor are connected with certain difficulties due to
the lack of very accurate and reproduced methods of its quantitative determination. These methods are extremely necessary for the
investigation of the chemical composition of this hormone, becau-

se it is necessary to identify the active substance from others
after separation and chromatography.

At the same time we still extrapolate the quantity of the natriuretic hormone on the natriuretic activity of the biological
substance under study on the grounds of its ability to increase
natriuresis in animals or change the short-circuit current in the
frog bladder or skin. But in all these cases it is said that the
natriuretic material is either present or absent in this biological substrate. And it is practically impossible to give its quantitative characteristic.

In this connection we have elaborated two simple methods of
quantitative bioassays of the natriuretic factor in experiments
on rats and on isolated segments of the rat's small intestine.

The assays carried out by us on rats will be described below.
Rats everaging I50 g in weight were allowed free acces to water
and fed sodium depleted diet for three days. The animals were
given 0.45% sodium chloride solution 3% of body weight by gavage.
Then one half of the rats (no less than 5 rats) was injected i.p.
0.3 ml of tested blood plasma or other tested material, and the
other half of the rats (as control) was injected the same volume
of isotonic saline. Then all the rats were placed in separate
cages with an accomodation for urine collection during one hour.
The sodium content was determined in hourly portions of urine
while the means and their standard errors were calculated by
standard statistical methods in every group of rats.

The quantity of the natriuretic factor was calculated in conditional units according to the formula

$$K = \frac{M_I \cdot M_2 - m_I \cdot m_2}{P \cdot (M_I^2 - m_I^2)}$$

where K - the quantity of the natriuretic factor in conditional
units per I ml, M_I - the mean of sodium excretion in control rats
m_I - the standard error of this value, M_2 - the mean of sodium
excretion in experimental rats, m_2 - the standard error of this
value, P - the volume of tested biological substance in ml infused i.p. to experimental rats.

One conditional unit is equal to such a quantity of the natriuretic factor which can increase the hourly natriuresis twice as much as compared to the control rats. The values of the natriuretic factor content in blood plasma of rats and rabbits are given in Table I.

Table I

THE CONTENT OF THE NATRIURETIC FACTOR IN BLOOD PLASMA OF RATS AND RABBITS (in conditional units per I ml)

Animals	Before expansion of extracellular space	After expansion of extracellular space	Significance
Rats	5.4±0.23	I0.6±0.5I	<0.00I
Rabbits	5.9±0.28	II.6±0.55	<0.00I

The quantitative determination of the natriuretic factor on the isolated rat's small intestine was assayed in the following way[7]. Rats were deprived of food at least I8 - 22 hours prior to the experiments, while water was allowed ad libitum. After decapitation a segment of the jejunum 4 - 5 cm long was isolated, a few segments being taken from the same rat. The isolated segment of the jejunum was turned out and tied up at both ends. The turned sack was incubated in aerated bicarbonate Krebs solution (in mmol/l: NaCl - I35; KCl - 4.5; $CaCl_2$ - 2.5; $MgSO_4$ - I.I8; $NaHCO_3$ - 5; NaH_2PO_4 - I.84; Na_2HPO_4 - 0.46; glucose - I2.2; pH - 7.4; at 37°C). It is necessary to prepare 3 - 4 such turned sacks

After incubation for I hour and subsequent weighing the tested material was added in the proportion of 0.0I - 0.2 ml per I0 ml of the medium. In 30 minutes of incubation it was weighed once more. The sacks were dried and the assessment of change in weight (either increase or decrease) was calculated per I g of the dried sack weight.

The results of these experiments were plotted on the diagram (Figure I), where changes of the sack weight were marked on the ordinate axis while the quantity of the tested material was plotted on the absciss axis. The results were expressed in intestinal units per I ml. One intestinal unit is equal to the same quantity of the natriuretic factor which can completely inhibit the transport by the isolated segment of the jejunum. This quantity corresponds to the point of intersection of the curve with the absciss. It is shown on Figure I.

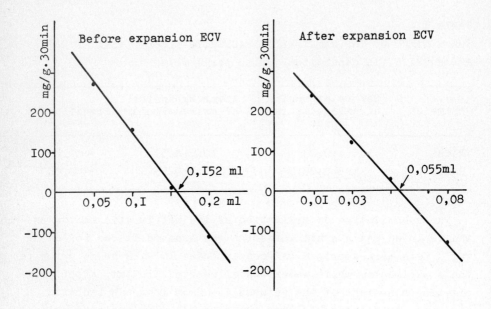

Fig. I. Circulation of the natriuretic factor content in blood plasma of rats. Explanation are in the text.

The quantity of the natriuretic factor per I ml of blood plasma was calculated in intestinal units according to the formula

$$K = \frac{I}{M}$$

where K - the quantity of the natriuretic factor in intestinal units per I ml, M - the value obtained from the diagram.

The quantity of the natriuretic factor in blood plasma of rats and rabbits expressed in intestinal units are presented in Table 2.

The natriuretic factor from the blood plasma of a dog assayed by these methods was inactivated in 2 - 3 days of storage at 4°C. This factor was preserved for 3 weeks after boiling or freezing

Table 2

THE CONTENT OF THE NATRIURETIC FACTOR IN BLOOD PLASMA OF RATS
AND RABBITS (in intestinal units per I ml)

Animals	Before expansion of extracellular space	After expansion of extracellular space	Significance
Rats	6.0±0.42	I5.6±I.I2	<0.00I
Rabbits	8.6±0.99	22.4±I.86	<0.00I

of blood plasma. The inactivation of the natriuretic factor was
mediated probably by enzymes of the blood plasma.

This factor remained unchanged quantitatively in the supernatant fluid after precipitation of plasma proteins by sulfosalicy-
lic or trichloracetic acids. It was inactivated after incubation
with the proteolytic enzymes (trypsin, chymotrypsin and thrombin).
Therefore the natriuretic factor may be regarded as a polypeptide
of a low molecular weight.

Subsequent deciphering of the chemical composition of the
natriuretic factor is difficult because it is very hard to accumulate this factor in sufficient supply, as it is quickly inactivated. We could preserve the concentrated natriuretic factor
during I year. For the preparation of this concentrate 30% solution of trichloracetic acid was added to the blood plasma (I6 ml
per I00 ml of plasma). After thorough mixing it was centrifuged.
Then the supernatant fluid was skimmed and washed clear from the
residuum of trichloracetic acid by ethyl ether. Then pH of the
supernatant was reduced to 7.3 by sodium hydroxide and afterwards
it was frozen and dried in vacuum. The activity of this natriuretic factor concentrate decreased only by 40 per cent after storage for a year.

Now I would like to turn to our investigations of column chromatography of this concentrate. These studies were performed on
2.5 x I00 cm Sephadex G-25 column. Optical density was monitored
in UV-absorbance at 280 nm. Figure 2 shows the general type of
chromatogram using 0.I M acetic acid as an eluent. We see 5 peaks
on this chromatogram. After the assay of their natriuretic activity by the above-mentioned methods we discovered that the natri-

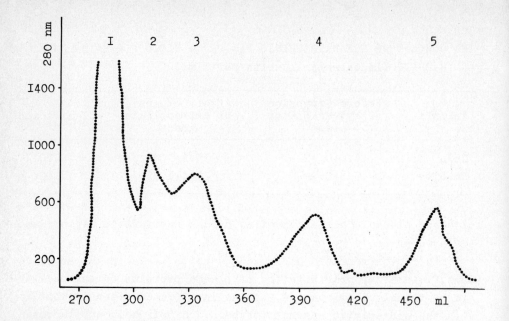

Fig. 2. Gel filtration of the natriuretic factor concentrate on
Sephadex G-25 column

uretic factor was present in the 2nd and 3rd peaks. There was no
natriuretic activity in other peaks.

Further separation of both peak concentrates by high-voltage
electrophoresis (3000 V and 200 mA) revealed that the composition
of these peaks was heterogeneous.

REFERENCES

1. Cort J.H., Lichardus B. (1968) Nephron, 5, 401-409.
2. Buckalew V.M. (1975) Proc.Soc.exptl.Biol., 149, 203-206.
3. Clarkson E.M. et al. (1976) Kidney Int., 10, 381-394.
4. Godon J.P. (1978) In: Natriuretic Hormone, ed. H.J.Kramer &
   F.Krück, Springer-Verlag, 88-100.
5. Ivanov Yu.I. (1973) Probl.endocrin. (Moscow), 19, 99-102.
6. Ivanov Yu.I. (1979) Endocrinol.exper., 13, 195-200.
7. Kosuba R.B., Ivanov Yu.I. (1978) Bull.exper.Biol. (Moscow),
   86, 624-625.

Hormonal Regulation of Sodium Excretion,
B. Lichardus, R.W. Schrier and J. Ponec, eds.
© 1980 Elsevier/North-Holland Biomedical Press

FURTHER STUDIES ON ISOLATION AND PURIFICATION OF A SMALL MOLE – CULAR WEIGHT NATRIURETIC HORMONE

HERBERT J. KRAMER, CHRISTIAN RIETZEL [+], DIETRICH KLINGMÜLLER, and RAINER DÜSING

Medizinische Universitäts-Poliklinik, Wilhelmstrasse 35-37,

5300 Bonn 1 (W-Germany)

INTRODUCTION

In previous studies we have shown that a small molecular weight fraction isolated from serum and urine of salt loaded rats, dogs, and healthy human subjects inhibits sodium transport of the isolated frog skin when added to the inside bathing Ringer solution. Using gel filtration techniques this fraction IV is eluted from a Sephadex G-25 column subsequent to inorganic salts[1]. In contrast to serum fractions from control rats, addition of this fraction isolated from serum of acutely saline loaded rats to the inside bathing Ringer solution resulted in an immediate and progressive fall in potential difference and short-circuit current of the isolated frog skin[2] as an indirect measure of net sodium transport[3]. These antinatriferic effects were also observed with serum fractions IV from healthy subjects under conditions of acute and chronic salt loading[1] and from patients with primary aldosteronism[1]. In addition, serum fractions IV from acutely saline loaded rats[2] and healthy human subjects[4] were shown to result in a significant natriuresis when injected into bioassay rats. We have further demonstrated that this antinatriferic and natriuretic action most likely results from inhibition of the Na-K-ATPase enzyme system[5,6,7] which mediates active transepithelial sodium transport[8].

In order to further explore the nature and identity of the natriuretic material it seemed necessary to have more ready access to larger amounts of source material for recovery and further identification of this yet unknown humoral agent.

In the present study we therefore investigated the presence of the natriuretic

[+] Pharmazeutisches Laboratorium der Röhm Chemie GmbH, Darmstadt, W-Germany

material in the urine of healthy subjects during normal salt intake, during dietary salt restriction and during high salt intake. We then attempted to further purify this natriuretic material by applying various chromatographic techniques.

MATERIAL AND METHODS

Urine collection during dietary changes in sodium balance

In healthy subjects (medical students) chronic changes in sodium balance were achieved by dietary salt restriction and high salt intake. On two preceeding days mean urinary sodium excretion amounted to 166 ± 46 and 159 ± 32 mEq/24 h, respectively. They were then placed on a low sodium intake of 34 mEq per day for five days and subsequently on a high dietary salt intake of 340 mEq per day again for five days.

During normal, low, and high salt intake urine was collected daily during 24-h periods and kept refrigerated until collection was completed. Aliquots of urine were lyophilized and the resulting powder was stored at -18° C until subjected to column chromatography. At this point samples were reconstituted in 10 ml of distilled water, pH was adjusted to 3.5 with concentrated acetic acid. Samples were then centrifuged at 3,000 rpm for 10 min at 5° C.

Chromatographic procedures

Supernates of acidified urine were applied to Sephadex G-25 columns using 0.1 N acetic acid (pH 3.5) as eluent. Descending flow rate averaged 2 ml/min. UV-absorbance at 280 nm was recorded automatically throughout fractionation. Single fractions of 2 to 4 ml which followed the elution of inorganic salts (Fraction III at a V_E/V_0-ratio of 2.2) between a V_E/V_0-ratio of 2.3 to 2.7 with a peak activity at 2.5 were pooled to fraction F IV (figure 1) and were subsequently lyophilized in siliconized glass containers at temperatures not exceeding 4° C. The resulting powder was stored at -18° C until further chromatographic separation and bioassay of natriuretic activity.

Bioassay

Bioassay of natriuretic activity of the various fractions was performed in female Sprague-Dawley rats weighing 206 to 250 g. They were previously fed a normal rat chow diet and had free access to food and water. On the day of study

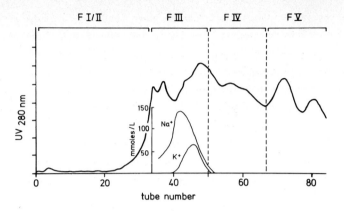

Fig. 1.   Elution patterns of human urine from Sephadex G-25 column with 0.1 N acetic acid as eluent. Indicated are UV_{280}-absorbance and elution of sodium and potassium. Single fractions (tubes) were pooled to fractions F I to F V.

animals were anesthetized with methohexital (50 mg/kg body weight intraperitoneally) and polyethylene catheters were inserted into the carotid artery, the jugular vein (PE 50) and transabdominally into the urinary bladder (PE 90). The animals were then placed in individual restraining cages mounted on a triple beam balance and were infused i.v. with 0.45% NaCl in 2.5% fructose at a rate of 33 to 62 μl/min in order to maintain body weight constant. 15-minute urine collection periods were started two hours after recovery from anesthesia and surgery and were continued throughout the entire study. When urinary sodium excretion was found stable during four consecutive collection periods each fraction was slowly injected in a random sequence into two bioassay animals. Test material was dissolved in the infusing solution containing Tris-HCl as buffer to maintain pH at 7.4. In the absence of natriuretic effects during six consecutive collection periods additional fractions were administered. With natriuretic fractions 15-minute urine samples were collected until baseline sodium excretion was again reached and infusion rate was adjusted to maintain body weight constant. Arterial blood pressure was monitored throughout the experiments by using a pressure transducer (Statham P-23-Db). Concentrations of sodium and potassium in serum and urine were determined by flame photometry.

Creatinine concentrations for calculation of endogenous creatinine clearance were determined enzymatically by the method described by Wahlefeld et al.[9] and phosphate concentrations were measured colorimetrically according to Taussky and Shorr[10]. Mean baseline urinary sodium excretion of bioassay rats averaged 0.730 ± 0.028 µEq/min. Within this range effects of natriuretic and of inactive fractions were well reproducible. Since a close linear relationship between the increase in cumulative sodium excretion and the maximum rise in sodium excretion above baseline was observed following injection of active fractions, peak increase in sodium excretion ($\Delta U_{Na} V$) above baseline was used to calculate specific natriuretic activity on the basis of the weight of material injected ($\Delta nEq\ Na^{+} \cdot min^{-1} \cdot mg^{-1}$). Data are presented as means $\pm$ S.E.M.

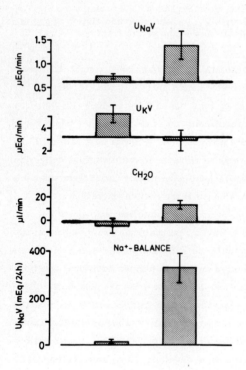

Fig. 2. Effects of fractions F IV of urine from healthy subjects obtained during dietary salt restriction and salt loading, resp., on urinary sodium ($U_{Na} V$) and potassium ($U_{K} V$) excretion and free-water clearance ($C_{H_2 O}$) when administered i.v. to conscious bioassay rats.

RESULTS

In eight healthy subjects mean urinary sodium excretion was 34 ± 7 mEq/24 h on the fifth day of low salt diet and 309 ± 61 mEq/24 h on the fifth day of high salt intake.

Fractions F IV of urine obtained during normal salt intake revealed some natriuretic activity ($\Delta U_{Na}V$: $+66.7 \pm 13.3\%$) and no significant natriuresis was observed with fraction F IV of urine obtained during salt restriction ($\Delta U_{Na}V$: $+25.0 \pm 0.8\%$), while these fractions caused a slight kaliuresis and negative free-water clearance (figure 2). Urine fraction F IV obtained on the fifth day of high salt intake resulted in a significant natriuresis ($\Delta U_{Na}V$: $+133.3 \pm 28.6\%$; $p < 0.01$ when compared to "low salt" fraction F IV) and increase in free-water excretion in bioassay animals without affecting urinary potassium excretion (figure 2).

For further purification of the natriuretic material fraction F IV was subjected to various chromatographic procedures including gel filtration, ion exchange chromatography and electrophoresis on thin layer plates. Rechromatography of salt-free fraction F IV using gel filtration resulted in further resolution into several peaks with distinct UV_{280}-absorbances. The chromatogram was subdivided accordingly into six fractions which were assayed for their natriuretic activity. A significant natriuresis was obtained after injection of the first fractions from urine of salt-loaded individuals designated as F IV$_A$ as shown in figure 3. This activity was either absent or significantly lower in identical fractions of urine obtained during salt depletion or normal salt intake, respectively.

Fractions F IV$_A$ were subsequently subjected to high pressure liquid chromatography using an ion exchange resin. The chromatogram was subdivided into four fractions according to UV-patterns and to fluorescence detection after labelling of substances containing primary amines. The early fractions designated as F IV$_B$ again revealed the natriuretic material as shown in figure 4. When compared to the original activity of F IV a 12-fold increase in specific activity of F IV$_B$ was observed.

Fraction F IV$_B$ was finally subjected to reverse phase chromatography. Of eight fractions obtained and subdivided according to the above criteria of UV-absorbance and fluorescence detection the natriuretic activity again was recovered in the early fractions (F IV$_C$) and is shown in figure 4. Specific activity was further increased 7-fold by this purification step. The activity of urine fraction F IV$_C$ from salt loaded individuals was more than 3-fold higher than that of urine obtained from subjects during dietary salt restriction.

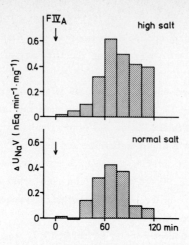

Fig. 3. Specific natriuretic activity of fractions F IV$_A$ (see text) obtained from healthy subjects during normal and high salt intake.

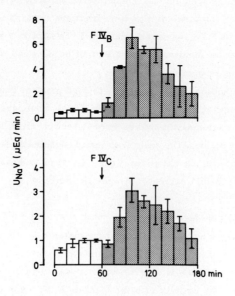

Fig. 4. Natriuretic activity of urine fractions F IV$_B$ and F IV$_C$ separated by high pressure liquid chromatography and reverse chromatography, respectively.

For further isolation urine fraction F IV was subjected to <u>ion exchange chromatography</u> using eluting buffers to achieve a <u>linear pH-gradient.</u> This resulted in excellent resolution into a number of distinct ninhydrin-positive peaks. Chromatograms were subdivided accordingly into six fractions. Natriuretic material with highest specific activity appeared in fraction F IV_D eluted in the weak acidic pH-range (pH 6.4 - 4.5) (figure 5). This was confirmed by <u>electrophoretic separation</u> of urine fraction F IV on thin layer plates when the various fractions obtained were eluted and tested for their natriuretic activity.

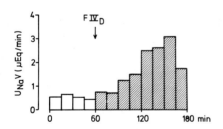

Fig. 5.   Natriuretic activity of urine fraction F IV_D eluted from ion-exchange column at pH 6.4-4.5.

DISCUSSION

We have previously demonstrated a natriuretic activity of small molecular weight (< 1,000 Daltons) in the serum of salt loaded individuals which may be derived from a circulating precursor substance of larger molecular size (> 10,000 Daltons)[11]. In the present study, the small molecular weight natriuretic material was also demonstrated in the urine of salt loaded healthy subjects and purified by various chromatographic steps to first result in 12-fold rise in specific activity which then further increased more than 7-fold by additional purification. The elution of this activity from the ion-exchange resin within a pH-range of 6.4 to 4.5 supports previous findings which suggest that the natriuretic activity is associated with a small acidic peptide.

Since the natriuresis after injection of active urine fraction F IV into bioassay animals was associated with an increase in free-water excretion in the absence of significant changes in potassium excretion it was assumed that its action within the nephron is located beyond the distal site of Na/K-exchange. However, injection of more purified active fractions resulted, in the absence of changes in endogenous creatinine clearance, in a significant increase in urinary phosphate and potassium excretion as well, suggesting inhibition of proximal tubular absorption. Since the rise in sodium excretion exceeded that in phosphate excretion by more than 30 percent in most assays (figure 6) it may be assumed that proximal as well as distal tubular effects of this material are responsible for the resulting natriuresis. We have previously observed an increase in renal cortical ATP- concentrations following acute saline loading[6] as well as an in vitro-inhibition of cortical Na-K-ATPase activity by active serum fractions F IV[5,7]. The present observation and these previous findings may therefore be compatible with an action of this peptide in cortical nephron segments, i.e. in proximal tubules as well as in distal cortical nephron segments where an ouabain-sensitive sodium transport system has also been demonstrated[12].

Assuming similar transport properties of collecting duct epithelium and amphibian membranes we have previously observed that antinatriferic fractions IV derived from five ml of serum from salt loaded individuals inhibit short-circuit current of the isolated frog skin by 20 to 30 percent. With a mean baseline short-circuit

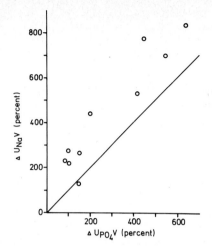

Fig. 6.   Correlation between increases in renal phosphate and in sodium excretion following injection of natriuretic fractions F IV$_C$.

current of 75 μA sec^{-1} cm^{-2} this degree of inhibition roughly corresponds to a decrease in net sodium transport of 0.5 to 0.6 μEq Na$^+ \cdot$ h$^{-1} \cdot$ cm^{-2}. These figures well agree with those reported by others, when this fraction of serum[13] or urine[14] from uremic patients was tested in vitro for inhibition of sodium transport using the isolated frog skin[13] or isolated cortical collecting duct[14] preparations, respectively. So far, however, the identity of these inhibitors isolated from serum and urine still remains a matter of speculation.

ACKNOWLEDGMENTS

The authors gratefully acknowledge the skillful technical assistance of Miss Angela Bäcker

REFERENCES

1.   Kramer, H.J., Bäcker, A. and Krück, F. (1977) Antinatriferic activity in human plasma following acute and chronic salt loading. Kidney Int., 12, 214-222.

2. Kramer, H.J., Gospodinov, B. and Krück, F. (1974) Humorale Hemmung des epithelialen Natrium-Transportes nach akuter Expansion des Extracellularvolumens: Weitere Untersuchungen zur Existenz eines natriuretischen Hormons. Klin.Wschr., 52, 801-808.

3. Ussing, H.H. and Zerahn, K. (1951) Active transport of sodium as the source of electric current in the short-circuited isolated frog skin. Acta Physiol. Scand., 23, 110-127.

4. Kramer, H.J. (1976) Natriuretic activity in plasma following extracellular volume expansion, In: Central nervous system control of Na$^+$ balance - relations to the renin-angiotensin system, edited by Kaufmann, W. and Krause, D.K., Thieme, Stuttgart, pp. 126-133.

5. Kramer, H.J., Gonick, H.C., Paul, W. and Lu, E. (1969) Third factor: Inhibitor of Na-K-ATPase ? Presented at the IV th Int.Congr.Nephrology, Stockholm, Abstract I (Free Communications), p.373.

6. Kramer, H.J. and Gonick, H.C. (1974) Effect of extracellular volume expansion on renal Na-K-ATPase and cell metabolism. Nephron, 12, 281-296

7. Gonick, H.C., Kramer, H.J., Paul, W. and Lu, E. (1977) Circulating inhibitor of sodium-potassium-activated adenosine triphosphatase after expansion of extracellular fluid volume in rats. Clin. Sci. Mol. Med., 53, 329-334.

8. Skou, J.C. (1965) Enzymatic basis for active transport of Na and K across cell membranes. Physiol. Rev., 45, 596-617.

9. Wahlefeld, A.W., Holz, G. and Bergmeyer, H.U. (1974) In: Methoden der enzymatischen Analyse, edited by Bergmeyer, H.U., Verlag Chemie, Weinheim, vol. 2, pp. 1834-1838.

10. Taussky, H.H. and Shorr, E. (1953) A microcolorimetric method for the determination of inorganic phosphorus. J. biol. Chem., 202, 675.

11. Kramer, H.J., Gonick, H.C. and Düsing, R. (1979) Nachweis und Charakterisierung natriuretischer Faktoren in Plasma und Urin (Abstract). Nieren- und Hochdruckkrankheiten, 8, 236.

12. Grantham, J.J., Burg, M.B. and Orloff, J. (1970) The nature of transtubular Na and K transport in isolated rabbit renal collecting tubules. J. Clin. Invest., 49, 1815-1826.

13. Flanigan, W.J., Anderson, D.S., Stout, K. and Koike, T.I. (1978) Site of action of a uremic serum fraction inhibiting sodium transport in frog skin. Nephron, 22, 117-123.

14. Fine, L.G., Bourgoignie, J.J., Hwang, K.H. and Bricker, N.S. (1976) On the influence of the natriuretic factor from patients with chronic uremia on the bioelectric properties and sodium transport of the isolated mammalian collecting tubule. J. Clin. Invest., 58, 590-597.

Hormonal Regulation of Sodium Excretion,
B. Lichardus, R.W. Schrier and J. Ponec, eds.
© 1980 Elsevier/North-Holland Biomedical Press

RELATIONSHIP BETWEEN TWO RENAL HORMONES : PROSTAGLANDINS AND THIRD FACTOR.

GODON, J. P. and CAMBIER, P.

Université de Liège, Département de Clinique et de Séméiologie médicales (Dir. :Prof. A. Nizet), Section de Néphrologie.

Since the work of Johnston et al.[1], numerous investigators have demonstrated that prostaglandins (PG) could be natriuretic. From all these studies, it was clear that a consistent natriuresis occured when PGE was infused into renal arteries[2-5]; what was not clear was the significance of such infusions since they used pharmacological and not intrarenal physiological doses of PG. Moreover, other non specific vasodilatators induced the same pattern of diuresis, natriuresis, increase in renal blood flow[6]. In another way, the use of PG synthesis inhibitors reached to the opposite results and therefore confirmed the conclusions obtained by the PG infusions[7-9].

Nevertheless, under some conditions, several authors have demonstrated an opposite effect of prostaglandins. On the amphibian epithelia, Fassina et al.[10], Barry and Hall[11], Lipson and Scharp[12] showed that PGE_1 increased short-circuit current and thus was natriferic.

Other experiments, performed on conscious dogs[13-14], hypophysectomized dog[15] or on blood perfused dog kidney[16] and using prostaglandin synthesis inhibitors evidenced the fact that PG might have an antinatriuretic role. One interpretation could be, of course, that these drugs, being potent inhibitors of numerous enzymes, might stimulate sodium reabsorption by another mechanism than the inhibition of prostaglandin synthesis.

Since the prostaglandins are known to mediate some physiological reactions, it was interesting to attempt to see if prostaglandins could be related to natriuretic hormone that we found previously to have a renal origin[17-19]. This relationship could represent an intrarenal control mechanism of sodium excretion.

Moreover, our experiments, being performed on an isolated rat kidney, could allow us to know if the natriuretic hormone is acting by itself or by mean of a substrate produced by another organ.

MATERIAL AND METHODS

Action of a natriuretic hormone on isolated rat kidneys.

a. Ten female Sprague-Dawley rats fed a salt rich diet ($\pm$ 9 meq NaCl a day) are bled and plasma extracts are prepared by ultrafiltration on Amicon filter and gel-filtration on a Sephadex G-100 column in order to select a 45.000 daltons fraction, as previously described[18,20,21]. We test the natriuretic activity of the extracts by administration to a cell free perfused rat kidney; each extract proceeds from 5 ml plasma, and after preparation is lyophilized and dissolved in 0.5 ml 9 %o saline. The kidneys are perfused according to Nishiisutsugi et al.[22] by a previously described technique[23], with a Krebs-Henseleit solution added with albumin, 60 g/l., glucose, 2 g/l., lactate 5.10^{-3} M and a polyfructosan as inulin * at a final concentration of 32 mg %. Kidneys are removed either from normal rats (n=11) (weight : 250-300 g) or from rats previously prepared by indomethacin (n=8); in this serie, 5 mg/kg and 2,5 mg/kg indomethacin are injected I.P. respectively one day and one hour prior to perfusion. As negative control of natriuretic extracts, we inject the solvent (0.5 ml 9 %o saline) to 5 normal kidneys and 6 Indomethacin pretreated kidneys.

b. A dose-response curve to natriuretic factor is performed using the same extracts but prepared from 1, 2.5, 5, 7.5, 10 ml of plasma and dissolved in 0.5 ml saline (n = 6, 6, 11, 3, 6, respectively).

Production of a natriuretic hormone by the isolated rat kidney.

Nine kidneys are removed from Sprague-Dawley female rats (weight 250-300 g) previously fed a salt poor diet ($<$ 0.1 meq Na / day) and perfused as described above. Perfusate samples are withdrawn before and 30 minutes after a 20 % (V/V') sodium chloride (conc. : 9 %o) load; these

---

* Inutest, Laevosan Gesellschaft, Linz, Donau, Österreich.

samples are prepared as the plasma samples in order to detect their
natriuretic activity. Nine other rat kidneys are isolated from rats fed
the same salt poor diet but previously injected by indomethacin (see   a)
and perfused similarly. Perfusate samples are also withdrawn before and
30 minutes after the same salt load and prepared as above. The natriuretic
activity of the extracts is tested in duplicate by administration to a normal
cell free perfused rat kidney (Diet : 2.5 meq Na / day); they proceed
from 5 ml perfusate and are dissolved in 0.5 ml saline.

General. The perfused rat kidney GFR is expressed by mean of
polyfructosan (Inutest) clearance. Absolute and fractional Na excretion
are calculated conventionnally. The natriuretic activity is expressed by
the mean differences $\pm$ S.E.M. of fractional or absolute Na excretion
calculated between the 10 minutes urine collection period   before and
the second 10 minutes urine collection period following the administration
of the extracts. Perfusate samples for Inulin , Na, proteins concentrations
are withdrawn at the mid-point of urine collection.

Statistical evaluation of the results are calculated according to
Student's " t " table for paired samples.

RESULTS.

Action of a natriuretic hormone on isolated rat kidneys.

a. The extracts processed from plasma of rats fed a salt rich diet
induced, when injected to the isolated kidney, a significant rise of absolute
and fractional Na excretion; the mean increase of fractional Na excretion
is + 6.01 $\pm$ 2.14 % compared to + 0.21 $\pm$ 2.15 % with the solvent alone
(P$<$ 0.02) (Fig. 1). The mean increase of absolute Na excretion is
+ 2.44 $\pm$ 1.66 μ eq / min with the natriuretic extracts and - 1.74 $\pm$ 1.52
μeq/min with the solvent alone. No significant modification of GFR,
perfusate flow rate and perfusion pressure is observed.

When the perfused kidney is removed from a previously Indomethacin
treated rats the same extracts induce a comparable rise of the fractional
or absolute Na excretion : + 4.09 $\pm$ 0.89 % and + 6.01 $\pm$ 2.14 μeq/min,
respectively. GFR and perfusate flow rate of such kidneys are statistically
comparable to normal ones.

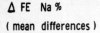

Influence of Indomethacin on the natriuretic factor activity.

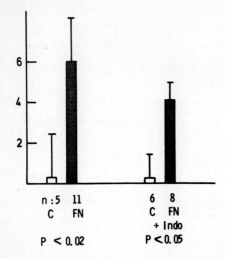

Fig. 1. Mean changes + S.E.M. of fractional sodium excretion (Δ FE Na %) in the isolated perfused rat kidney after the injection of natriuretic factor (F.N.) compared with the administration of the extract solvent (C). + Indo : same parameter in kidney isolated from Indomethacin pre-treated rats.

b. A linear dose-response curve is obtained when the plasma extracts are processed from 1 to 10 ml of plasma. The mean increase of fractional Na excretion (calculated by the mean differences between the periods after and before extracts injections) evolves from 1.86 + 1.62 % to 12.63 + 2.05.(Fig. 2).

Production of the natriuretic hormone by the isolated rat kidney.

Inhibition of its production by Indomethacin. The extracts prepared from the fluid perfusing the " salt depleted kidneys " do not induce a significant natriuresis; expressed as well in fractional as in absolute values, this natriuresis does not differ from solvent injection : thus, no natriuretic activity is detectable. Conversely, the perfusate extracts obtained after the salt loading induce an important rise in the fractional Na excretion : + 6.05 + 1.92 %; this natriuresis is significantly different from the former ($P < 0.02$) (Fig. 3).

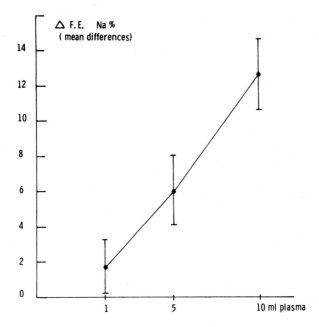

Dose - response curve of the natriuretic activity.

Fig. 2. Dose-response curve obtained by the injection into isolated rat kidneys of extracts proceeding from increasing samples of rat plasma. In ordinate are shown the mean changes in fractional sodium excretion ($<$ FE Na).

When the perfused kidney is isolated from a salt deprived, Indomethacin pretreated rat, no natriuretic activity can be detected in the perfusate extracts after the salt load (Fig. 3), the results being expressed as well in absolute or fractional values. GFR and perfusate flow rate are not modified by the extracts.

328

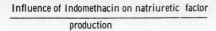

Influence of Indomethacin on natriuretic factor
production

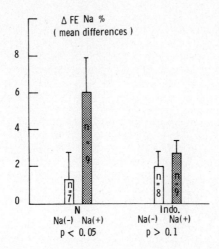

Fig. 3. Mean changes + S.E.M. in fractional sodium excretion (Δ FE Na) in the isolated perfused rat kidneys after the injection of perfusate extracts from normal rats (N) before (Na(-)) and after saline load (Na(+)) and after the injection of perfusate extracts from Indomethacin (Indo) pretreated rats before (Na (-)) and after saline load (Na (+)).

DISCUSSION.

The production or the release of the natriuretic factor by a totally isolated dog[21] or rat kidney demonstrate that its origin could be renal or that it can be released by the kidney when it is stored in it. Our previous experiments had demonstrated that this factor disappears from plasma and urine of rats or men with induced or spontaneous glomerulonephritis[18,20,24] in which the only injury is renal and that this factor can be produced by cultured renal tubular cells[19]. Therefore, we think that it is really synthesized by the kidney itself.

This work demonstrates that this natriuretic factor is active on a totally isolated rat kidney. Since this kidney is perfused by an artificial solution, the natriuretic factor does not need any extra-renal substrate for its action (unlike angiotensinogen in renin - angiotensin system). Moreover, there is a linear relationship between the injected amount of natriuretic factor and the natriuretic response of the kidney. Since, we know its site of production, its target organ and since we show a dose-response curve, we can assert that this factor is a true hormone necessary, at least for one part, to regulate the sodium transport.

The natriuretic role of prostaglandins is still to be considered since there are controversial opinions about it [1-16]. Nevertheless, it seems that infusion of PG of A and E series induce a marked diuresis and natriuresis [1-5] accompanied by an increased renal blood flow with redistribution of flux from medulla to cortex as seen after saline loading or furosemide administration but also after infusion of various vasodilatators [6].

The use of PG synthesis inhibitors reduces renal blood flow in the dog [14], decreases the enhanced renal blood flow induced by ethacrynic acid [26] and blunts the natriuretic effect of furosemide for Patak et al. [27], for Nizet (personnal communication), indomethacin does not influence the natriuretic effect of furosemide on blood perfused dog kidney. Moreover, Düsing et al. [8] have evidenced the role of PG as a mediator of natriuresis following acute E.C.V. expansion with blood dilution by saline; in their experiments, the PG synthesis inhibition reduces significantly the diuresis and the fractional Na excretion without changes in GFR; they conclude that " in addition to the natriuretic humoral activities , the prostaglandin system must be considered as an additional mediator of the natriuresis following acute expansion of the extracellular fluid volume." We think that prostaglandins are not an additional mediator but participate to the natriuretic response of the kidney after a salt load, inducing or allowing natriuretic hormone synthesis.

The present work shows that natriuretic hormone does not need prostaglandins to be active; however, the presence of renal prostaglandins seems to be a prerequisite for the production of the natriuretic hormone by the kidney. This establishes a linkage between two control systems of the renal sodium excretion : prostaglandins and natriuretic hormone.

REFERENCES.

1. Johnston, H.H., Herzog, J.P. and Lauler, D.P. (1967). Effect of prostaglandin E_1 on renal hemodynamics, sodium and water excretion. Am. J. Physiol. 213, 939-946.

2. Martinez-Maldonado, M., Tsaparaz, N., Eknoyan, G. and Suki, W.N. (1972). Renal actions of prostaglandins : comparison with acetylcholine and volume expansion. Am. J. Physiol., 222, 1147-1152.

3. Gross, J.B. and Bartter, F.C. (1973). Effects of prostaglandins : comparison with acetylcholine and volume expansion. Am. J. Physiol. 225, 218-224.

4. Strandboy, J.W., Ott, C.E., Schneider, E.G., Willis, L.R., Beck, N.P., Davis B.B., Knox, F.G. (1974). Effect of prostaglandins E_1 and E_2 on renal sodium reabsorption and starling forces. Amer. J. Physiol., 226, 1015-1021.

5. Arendshorst, W.J., Johnston, P.A. and Selkurt, P.E. (1974). Effect of prostaglandins E_1 on renal hemodynamics in non diuretic and volume - expanded dogs. Am. J. Physiol., 226, 218-225.

6. Stein, J.H., Ferris, T.F., Hupsich, E., Smith, T.C. and Osgood, R.W. (1971). Effect on renal vasodilatation on the distribution of cortical blood flow in the kidney of the dog. J. Clin. Invest. 50, 1429-1438.

7. Feigen, L.P., Klainer, E., Chapnick, B.M. and Kadowitz, P.J. (1976). The effect of indomethacin on renal function in pentobarbital-anesthetized dogs. Pharmac. Exp. Ther., 198, 457-463.

8. Düsing, R., Opitz, W.D., Kramer, H.J. (1977). The role of prostaglandins in the natriuresis of acutely salt-loaded rats. Nephron, 18, 212-219.

9. Barthe, J. (1977). Effect on indomethacin on renal function in anesthetized dogs. Int. Urol. Nephrol., 9, 81 - 90.

10. Fassina, G., Carpenedo, F., Santi, R. (1969). Effects of prostaglandin E_1 on isolated short-circuited frog skin. Life Sci., 8, 181 - 187.

11. Barry, E. and Hall, W.Y. (1969). Stimulation of sodium movement across frog skin by prostaglandin E_1. J. Physiol., Lond., 200, 83-84.

12. Lipson, L.C. and Scharp, G.W.G. (1971). Effect of prostaglandin E_1 on sodium transport and osmotic water flow in the Am. J. Physiol., 220, 1046-1052.

13. Zins, G.R. (1975). Renal prostaglandins. Am. J. Med., 58, 14-24.

14. Kirschenbaum, M.A. and Stein, J.H. (1977). The effect of prostaglandin inhibition on sodium excretion during expansion of the extracellular fluid volume. J. Lab. Clin. Med. , 90, 46-56.

15. Gill, J.R. , Alexander, R.W. , Halushka, P.V. , Pisano, J.J. and Keiser, H.R. : Indomethacin inhibits distal sodium reabsorption in the dog. Clin. Res. 23, 431 A.

16 Vanherweghem, J.L. , Ducobu, J. , D'Hollander, A. (1975). Effects of Indomethacin on renal hemodynamics and on sodium and water excretion by the isolated dog kidney. Pflugers Arch. , 357, 243-252.

17. Godon, J.P. and Nizet, A. (1974). Release by isolated dog kidney of a natriuretic material following saline loading. Arch. Intern. Physiol. Bioch. , 84, 309 - 311.

18. Godon, J.P. (1978). Renal origin of natriuretic hormone in " Natriuretic Hormone ", Kramer, H.Y. Krück, F. , ed. Springer Verlag, Berlin, 88 - 100.

19. Godon, J.P. and Dechenne, C. (1978). In vitro production of a natriuretic material of renal origin. Renal Phys. , 1, 201 - 210.

20. Godon, J.P. (1978). Evidence of increased proximal sodium and water reabsorption in experimental glomerulonephritis. Role of a natriuretic factor of renal origin. Nephron,21, 146-154.

21. Godon, J.P. and Nizet, A. (1974). Release by isolated dog kidney of a natriuretic material following saline loading. Arch. Int. Physiol. Bioch. , 84, 309 - 311.

22. Nishiisutsugi-Uwo, J.M. , Ross, B.D. , Krebs, H.A. (1967). Metabolic activities of the isolated perfused rat kidney. Biochem. J. , 103, 852 - 862.

23. Cambier, P. , Godon, J.P. (1979/80). Dissociation of sodium and glucose transport in the isolated perfused rat kidney : Effect of lactate as a substrate. Renal Physiol. , 2, 12-20.

24. Godon, J.P. (1975). The oedematous phase of acute human glomerulonephritis is due to the disappearance of a natriuretic factors which reappears during recovery. Dialysis, Transplantation, Nephrology, 12, 330 - 337.

25. Birtch, A.G. , Zakheim, R.M. , Jones, L.G. and Berger, A.C. (1967). Redistribution of renal blood flow produced by furosemide and ethacrynic acid. Circulation Res. , 21, 869 - 878.

26. Williamson, H.E. , Bourland, W.A. and Marchand, G.R. (1974). Inhibition of ethacrynic acid induced increase in renal blood flow by indomethacin. Prostaglandins 8, 297-301.

27. Patak, R.V. , Mookerjec, B.K. , Bentzel, C.J. , Hysert, P.E. , Babej, M. and Lee, J.B. (1975). Antagonism of the effects of furosemide by indomethacin in normal and hypertensive men. Prostaglandins, 10, 649-659.

Hormonal Regulation of Sodium Excretion,
B. Lichardus, R.W. Schrier and J. Ponec, eds.
© 1980 Elsevier/North-Holland Biomedical Press

CHEMICAL PROPERTIES, PHYSIOLOGICAL ACTION & FURTHER SEPARATION OF A LOW
MOLECULAR WEIGHT NATRIURETIC SUBSTANCE IN THE URINE OF NORMAL MAN

EVELYN M. CLARKSON, DAVID R. YOUNG, SHEELAGH M. RAW and HUGH E. de WARDENER
Department of Medicine, Charing Cross Hospital Medical School, Fulham Palace
Road, London W6 8RF, England

Human urine contains a low molecular weight natriuretic substance which is
present in greater amounts during salt loading but is also present during salt
deprivation[1].   Thus the large quantities of urine required to isolate and
characterise the natriuretic substance can be obtained without salt loading,
from normal man on a normal diet.   In the work to be described, 400 l of urine
were used to determine some chemical and physical properties of the natriuretic
substance while another 200 l have been used to purify the natriuretic material
further.

The urine was obtained over several months during the day.   Normal subjects
micturated in a cold room at $4^{o}C$.   The urine contained about 200 mEq of sodium
per 2g creatinine.   After screening for the presence of organisms, it was
stored at $-15^{o}C$ and freeze dried commercially.   The average 24 h excretion of
creatinine was previously found to be about 2 g[2].   Therefore in order that
results obtained with extracts prepared from day urine could be compared with
those obtained with 24 h urine, the amount of freeze dried urine which contained
2g of creatinine was taken to represent 24 h of urine.   Until a very late stage
in the purification procedures when a cytochemical assay was used[3] all extracts
were assayed in the conscious rat infused at 0.2 ml/min with 10 mEq NaCl and 5%
dextrose (dextrose saline) via a needle in the tail vein, by a technique which
has been described previously[4].   Each rat received extract equivalent to 7 min
to 4 h of original urine dissolved in 1 ml of dextrose saline.   The natriuretic
activity of each extract was assessed by comparing the mean urinary sodium
excretion during the 40 mins before an injection with that during the 20 min
after.   The change in urinary sodium excretion due to an injection of extract
was compared with the change in sodium excretion of rats which received an
injection of dextrose saline alone.

The first stage in the separation of the natriuretic substance was accomplished by gel filtration on G25 Sephadex, 24 h aliquots of freeze dried urine
dissolved in water were fractionated on columns 5 x 90 cm, using 0.01 M ammonium
acetate as eluent.   The natriuretic fraction (F4) emerged immediately after the
salts, and was freeze dried.   1 h of urine yielded 8 to 10 mg of this material.

334

Ultrafiltration was used as a means of determining the approximate molecular weight of the natriuretic substance in F4. The natriuretic activity was found to be ultrafiltrable through a membrane (Amicon UM05) with a molecular weight cut off of 500. The molecular weight is therefore unlikely to be more than 1000. The solubility of F4 in various organic solvents was next studied. The natriuretic activity was found to be totally soluble in glacial acetic acid, phenol, ethanol and 95% acetone. It was variably soluble in 100% acetone, iso-propanol and isobutanol and insoluble in ethyl acetate, chloroform and ether. Thus the natriuretic substance is polar. Moreover, extraction with 95% acetone removed 50% of material which was not natriuretic. In the following account of our attempts to destroy the natriuretic material by chemical and enzymatic methods, and of the experiments to determine it's physiological action, the material used was 95% acetone soluble F4. This is referred to throughout as 95% ASF4.

CHEMICAL PROPERTIES

The first experiments were aimed at finding out whether the substance was a peptide. The material was therefore incubated with proteolytic enzymes and

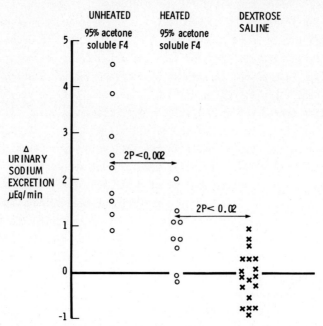

Fig. 1. Changes in urinary sodium excretion of rats given 95% ASF4 (o) equivalent to 2 h of original urine before and after heating at 100° for 1 h at pH 10, and of rats given dextrose saline (x). (Reproduced with permission of Kidney Int².).

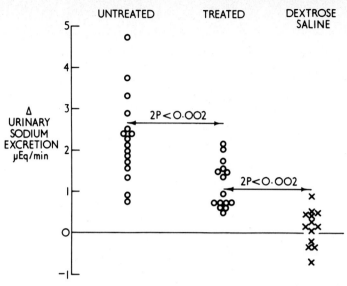

Fig. 2. Changes in urinary sodium excretion of rats given 95% ASF4 (o) equivalent to 3 h of original urine before and after heating in 6N HCl at 110° for 22
to 90 h, and of rats given dextrose saline (x). (Reproduced with permission
of Kidney Int[2]).

subjected to heat at high and low pH. Initially the enzymes used were pepsin,
subtilysin and leucine aminopeptidase. Incubation was carried out at 37°C
under confirmed sterile conditions at a pH appropriate for each enzyme. The
ratio of enzyme to 95% ASF4 ranged between 1/10 and 1/50. Control solutions of
95% ASF4 containing no enzyme were incubated simultaneously and after incubation
all the solutions were refractionated on G25 Sephadex in order to remove buffer,
enzyme and any contaminants in the enzyme preparation. None of these enzymes
destroyed the natriuretic activity of 95% ASF4. The stability to heat at pH 10
of the natriuretic substance in 95% ASF4 (Fig 1) was studied as follows. One
half of a solution of the material was heated at pH 10 for 60 min and compared
with the other control half which was not heated. Care was taken that the
sodium concentration and osmolality of the 2 samples were the same. The natriuretic activity was considerably diminished by heating at pH 10 ($2P < 0.002$)
but was not totally destroyed ($2P < 0.02$). To determine the effect of heating
at low pH (Fig. 2) 95% ASF4 equivalent to 15 h of original urine was heated
anaerobically in 6N HCl at 110°C for 22 to 90 h. The bulk of the acid was
removed by evaporation and freeze drying and the remainder neutralised with
NaOH. The hydrolysed material was then refractionated on G25 Sephadex in order
to remove sodium added during neutralising and some products of hydrolysis. The

natriuretic activity of the refractionated hydrolysed 95% ASF4 was compared with refractionated but unhydrolysed 95% ASF4. Hydrolysed and unhydrolysed material was assayed in amounts equivalent to 3 h original urine. Anaerobic acid hydrolysis significantly reduced (2P< 0.002) but did not totally destroy the natriuretic activity of 95% ASF4 (2P<0.002).

The resistance of the natriuretic material to destruction by the proteolytic enzymes and its relative stability to heat at high and low pH do not support the substance being a peptide and the effect of nitrous acid was investigated (Fig. 3). 95% ASF4 equivalent to 15 h of original urine was dissolved in acid and treated with sodium nitrite at 5°C. The treated material was then freeze dried, refractionated on G25 Sephadex and its natriuretic activity compared with re-fractionated untreated 95% ASF4. Each rat received material equivalent to 3 h original urine. Nitrous acid totally destroyed the natriuretic activity of 95% ASF4. The urinary sodium excretion of rats which received 95% ASF4 treated with nitrous acid was not different from that of rats which received dextrose saline alone. These results suggested that the natriuretic activity was dependant on an amine group and the next set of experiments were directed at finding out whether the natriuretic substance was a catecholamine.

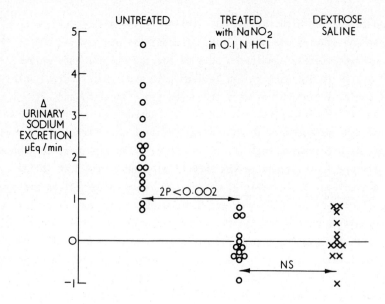

Fig. 3. Changes in urinary sodium excretion of rats given 95% ASF4 (0) equivalent to 3 h of original urine before and after treatment with nitrous acid at 5 to 10° for 45 min, and of rats given dextrose saline (X). (Reproduced with permission of Kidney Int[2]).

95% ASF4 equivalent to 15 h of original urine was dissolved in phosphate
buffer, pH 7.4, and incubated for 45 min at 37° with monamine oxidase. Oxygen
was bubbled through the solution throughout the period of incubation. A control
solution of 95% ASF4 containing no enzyme was incubated simultaneously in the
same way. The sterility of the solutions was confirmed by culture at the end
of the incubation, and all solutions were freeze dried and refractionated on
G25 Sephadex before assaying. In case the natriuretic activity was due to conjugated catecholamine, experiments with monamine oxidase were also performed
with 95% ASF4 which had already been incubated either with β-glucuronidase or
aryl sulphatase. The natriuretic activity of 95% ASF4 was not destroyed or
impaired by any of these procedures. It is concluded that the natriuretic
activity is not due to free or conjugated catecholamine.

In a final attempt to characterise the natriuretic substance the effect of
incubating with another group of proteolytic enzymes was investigated. The
enzymes used were amino peptidase M, carboxypeptidase A & B and prolidase.
Experimental procedures were as described for the previous set of enzymes.
Prolidase was supplied as a suspension in 2.7 M ammonium sulphate and in experiments with this enzyme, either boiled enzyme or 2.7M ammonium sulphate was
added to the control solution of 95% ASF4 before incubation. The natriuretic

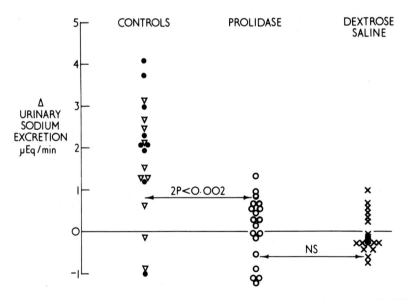

Fig. 4. Changes in urinary sodium excretion of control rats given 95% ASF4
incubated with either ammonium sulphate (▼) or with the supernatent from boiled
prolidase (●) and of rats given 95% ASF4, incubated with prolidase (o). Values
for rats given dextrose saline are denoted by the symbol X. (Reproduced with
permission of Kidney Int[2]).

338

activity of 95% ASF4 was not affected by carboxypeptidase A or B or by amino-
peptidase M, but was totally destroyed by prolidase. This finding suggests
that the natriuretic substance is a peptide containing proline. Several pre-
cautions were taken to try to ensure that this effect was not an artefact.
Sterility was ensured by culture at the end of incubation. Sodium azide in the
reconstituted extract can prevent the natriuretic response but this was not
used. The addition of boiled enzyme suspension to the control solutions makes
it unlikely that any inorganic material (e.g. manganese) in the enzyme preparation caused the loss of natriuretic activity. The evidence that the natriuretic substance is a peptide however is based on the effect of only one proteolytic enzyme (prolidase). The other findings, such as the stability of the
substance to heating at pH 10 and to acid hydrolysis do not support this conclusion. Alternative explanations of the effect of prolidase on the natriuretic
activity are 1, as the enzyme preparation, obtained from pig kidney was not pure,
the inactivation of the natriuretic substance was brought about by a non proteolytic enzyme, or 2, the natriuretic substance is destroyed by prolidase though
it is not a peptide, because it contains a proline residue.

PHYSIOLOGICAL ACTION

A bolus I.V. injection of 95% ASF4 into a rat produced a natriuresis which
occurred mainly in the first 20 min after the injection. Fig. 5 illustrates
the change in urinary sodium excretion which occurred in the first 20 min after
the injection of various quantities of 95% ASF4. The least quantity of extract
which produced a detectable natriuresis was 600 µg corresponding to 7 min of
original urine. The maximum response was obtained with 2.5 mg corresponding to
30 min of urine. This pattern of response to increasing quantities of natriuretic material suggests the saturation of receptor sites, and is in contrast to
the type of response to a toxic substance such as vanadate. The administration
of increasing quantities of vanadate cause a continuous increase in urinary
sodium excretion until the concentration of sodium in the urine equals that of
the plasma (I.M. Glynn, personal communication).

The effect of 95% ASF4 on sodium transport *in vitro* was carried out using red
cells. Normal human red cells which had been loaded with ^{22}Na were incubated
at 37^0 for 5 h in tissue culture medium containing 95% ASF4 equivalent to 1 h
of original urine per ml. Intracellular Na and the rate constant for total ^{22}Na
efflux from the cells was compared with that of cells incubated simultaneously
in medium containing no 95% ASF4. In six experiments the intracellular sodium
of cells incubated with 95% ASF4 rose from a mean of 7.4 to 8.8 mEq/l cells
($P<0.05$) and the rate constant for total sodium efflux fell from a mean of

0.40 to 0.32 h $^{-1}$ (P<0.05).   In addition Glynn (personal communication) has found that 95% ASF4 inhibits kidney Na-K-ATPase *in vitro*, and that this inhibition is not due to vanadate.

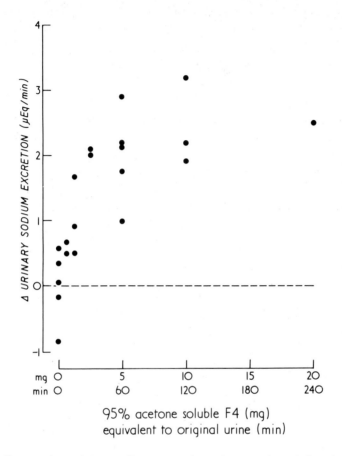

Fig. 5.   Changes in urinary sodium excretion of rats given bolus I.V. injection of 0.6 mg of 95% ASF4 equivalent to 7 to 240 min of original urine.   Each point represents the mean urinary sodium excretion of 2 to 5 rats.   (Reproduced with permission of Kidney Int.[2]).

FURTHER SEPARATION PROCEDURES

Further purification was achieved by refractionating the 95% ASF4 on G25 Sephadex in 0.01 M ammonium acetate.   By this means the weight of natriuretic material obtained from 1 h of urine was reduced to about 2 mg with no loss in activity.

The refractionated 95% ASF4 was next subjected to large scale paper chromatography using n-butanol-acetic acid water (4:1:5) as solvent).   The natriuretic fraction 7 was eluted with water and contained about 400 μg/h of original urine.   The activity was reduced to about a half.

By fractionating this material further using ion exchange chromatography (CM Sephadex) and an ammonium acetate gradient the natriuretic fraction 5 was reduced in weight to 3 μg/h of original urine and a marked natriuresis was produced by the injection of material equivalent to 2 to 3 h of urine.   With these three further separation procedures it is possible to obtain an extract with specific activity which is x 500 that of the original 95% ASF4.   Fractionation of this extract using thin layer silica gel chromatography followed by high performance liquid chromatography has produced further increases in specific activity.   The small amounts of material obtained in this manner are difficult to weigh but 1 h of the active fraction now weighs less than 100 ng.

REFERENCES

1.   Clarkson, E.M., Raw, S.M. and de Wardener, H.E. (1976) Kidney Int, 10, 381-394.

2.   Clarkson, E.M., Raw, S.M. and de Wardener, H.E. (1979) Kidney Int, 16, 710-721.

3.   Alaghband-Zadeh, J., Fenton, S., Clarkson, E., MacGregor, G.A. and de Wardener, H.E. (1980) Symposium on Regulation of Renal Sodium Excretion by Hormones, Elsevier/North-Holland, Amsterdam.

4.   Brown, P.R., Koutsaimanis, K.G. and de Wardener, H.E. (1972) Kidney Int, 2, 1-5.

Hormonal Regulation of Sodium Excretion,
B. Lichardus, R.W. Schrier and J. Ponec, eds.
© 1980 Elsevier/North-Holland Biomedical Press

341

PRELIMINARY STUDIES FOR THE POSSIBLE DETECTION IN PLASMA OF THE SMALL MOLECULAR
WEIGHT URINARY NATRIURETIC MATERIAL

JAMSHID ALAGHBAND-ZADEH, STEPHEN FENTON, EVELYN CLARKSON, GRAHAM A. MacGREGOR
AND HUGH E. de WARDENER
Department of Chemical Pathology and Department of Medicine, Charing Cross
Hospital Medical School, Fulham Palace Road, London W6 8RF, England

The technique reported below describes a sensitive quantitative method for
the detection of a substance which is present in a highly purified urinary
natriuretic extract and in plasma.

MATERIALS AND METHODS

The urinary natriuretic extract (F4) was obtained from a Sephadex G25 fractionation.   It contains the low molecular weight (<500) natriuretic substance
and produces a transient natriuresis when injected I.V. into rats.   The properties of this substance have been reported by Clarkson et al (1979)[1].   The
cytochemical techniques used were those described by Chayen et al (1973)[2].   In
principle the one described below consists of measuring glucose-6-phosphate
dehydrogenase (G6PD) activity in segments of guinea-pig kidney.

Male guinea pigs (Dunkan Hartley strain) 250g maintained on a normal guinea
pig diet were killed by dislocating the neck.   The kidneys were removed by dissection, trimmed of excess fat and decapsulated.   The kidneys were then halved
sagitally and segments approximately 2 mm thick were produced.   Each segment
was maintained separately in a sealed culture chamber in an atmosphere of 95%
O_2 : 5% CO_2, the segments being exposed to a non-proliferative culture medium
(Minimum Essential Medium) at $37^{o}C$ for 5 h.   The culture medium was then
removed and replaced by fresh culture medium containing dilutions of the test
material or plasma.   The segments were exposed for an optimum time then rapidly
chilled to $-70^{o}C$ and stored at this temperature until required.   G6PD activity
was then measured in the following way.   Each segment was mounted separately
and sectioned at 16 μ in a refrigerated Cryostat at $-30^{o}C$.   The sections were
'flash dried' by apposing a warm microscope slide close to the supercooled
section.   The sections were then warmed to $37^{o}C$ and exposed to the reaction
medium to demonstrate the activity of the enzyme G6PD, Chayen et al (1973)[2].
The cytochemical reaction for G6PD produces an insoluble and highly localised
Formazan deposit throughout the nephron.   The amount of Formazan deposit which
represents the activity of the G6PD was quantified with a Vickers M85 scanning

and integrating microdensitometer in the appropriate cells in the nephron (see below).   The results are expressed as mean integrated extinction x 100.

RESULTS

   When segments were exposed to culture medium alone little G6PD activity was observed in any part of the nephron.   Dilutions of a relatively pure preparation of the low-molecular weight natriuretic substance (F4) gave a marked increase of G6PD activity in the proximal convoluted tubules adjacent to the glomeruli in the outer cortex, in the straight tubules near the medullary cortex (juxtamedullary tubules), and in the collecting ducts.

The optimisation of the time of response of G6PD activity when the segment of kidney is exposed to F4

   Two dilutions of F4 were made.   A number of segments of guinea-pig kidney were then exposed to these 2 dilutions for 2 to 20 min.   The G6PD activity was quantitated by microdensitometry in the proximal tubules, the juxtamedullary tubules, and the distal tubules of these segments.   Although the collecting ducts showed the greatest G6PD activity, in most of the sections the collecting ducts had been lost during sectioning.   In addition the amount of Formazan deposit in collecting ducts was too great for quantification by microdensitometry.   Because of these technical difficulties it was not possible to demonstrate a time response in the collecting ducts as satisfactorily as in other parts of the tubules.   Two peaks of G6PD activity were observed, at 2 min and at 18 min, in the proximal tubules and the juxtamedullary tubules at both concentrations of F4 (Fig.1).   The distal tubule also showed peaks at 2 min and 18 min of G6PD activity but at higher concentrations of F4.

Evidence that F4 induces the enzyme glucose-6-phosphate dehydrogenase

   The enzyme G6PD requires both substrate (glucose-6-phosphate) and co-enzyme (NADP) to show activity and generate hydrogen.   The hydrogen then reduces the Neotetrazolium salt (NT) in the reacting medium to an insoluble Formazan dye which appears as blue granules.   It was possible, however, that F4 might liberate hydrogen by a non-enzymatic reaction.   In order to prove enzyme activity two segments of the kidney were cultured as before.   One was exposed to culture medium alone, and the other was exposed to an F4 preparation for 2 min as follows.   Eight serial sections were taken from each block and two sections were reacted in presence of substrate, co-enzyme and Neotetrazolium salt; two in the presence of co-enzyme and Neotetrazolium and finally two in the presence of Neotetrazolium alone.   The effect of F4 on the increase in Formazan deposit was observed only in those sections reacted in the presence of substrate co-enzyme and Neotetrazolium (Table 1).   Thus it can be concluded that F4 stimulates G6PD activity.

TABLE 1

G6PD ACTIVITY IN THE NEPHRON

Formazan deposit was seen only in the sections reacted in the presence of the substrate: glucose-6-phosphate dehydrogenase (G6PD), the co-enzyme: nicotmamide adenine dinucleotide (NADP) and the hydrogen acceptor neotetrazolium (NT). This Formazan deposit was pronounced in the sections from the segment exposed to F4.

Segment	Treatment	G6PD+NADP+NT	G6PD+NT	NADP+NT	NT
1	F4	+++	-	-	-
=	Culture medium	+	-	-	-

+ : Positive Formazan deposit; - : Negative Formazan deposit

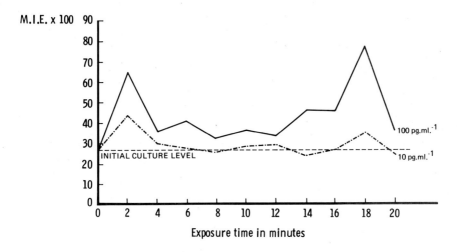

Fig.1. Glucose-6-phosphate dehydrogenase activity in the proximal tubules of segments of guinea pig kidney exposed to 10 Pg/ml of F4 for 2 to 20 min.   The G6PD activity is expressed as Mean Integrated Extinction (MIE) on the Y axis and the time in minutes of the X axis.   The broken line illustrates the G6PD activity produced by the culture medium alone.   10Pg F4 ≡1/100h collection of urine.

Dose response
    The dose response of G6PD activity to F4 in the proximal tubules, the juxta-medullary tubules, the distal tubules, and the collecting ducts was measured at 2 min and 18 min.   The 18 min peak did not show a linear response in any part

344

of the tubule and was not considered further.   The distal tubule was excluded
because large amounts of F4 were required to elicit a response and also because
it is a known site of action of parathyroid hormone.   The collecting duct was
excluded because of the technical difficulties mentioned above, and because it
is a known site of action of antidiuretic hormone.

   Initial results showed that both the proximal tubules and the juxtamedullary
tubules appeared to give a linear dose response to F4 at 2 min.   As it was much
easier to identify and thus quantitate the Formazan deposits in the proximal
tubule cells adjacent to the glomeruli in the outer cortex, these were chosen to
obtain a definitive dose response.   These cells also had the added advantage
that they are least likely to suffer from interference from circulating hormones.

   Segments from a guinea-pig kidney were exposed to three dilutions of F4 for
2 min.   The dilutions were 1/1000; 1/10,000 and 1/100,000 of an amount of F4
obtained from a 1 h collection of urine.   Another three segments were exposed
to dilutions of plasma from a normal individual at 1/100; 1/1000 and 1/10,000
for 2 min.   G6PD in these segments were then quantified in duplicate (Fig. 2).

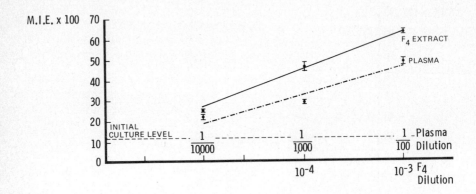

Fig. 2. Glucose-6-phosphate dehydrogenase activity in the proximal tubules after
2 min exposure to dilutions of F4 and plasma represented as mean integrated
extraction x 100 (M.I.E. x 100) on the Y axis.   The standard response: three
concentrations of F4 were used; 1/1000, 1/10,000 and 1/100,000 dilutions of F4
obtained from 1 h of urine.   Dilutions of plasma: Three dilutions of plasma
(1/100, 1/1000, 1/10,000) were used.   The vertical bars join duplicate results.
The lower broken line illustrates G6PD activity in the proximal tubules from a
segment exposed to culture medium alone for 2 min.

There was a log linear increase of G6PD activity with increasing concentrations
of F4.   The plasma dilutions also showed a positive log linear increase of
G6PD activity.   There was no divergence from parallelism (P<0.5) between the
4 and the plasma response.   If it is assumed that the G6PD activity produced

by a 1/100 dilution of F4 is equivalent to 100 arbitrary units then the potency estimate for the normal plasma was 8.15 units. The index of precision (λ) was 0.07 with Fiducial limits of 61% to 106%.

Specificity of the 2 min peak of G6PD activity in the proximal tubules induced by F4 and plasma

Known hormones acting on the nephron were put on to kidney segments at normal circulating concentrations, and at x100 their circulating levels. The following hormones did not induce any change in G6PD activity in the proximal tubules at 2 min:- Parathyroid hormone; Aldosterone; Angiotensin II; Calcitonin; 1,25 dihydroxy vitamin D; 24,25 dihydroxy vitamin D; 25 hydroxy vitamin D; Dopamine; Adrenaline; Noradrenaline; A non-natriuretic G25 fraction of urine (FIII) also had no effect. Arginine Vasopressin at a concentration of 2μU/ml showed some inhibition of G6PD in all parts of the tubules and the collecting ducts at 2 min. The inhibition was more marked in the collecting ducts and distal tubules than in the proximal tubules and the juxtamedullary tubule. At the usual physiological range of plasma ADH of 0.5 to 10 μU/ml, dilutions of plasma 1/100 and 1:1000 prevent interference from ADH in the G6PD assay.

The effect of sodium intake on the capacity of plasma from normal subjects to induce G6PD activity in the proximal tubules at 2 min.

Five normal male subjects, mean age 22 yr, were studied on the 7th day of a 10 mmol sodium intake per day, and on the 7th day of a 350 mmol sodium intake per day. Twenty-four hour urinary sodium excretion, weight, and blood pressure were measured daily. Heparinised blood was taken on the 7th day of each type of sodium intake after sitting the subject upright for 10 min between 10.00 h and 12.00 h. It was immediately spun in a cold room at +4°C and the plasma stored at -20°C until the assay.

Segments of guinea-pig kidney were exposed to three dilutions of a highly purified F4 (equivalent to 1 h collection) at dilutions of 1/100, 1/1000, 1/10,000 and dilutions of plasma at 1/100, and 1/1000 for 2 min. The F4 extract used was that obtained after 6 consecutive extraction procedures (see Clarkson et al same symposium)[3]. The G6PD activity was quantitated in the proximal tubule in duplicate; the samples and the standards having been labelled at random. The plasma and F4 dilutions showed parallel G6PD responses. The plasma from normal subjects on a low salt diet stimulated G6PD activity less than the plasma from the same subjects on a high sodium diet (Fig. 3).

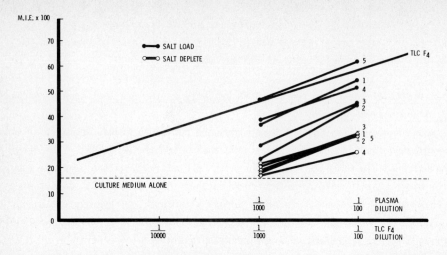

Fig. 3. G6PD activity of proximal tubules after incubation in dilutions of F4 and of plasma from normal subjects (No. 1 to 5) on high and low salt diets. Lower broken line; G6PD activity produced by culture medium alone. Solid line; F4 response at 1/100, 1/1000, 1/10,000 dilution (TLC F4 ≡ the F4 fraction obtained from thin layer chromatography)● ●G6PD activity of the normal subjects on a high salt diet at 1/100, 1/1000 dilution.○ ○G6PD activity of the same normal subjects on a low salt diet at 1/100, 1/1000 dilution.

TABLE 2

F4-LIKE BIOACTIVITY OF NORMAL PLASMA

The capacity of the plasma from five normal subjects on high and low salt diets to induce G6PD activity in the proximal tubules at 2 min are expressed in arbitary F4 units where 100 units of F4 activity ≡ 1/100 dilution of F4 from 1h of urine.

Normal Subject	Urinary Na$^+$ mmol/24h	Salt loaded plasma	Salt depleted plasma
			Units of F4 activity
1. M.C.	15.04 257.00	2.01 ----	---- 11.1
2. P.S.	10.50 310.00	0.16 ----	---- 8.1
3. J.D.	2.44 308.00	0.22 ----	---- 12.0
4. S.M.	10.61 380.00	0.73 ----	---- 10.5
5. C.H.	2.40 413.00	0.16 ----	---- 61.7

If the effect of plasma on G6PD activity is defined in arbitrary units, where the effect on G6PD activity of 1/100 dilution of F4 derived from 1 h of urine represents 100 units, the effect of plasma from the subjects when salt loaded was approximately x 10 to x 50 greater than when salt depleted (Table 2).

DISCUSSION

The sensitive cytochemical techniques of Chayen et al (1973)[2] have made it possible to observe and measure the induction of G6PD activity which is produced by a highly purified urinary extract (F4) known to contain a small molecular weight natriuretic substance. The results also demonstrate that normal plasma contains a substance which has similar cytochemical G6PD inducing characteristics as that which stimulates G6PD in F4. And that the plasma concentration of this substance is directly related to sodium intake.

It is likely that the increase in G6PD activity by F4 and plasma is due to inhibition of Na^+-K^+-ATPase. It is known that inhibition of Na^+-K^+-ATPase is associated with stimulation of the pentose shunt pathway and thus an increase in G6PD activity (Dikstein, 1971)[4]. In keeping with this observation when a segment of guinea-pig kidney was exposed to Ouabain at a concentration of 10^{-4} molar for 2 min there was a rise of G6PD activity in the proximal tubules by the cytochemical technique described here. Furthermore I. Glynn (personal communication) has recently shown that F4 inhibits a preparation of the Na^+-K^+ ATPase *in vitro*. Finally using a technique developed by Chayen and Bitensky (Personal Communication) for the quantitative measurement of the Na^+-K^+-ATPase in kidney segments we have recently demonstrated that F4 not only increases G6PD activity, but also inhibits Na^+-K^+-ATPase activity in the proximal tubules, and the thick ascending limb of the loop of henle (unpublished observations). It is thus probable that the substance in plasma which is detected by the G6PD assay described above is a circulating Na^+-K^+-ATPase inhibitor.

ACKNOWLEDGEMENT

We wish to thank Drs. J. Chayen and L. Bitensky at the Kennedy Institute of Rheumatology for their advice and encouragement and the Medical Research Council for financial support.

REFERENCES
1.   Clarkson, E.M., Raw, S.M. and de Wardener, H.E. (1979) Kidney Int. 16, 710-721.

348

2.   Chayen, J., Bitensky, L. and Butcher, R.G. (1973) Practical Histochemistry,
     John Wiley and Sons, London and New York.

3.   Clarkson, E.M., Young, D.R., Raw, S.M. and de Wardener H.E. (1980)
     Symposium on regulation of renal sodium excretion in hormones. Elsevier,
     North Holland, Amsterdam.

4.   Dikstein, S. (1971) Naturwissenschaften, 58,439-443.

EVIDENCE THAT NATRIURETIC FACTOR IS A CASCADING PEPTIDE HORMONE SYSTEM.
Kenneth A. Gruber and Vardaman M. Buckalew, Jr., Departments of Medicine and
Physiology & Pharmacology, Bowman Gray School of Medicine, Winston-Salem,
North Carolina 27103 USA.

Introduction

While considerable physiological evidence exists to support the concept of
a humoral natriuretic factor [1,2,3], there has been difficulty in confirming
reports of its detection in plasma of volume-expanded (V-E) subjects [4,5,6].
For the past four years, our laboratories have collaborated on the isolation of
this putative hormone from plasma of V-E dogs. In this review, we present
evidence that natriuretic factor is a small molecular weight peptide derived
from a circulating precursor, and is recognized by antibodies to sodium-
potassium adenosine triphosphatase ($[Na^+ + K^+]$ ATPase) inhibitors.

Initial Isolation

Buckalew et al. [7,8] have previously demonstrated that plasma of V-E dogs
contains a factor which inhibits sodium transport in anuran bladders (antinatriferic activity) and causes an immediate natriuresis in assay rats. The
toad bladder assay system is an analog of the distal renal tubule and collecting
duct. A similar activity has been demonstrated by other investigators in V-E
human plasma, dog urine and rat kidney [9,10,11]. In a previous communication
[12], it was demonstrated that this activity could be isolated on a Biogel P-2
column in a U-V positive post-salt fraction (IV). More recently [13], we have
separated Biogel fraction IV on a high performance cation-exchange chromatography column (Figure 1). The column effluent was monitored by a preparative
fluorescamine detection system, and antinatriferic activity (expressed as percent inhibition of short circuit current [SCC]) appeared in a fluorescamine-
positive peak in the column void volume (Figure 2). The elution of the activity in a column fraction which reacts with the reagent fluorescamine suggested
the possibility that the antinatriferic factor (AF) contains a free primary
amino group.

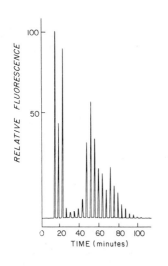

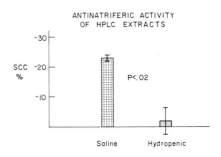

Figure 2. Antinatriferic activity in
V-E and hydropenic samples after separation on Partisil SCX.

Figure 1. Separation of Biogel IV on a Partisil
SCX column. The column effluent was monitored by
a preparative fluorescamine system; this results
in the discontinuous appearance of the chromatogram. Each line represents one
sampling period. Antinatriferic activity is found in the void volume peak (first
two sampling periods). (Permission of Soc. for Exper. Biol. and Med., [13].)

To further investigate this possibility, we tested our cation-exchange extract with the reverse-phase peptide assay of Gruber et al. [14]. In this procedure a small aliquot of each bioassayed sample was reacted with fluorescamine at pH 7. Under these reaction conditions fluorescamine preferentially forms fluorophors with peptides [15], while amino acids require a high pH to maximally form the characteristic fluorophor. The derivatized peptide can then be separated on a reverse-phase high performance liquid chromatography (HPLC) column. Figure 3 shows the separation of a cation-exchange column void volume fraction, from plasma of a V-E dog, on a reverse-phase column. Two unique peaks were seen which were not present in hydropenic plasma samples.

Evidence for a Circulating Precursor

In an attempt to achieve better recovery of the antinatriferic factor, we collected dog blood in the presence of the enzyme inhibitor bacitracin, and isolated our plasma more rapidly. To our surprise, this results in consistently decreased activity in our V-E plasma extracts.

We felt that there were several possibilities to account for these results. The first was that the factor was not stable to the heat precipitation step. A second possibility was that the factor circulated as an inactive precursor which was converted to the active molecule during the isolation and processing of the plasma.

To investigate these possibilities, we performed the following experiment. Blood from V-E dogs was split into two paired samples and processed by different protocols. In the first (fast processing) method, the blood was collected over bacitracin in iced heparinized syringes, the plasma isolated in a refrigerated centrifuge, and its proteins heat precipitated. The total elapsed time for this procedure was 15 minutes. The second (slow processing) method involved collecting the blood without bacitracin or ice, isolating the plasma, and incubating it at 22°C for 30 minutes before the heat precipitation step. Appropriate

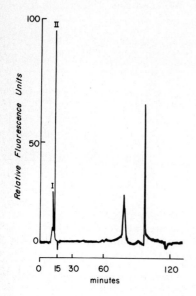

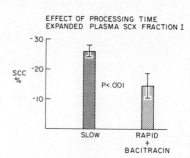

Figure 4. Comparison of the antinatriferic activity found in the two types of plasma processing protocols.

Figure 3. Separation on Partisil ODS (reverse-phase column) of a fluorescamine derivatized aliquot of the Partisil SCX void volume peak from a V-E sample. Note first two peaks. (Permission of the Society for Experimental Biology and Medicine, [13].)

controls demonstrated that bacitracin itself would not affect the biological activity.

The results of this experiment are seen in Figure 4. Slow processed samples had approximately twice the activity of their fast processed pairs. Since both groups were subjected to heat precipitation, we felt that this experiment provided evidence for a precursor in the formation of this factor. In addition, these findings provided a possible explanation for the difficulty of some investigators to consistently recover antinatriferic activity in plasma of V-E subjects [4,5,6].

Evidence that this factor is a small peptide was provided by the reverse-phase HPLC assay of fast and slow processed samples. The peak heights of the two peaks unique to V-E samples were increased in the slow processed group, suggesting that they might be associated with the increased antinatriferic activity. To pursue this, we plotted the height of each peak against the antinatriferic activity in the sample from which it was taken. The results (Figure 5) demonstrated a linear relationship between reverse-phase peak height and antinatriferic activity. Since both peaks showed this relationship, it was possible that they were breakdown products of the precursor, with at least one of them representing a peptide with antinatriferic properties.

Additional proof that antinatriferic activity was due to a peptide was provided by enzyme digestion experiments. An HPLC extract derived from 30 mls of V-E plasma was dissolved in phosphate buffer (pH 7) and divided into three paired aliquots. One sample was treated with 5 units of immobilized trypsin, another with 5 units of immobilized chymotrypsin, while the third served as a control. All samples were incubated for 30 minutes at 37°C, the enzyme separated by centrifugation, and the supernatant assayed for antinatriferic activity. The results (Figure 6) indicate that the activity is trypsin sensitive, but chymotrypsin insensitive.

Detection of the Putative Precursor to Antinatriferic Factor

Sealy et al. [16] were the first to detect a natriuretic factor with delayed

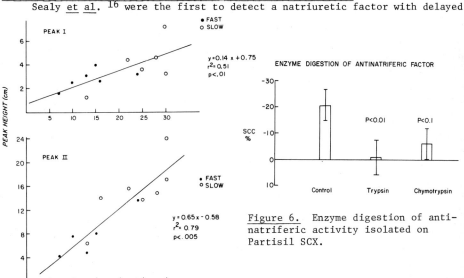

Figure 6. Enzyme digestion of anti-natriferic activity isolated on Partisil SCX.

Figure 5. Reverse-phase peak height of fast and slow V-E samples plotted against the sample's antinatriferic activity. (Permission of Soc, for Exper, Biol, and Med, [13].)

activity in V-E subjects. While several groups have confirmed that the anti-natriferic factor has immediate natriuretic activity [8,17], there have been no studies on the effect of the former factor on toad bladder sodium transport. Clarkson et al. [18] proposed that the factor with delayed natriuretic activity might be the precursor to the more commonly detected immediate natriuretic or antinatriferic factor.

In an attempt to directly confirm this hypothesis, we attempted to isolate the factor described by Sealy et al. [16] to test its activity in the anuran bladder assay. To detect this factor in plasma extracts, we developed a rat bioassay preparation. Rats were anesthetized with pentobarbital and a steady state of anesthesia was maintained by giving a continuous intravenous infusion of pentobarbital. The rats were made modestly diuretic by the IV infusion of 0.45% saline at 100 µl/min. This preparation has an extremely steady baseline and small changes in sodium excretion can be detected (Buckalew and Gruber, paper in preparation).

Initial attempts to isolate this factor involved the use of Diafiltration[R] combined with isolation of the presalt fraction off of a Biogel P-2 column. Preliminary experiments showed a factor causing prolonged natriuretic activity (Figure 7). However, additional isolation experiments revealed steadily decreasing amounts of activity.

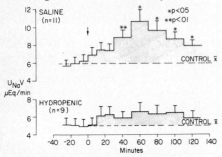

Figure 7. Effect of a Biogel P-2 extract on sodium excretion in the rat. Onset of effect is delayed by 10-20 minutes, and the natriuresis lasts more than two hours.

Since we were confident about the reliability of our Diafiltration step, we focused our suspicions on the Biogel P-2 column. To examine the possibility that deteriorating column performance could cause some peptides to elute in the salt peak, we monitored the Biogel P-2 column effluent with a preparative fluorescamine detection system. The chromatogram obtained revealed a large amount of fluorescamine-positive material eluting in the salt peak. When the salt peak was collected and chromatographed on the cation-exchange column, delayed natriuretic activity was detected at an elution time of 24-52 minutes, while all the salt eluted in the void volume peak.

However, since the Biogel P-2 column was not providing us with a reproducible isolation technique, we eliminated that step and separated plasma diafiltrates on cation-exchange HPLC. Delayed prolonged natriuretic activity eluted at 24-52 minutes (Fraction II) (Buckalew and Gruber, paper in preparation).

To test the hypothesis that this natriuretic factor was the precursor to antinatriferic factor, HPLC Fraction II was tested for antinatriferic activity before and after treatment with immobilized trypsin. Trypsin was chosen as the enzyme most likely to cleave a possible precursor since it has been demonstrated that many peptide hormone precursors are trypsin sensitive [19,20,21], apparently due to paired basic amino acid residues [22].

Prior to enzyme digestion, Fraction II has no antinatriferic activity. Preliminary experiments [23] have demonstrated that trypsin digestion of Fraction II results in the production of an antinatriferic peptide. The HPLC retention time of this peptide is similar to the naturally occurring anti-natriferic factor (vide supra). Experiments are currently in progress to extend these observations (Whitaker, et al., paper in preparation).

These experiments suggest that the delayed natriuretic factor may be the precursor to the antinatriferic peptide.

Digitalis-Like Properties of Natriuretic Hormone

During the course of our initial isolation experiments, it became quite
obvious that we needed a more sensitive and dependable assay for the putative
natriuretic hormone to make more rapid progress toward its characterization.
The possibility of using subcellular particles in an enzymatic or binding assay
was particularly interesting to us.

Gonick's laboratory was the first to suggest that the mechanism of action
of natriuretic factor was inhibition of renal Na-K ATPase [17]. They demonstrated
that a factor which could inhibit both renal Na-K ATPase and anuran bladder
sodium transport could be isolated from the kidneys of V-E rats. This was
certainly a logical proposal since stimulation of the production of this enzyme
by aldosterone is responsible for renal sodium retention. In addition, there
is evidence that inhibition of toad bladder sodium transport can be due to
inhibition of Na-K ATPase [24].

As a unique approach to investigating the question of the Na-K ATPase inhibiting properties of natriuretic hormone, we decided to test our plasma extracts with antibodies to a known Na-K ATPase inhibitor. The basis for our
experiment was an approach first used by Sidney Spector and his associates.
They proposed that some antibodies to drugs might recognize endogenous substances which act at the same receptor [25], presumably due to similarities in
the antibody and receptor binding sites.

This technique has allowed Asano and Spector [26] to demonstrate that antibodies to benzodiazepams will also recognize purines, substances which will
displace benzodiazepams from their putative receptors in brain. These findings
have substantiated the proposal that purines may function as endogenous benzodiazepams in the central nervous system [27].

The more readily obtained antibodies to a known Na-K ATPase inhibitor were
to the cardiac glycoside digoxin. We obtained a clinical digoxin radioimmunoassay kit (New England Nuclear) to test our plasma diafiltrates and HPLC extracts. Using this assay, we were able to detect an endogenous digoxin-like
substance in plasma diafiltrates (Figure 8) and HPLC extracts [28]. We could
detect endogenous immunoreactivity in the void volume of the cation-exchange
column, and at an elution time of 30 minutes. These are the same areas of the
column effluent in which we find the antinatriferic factor and its putative
precursor (Gruber, Whitaker and Buckalew, submitted for publication).

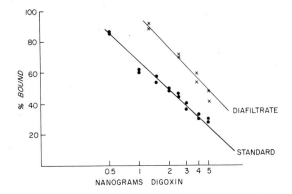

Figure 8. These curves
represent competition be-
tween a digoxin standard
or a V-E dog plasma dia-
filtrate, and I[125] digoxin
for binding to an anti-
digoxin antibody. The
points on the diafiltrate
curve represent volumes of
plasmas ranging from .8 to
3.2 mls.

We used the approach of immunoprecipitation to further purify the endogenous digoxin immunoreactivity detected in the SCX void volume. Immunoprecipitation of V-E plasma diafiltrates was performed using an antidigoxin antibody
precipitated by a second antibody. Release of the endogenous digoxin-like

354

substance was by mild acidification of the precipitant. This approach resulted in the isolation of a substance with antinatriferic activity similar to that isolated by our chromatographic technique (vide supra, [13]).

In a preliminary communication [28], we have reported the ability to detect, by radioimmunoassay, endogenous digoxin immunoreactivity in plasma extracts of dog, sheep, and man [28].

Summary

The data reported in this paper provides evidence to support the hypothesis that the putative "natriuretic hormone" is a peptide cascade, the active component(s) of which are recognized by antibodies to the known $[Na^+ + K^+]$ ATPase inhibitor digoxin.

In an attempt to demonstrate the precursor of the active hormone, we have partially purified the delayed natriuretic substance described by Sealy et al.[16]. The pattern of natriuresis shown in Figure 7 is characterized by a 10-20 minute delay in onset, with a prolonged effect lasting more than two hours. The natriuretic effect of this factor is suggestive evidence that it could be a precursor to the shorter acting substance. The HPLC retention times of these two factors indicates that the substance with delayed natriuretic activity has the larger molecular weight. Preliminary studies have shown that the HPLC fraction containing this factor does not inhibit anuran membrane sodium transport. However, trypsin digestion of this fraction releases a substance with antinatriferic activity.

While developing a more rapid assay for natriuretic hormone we investigated the possibility that it might be an endogenous digitalis-like substance. The data presented shows that V-E plasma extracts contain a substance which competes with digoxin for binding to antidigoxin antibodies. Isolation of this substance by immunoprecipitation has shown that it can inhibit toad bladder sodium transport.

Further studies are in progress to complete the isolation of natriuretic factor and demonstrate its effect on Na-K ATPase activity

Acknowledgements

This work was supported in part by NIH Grant AM 17341, NSF Grant BN5 77-25988, and a Grant from Wyeth Pharmaceuticals.

References

1. DeWardener, H.E. et al. (1961) Clin. Sci, 21, 249-258.
2. Kaloyanides, G.J. and Azer, M. (1971). J. Clin. Invest, 50, 1603-1612.
3. Blythe, W.B. (1971). Circulation Res 28, II-21 - II-31.
4. Brown, D.C. et al. (1974). Kidney International 6, 388-395.
5. Schrier, R.W. et al. (1973). In: Handbook of Physiology, Waverly Press, Baltimore, pp 708.
6. Wright, F.S. et al. (1969). J. Clin. Invest. 48, 1107-1113.
7. Buckalew, V.M., Jr. et al. (1970). J. Clin. Invest, 49, 926-935.
8. Buckalew, V.M., Jr. and Nelson, D.B. (1974). Kidney International 5, 12-22.
9. Kramer, H.J. et al. (1977). Kidney International 12, 214.
10. Favre, H. et al. (1975). J. Clin. Invest, 56, 1302-1311.
11. Gonick, H.C. and Saldanha, L.F. (1975). J. Clin. Invest. 56, 247-255.
12. Buckalew, V.M., Jr. (1978). In: Natriuretic Hormone, edited by H.J. Kramer and F. Kruck, Springer-Verlag, Berlin, Heidelberg, pp 131-141.
13. Gruber, K.A. and Buckalew, V.M., Jr. (1978). Proc. Soc. Exp. Biol. Med, 159, 463-467.
14. Gruber, K.A. et al. (1976). Proc. Nat. Acad. Sci, USA 73, 1314-1318.
15. Udenfriend, S. et al. (1972). Science 178, 871-872.
16. Sealy, J. et al. (1969). J. Clin. Invest. 48, 2210-2224.

17. Hillyard, S.D. et al. (1976). Circulation Res. 38, 250-255.
18. Clarkson, E.M. et al. (1976). Kidney International 10, 381-394.
19. Steiner, D.F. et al. (1967). Science 157, 697-706.
20. Kemper, B. et al. (1972). Proc. Nat. Acad. Sci., USA 69, 643-647.
21. Gruber, K.A. and Morris, M. (1980). Endocrine Res. Comm. 7, 45-59.
22. Chretien et al. (1979). Canadian J. Biochem. 57, 1111-1121.
23. Gruber, K.A. and Buckalew, V.M., Jr. (1978). Circulation 58, 214.
24. Kaplan, M.A. et al. (1974). J. Clin. Invest. 53, 1568-1577
25. Ginzler, A. et al. (1976). Proc. Nat. Acad. Sci., USA 73, 2132-2136.
26. Asano, T. and Spector, S. (1979). Proc. Nat. Acad. Sci., USA 76, 777-779.
27. Tallman, J.F. et al. (1980). Science 207, 274-281.
28. Gruber, K.A. et al. (1979). Proc. Amer. Soc. Neph., Abstract 47A.

Hormonal Regulation of Sodium Excretion,
B. Lichardus, R.W. Schrier and J. Ponec, eds.
© 1980 Elsevier/North-Holland Biomedical Press

SITE OF ACTION OF PLASMA NATRIURETIC FACTOR IN THE RAT KIDNEY

H. SONNENBERG, C.K. CHONG, S. MILOJEVIC AND A.T. VERESS
Department of Physiology, University of Toronto, Toronto, Ontario, Canada
M5S 1A8

INTRODUCTION

Following the classic demonstration that acute saline infusion resulted in partial inhibition of proximal tubular fluid absorption,[1] it seemed that the intrarenal site of 'volume natriuresis' had been discovered. However, it soon became evident that proximal transport inhibition was not a requisite for the renal volume response: Intravenous infusion of iso-oncotic solution did not reduce proximal tubular reabsorptive capacity, even though a homeostatically effective natriuresis was observed.[2] Conversely, renal intra-arterial infusion of saline did not result in natriuresis, although proximal reabsorption was reduced.[3] Therefore, infusion of donor blood was used to study sequential changes of transport along the nephron during hypervolemia.[4,5] No inhibition of reabsorption was found in proximal tubules, loops of Henle, or distal tubules of surface nephrons, indicating that the collecting duct system and/or deep nephrons inaccessible to micropuncture were the intrarenal sites of reduced sodium transport. Direct microcatheterization of medullary collecting ducts demonstrated complete inhibition of normal sodium reabsorption in this nephron segment following intravascular volume expansion, and also suggested that the resulting natriuresis could be modified by altered delivery of tubular fluid from deep nephrons.[6]

We have previously shown that the renal response to blood infusion is[7] associated with release of a humoral natriuretic factor into the circulation. This factor can be extracted from the plasma of blood-volume-expanded rats, and has been partially purified.[8] In the experiments to be reported we used micro-catheterization to study the effect of this plasma factor on delivery to, and transport in the medullary collecting duct system of bioassay rats.

METHODS

Bioassay procedure. Male Sprague-Dawley rats (weight range: 281-383 g) were anaesthetized with Nembutal (50 mg/kg) and received supplementary doses of the drug as required. They were prepared for microcatheterization as previously described.[6] On completion of surgery an intravenous priming dose (0.5 ml/100g body weight) of 2/3 Ringer's solution and 1/3 homologous rat plasma[9] was administered in 20 min, followed by constant infusion of the same solution at a rate of 0.5 ml/100 g body weight·hr. The solution contained ^{3}H inulin (16 µc/ml). After an equilibration period of 45 min, a 30 min urine sample was collected. Test material (see below) was then injected[8]. Allowing a further 30 min for development of the renal response, collecting duct samples were taken over the subsequent 2 hrs. Urine collections were continued during this time. Arterial blood samples (5 - 10 µl) were withdrawn at the midpoint of each urine collection. Pairs of collecting duct fluid samples were obtained by inserting a catheter into a given duct system first to a point near the opening onto the papillary tip and then to a point near the cortico-medullary border. An average of 3 different duct systems was used per animal. Concentrations of ^{3}H inulin and of sodium were measured in tubular fluid, plasma and urine[6]. Mean data per animal was calculated, and statistical significance of differences was assessed using paired and unpaired t-tests.

Test materials. Natriuretic plasma factor was obtained from plasma of hypervolemic rats as described previously[8]. After column chromatography on Sephadex G-200 a small-molecular-weight fraction was desalted and lyophylized. The fraction was reconstituted in 1 ml H_2O and brought to isotonicity by addition of NaCl prior to intravenous injection into bioassay rats. Six animals were used to test the effects of fractions from hypervolemic donors. Plasma factor obtained by the identical method from isovolemic donor rats was injected into 5 rats. A further group of 4 animals received reconstituted eluate subjected to the same extraction procedures as plasma. The latter 2 groups showed no differences in renal or collecting duct function and were therefore pooled into a common control group for statistical comparison with the first set of bioassays.

RESULTS

Average cardiovascular data for the two groups of rats before and after injection of test substances is given in Table 1. There were no significant differences in any of the measured variables between the two groups, nor were there any changes within groups as a result of the injection.

Changes in kidney function are shown in Table 2. Both types of injection were associated with significant increases in urine volume and sodium excretion, while filtration rates remained unchanged. However, administration of plasma factor derived from hypervolemic rats resulted in highly significant enhancement of diuresis and natriuresis, compared to factor from normovolemic donors

TABLE 1

BLOOD VARIABLES IN BIOASSAY RATS BEFORE AND AFTER INJECTION

Injection	Blood Pressure mmHg		Hematocrit %		Plasma sodium meq/l		Plasma potassium meq/l	
	before	after	before	after	before	after	before	after
Control (n=9)	143±3	136±2	45±1	44±1	140±1	141±1	4.5±.1	4.2±.1
Hypervol-derived (n=6)	145±4	141±6	46±1	45±1	142±2	140±1	4.3±.2	3.9±.1

TABLE 2

RENAL FUNCTION IN BIOASSAY RATS BEFORE AND AFTER INJECTION

Injection	Urine volume μl/min·gkW[a]		Sodium excretion meq/min·gkW		Filtration rate ml/min·gkW	
	before	after	before	after	before	after
Control (n=9)	4.0±4	6.6[b,c]±.6	124±23	392[b,c]±89	0.80±.02	0.78±0.2
Hypervol-derived (n=6)	4.5±5	13.4[b]±.6	214±42	1496[b]±150	0.85±.04	0.89±.06

[a]Values expressed per gram experimental kidney weight
[b]Statistically significant difference (p = 0.05 or less) within each group
[c]Statistically significant difference (p = 0.05 or less) between two groups
or to vehicle injection.

After injection of test substance the fraction of filtered fluid remaining in the catheterized collecting duct systems near the cortico-medullary border and the papillary tip were calculated from tubular fluid-to-plasma inulin concentration ratios, and were averaged in each animal. Results for the two groups are shown in Fig. 1. As expected from the urinary data (Table 2) fractional volumes at the end of the duct were significantly greater in the group receiving hypervolemic-derived plasma factor (p < 0.05). Similarly, the delivery of fractional volume to the medullary collecting system was also enhanced (p < 0.02).

An analogous plot of the fraction of filtered sodium remaining in the duct is shown in Fig. 2. Again, fractional sodium remainder was significantly higher after injection of hypervolemic-derived factor, both at the beginning (p < 0.05) and end (p < 0.01) of the collecting duct.

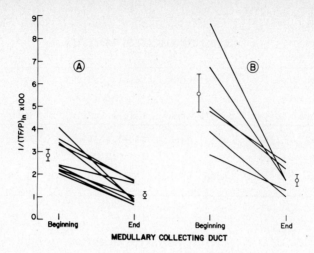

Fig. 1. Percentage of filtered fluid remaining in medullary collecting duct of (A) animals injected with control solutions and (B) animals injected with plasma factor from hypervolemic rats. Group averages ± S.E. are indicated by open circles; solid lines connect data from individual rats.

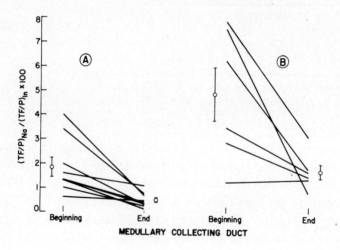

Fig. 2. Percentage of filtered sodium remaining in medullary collecting duct in individual rats. Symbols and explanations as for Fig. 1.

To determine whether transport of salt and water along the duct itself was affected by the natriuretic plasma factor, reabsorption was calculated as the difference in each animal of deliveries to beginning and end of the collecting system. Results are shown in Fig. 3.

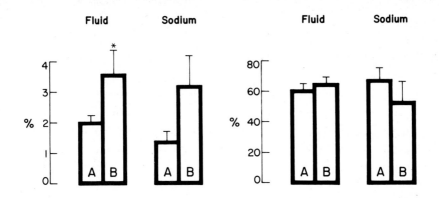

Fig. 3. Reabsorption of fluid and sodium in the medullary collecting duct after injection of control solutions (A) and hypervolemic-derived factor (B). Left panel: absolute reabsorption; right panel: percent reabsorption of load delivered to the duct.

As can also be seen from Figs. 1 and 2, absolute collecting duct reabsorption of fluid and sodium was actually increased in animals receiving the plasma factor derived from hypervolemic donor rats. However, when expressed as a function of flow into the duct no difference in reabsorption was found, demonstrating that salt and water transport was proportional to delivered load.

DISCUSSION

Our earlier segmental analysis of the intrarenal site of transport inhibition following blood volume expansion[4,5,6] suggested that 'natriuretic hormone' could either increase delivery of salt and water to the medullary collecting duct, presumably from deep nephrons, or it could directly inhibit normal reabsorption in the duct itself. The present results demonstrate that a humoral factor, extracted from the plasma of hypervolemic rats, enhanced the tubular load of sodium and fluid entering the medullary duct. Associated with this elevated delivery was an increased reabsorption in the collecting system.[10] Such load-dependency of collecting duct transport has been found previously, indicating the contribution of this part of the nephron to overall glomerulo-tubular balance. These findings explain the relatively small natriuresis due to circulating humoral factor compared to the total renal volume response: for full expression of the excretory effect of natriuretic factor a simultaneous inhibition of collecting duct reabsorption, presumably by non-hormonal means, is also required.[7]

In earlier experiments we have shown that rats fed a salt-poor diet had a reduced natriuretic response to blood volume expansion, compared to animals fed a salt-rich diet.[11] Prior cross-circulation of two such rats increased a subsequent volume response of the salt-deprived animal to the level of its high-salt partner, demonstrating the existence in the latter of transferable humoral natriuretic factor, which was present before acute blood volume expansion.[11] It was also found that the difference in volume natriuresis between salt-deprived or salt-loaded rats was due to a difference in fluid and sodium delivery to the collecting duct system, both groups showing identical inhibition of collecting duct transport per se.[6] Together with the finding that in normal animals natriuretic hormone could only be detected when acute hypervolemia was sustained,[7] these results suggest that the physiological role of natriuretic hormone is in long term regulation of body fluid volume.

In agreement with earlier findings,[8] plasma extract from normovolemic donor rats also increased salt and water excretion in the present study. In contrast to the hypervolemic-derived factor, however, reduced reabsorption in the collecting duct itself would seem responsible for this effect, since fractional reabsorption of delivered load was less than that of normal antidiuretic rats.[10] In any case, the similar transport reduction obtained with reconstituted eluate alone suggests that this is an artifact of our extraction procedure.

In summary, natriuretic factor extracted from plasma of hypervolemic rats acts by increasing tubular delivery of salt and water to the medullary collecting duct system. The effect on urinary excretion remains limited, if reabsorption in the duct itself is normal. Should duct transport be inhibited, however, as in acute hypervolemia, the presence of the factor results in enhanced diuresis and natriuresis.

ACKNOWLEDGEMENTS

Supported, in part, by a grant from the Ontario Heart Foundation.

REFERENCES

1. Dirks, J.H., Cirksena, W.J. and Berliner, R.W. (1965) J. Clin. Invest. 44, 1160-1170.

2. Sonnenberg, H. and Solomon, S. (1969) Can. J. Physiol. Pharmacol. 47, 153-159.

3. Knox, F.G., Howards, S.S., Wright, F.S., Davis, B.B. and Berliner, R.W. (1968) J. Clin. Invest. 47, 1561-1572.

4. Sonnenberg, H. (1971) Can. J. Physiol. Pharmacol. 49, 525-535.

5. Sonnenberg, H. (1972) Am. J. Physiol. 223, 916-924.

6. Sonnenberg, H. (1976) Circul. Research 29, 282-288.

7. Sonnenberg, H., Veress, A.T. and Pearce, J.W. (1972) J. Clin. Invest. 51, 2631-2644.

8. Veress, A.T., Milojevic, S. and Sonnenberg, H. (1980) Clin. Sci., in press.

9. Maddox, D.A., Price, D.C. and Rector, F.C.Jr. (1977) Am. J. Physiol. 233, F600-F606.

10. Sonnenberg, H. (1978) New Aspects of Renal Function, Excerpta Medica, Amsterdam-Oxford, pp. 175-180.

11. Pearce, J.W., Sonnenberg, H., Veress, A.T. and Ackermann, U. (1969) Can. J. Physiol. Pharmacol. 47, 377-386.

Hormonal Regulation of Sodium Excretion,
B. Lichardus, R.W. Schrier and J. Ponec, eds.
© 1980 Elsevier/North-Holland Biomedical Press

SODIUM AND CHLORIDE PERMEABILITY OF COLLECTING DUCTS AND THE EFFECT OF SALT LOADING STUDIED *IN VITRO*

CHERYL RAY and TREFOR MORGAN
Faculty of Medicine, University of Newcastle, N.S.W., Newcastle (Australia)

INTRODUCTION

The mechanism that controls the excretion of sodium is not completely understood. In addition to the control exerted by aldosterone and glomerular filtration rate there is evidence that a "third" factor is involved in the control of salt excretion[1,2]. Early work demonstrated that following massive volume expansion proximal tubule reabsorption of salt and water was depressed[3] and subsequent work indicated that this was due to depression of plasma protein[4]. Howards *et al* in 1968[5] clearly demonstrated that the effects of volume expansion with albumin differed from expansion with saline and while volume expansion with albumin depressed proximal tubule absorption it had little effect on net sodium excretion compared to the massive natriuresis induced by similar volume expansion with saline. Thus saline infusion had an additional effect on sodium reabsorption beyond the proximal tubule. Morgan and Berliner[6] in 1969 showed in a microperfusion study that this effect did not take place in the loop of Henle or distal tubule and postulated that the effect was a depression of sodium reabsorption in the collecting duct.

Various assays have been developed for assaying a natriuretic factor present in plasma and urine. The one developed by Sealey *et al*[7] and a similar assay used by Brown *et al*[8] showed that in a rat in water diuresis the sodium concentration in the rats urine altered with little change in volume flow. This effect suggested an inhibition of sodium transport out of the collecting ducts or an increase in the permeability of collecting ducts to sodium allowing entry of sodium into the urine from the interstitium of the papilla.

This study was planned to investigate in an isolated rat papilla the sodium and chloride permeability of the papillary collecting duct and its response to various substances.

MATERIALS AND METHODS

Papillae were obtained from the kidneys of Wistar rats and collecting ducts were perfused as described previously[9,10]. $^{22}Na^+$ and $^{36}Cl^-$ were added to the perfusate and the diffusional permeability of these two substances were measured simultaneously.

The effects of ADH, aldosterone, prostaglandin E_2, indomethacin, plasma from volume expanded rats, extract of "natriuretic hormone" from human urine[11] on the diffusional permeability of $^{22}Na^+$ and $^{36}Cl^-$ were measured. In separate experiments the animals from which the papillae were to be removed were pretreated with different salt diets, with aldosterone or by adrenalectomy and the effects of these manoeuvres on the diffusional permeability to $^{22}Na^+$ and $^{36}Cl^-$ were measured.

Many studies were recollection studies[10] from the same collecting duct. Such studies were analysed using a "paired" and also unpaired "t" test. Other studies were analysed using an unpaired student "t" test.

RESULTS

The diffusional permeability of papillary collecting ducts to $^{22}Na^+$ and $^{36}Cl^-$ were 0.47 ± 0.03 μm sec^{-1} and 0.76 ± 0.05 μm sec^{-1} respectively (n=120). These values were significantly different and in only one papillary collecting duct was the diffusional permeability to $^{22}Na^+$ higher than the value found for $^{36}Cl^-$. The ratio of Cl^- to Na^+ permeability was 1.62 ± 0.05. In subsequent results the diffusional permeability of the collecting duct to $^{22}Na^+$ and $^{36}Cl^-$ refer to the values for controls determined at the same time as the experimental manoeuvres were being undertaken.

Rats were placed on diets of different sodium content and the 24 hour urine excretion of Na^+ was 0.15 mmol/day, 1.0 mmol/day, 4.0 mmol/day in the low, normal and high salt intake groups. The diffusional permeability of the papillary collecting ducts to Na^+ and Cl^- did not differ between the groups (table 1); though the value on the high salt diet was greater this failed to reach significance.

TABLE 1

EFFECT OF DIET ON DIFFUSIONAL PERMEABILITY TO $^{22}Na^+$ and $^{36}Cl^-$

| | n | Diffusional Permeability µm sec^{-1} | | Ratio |
		$^{22}Na^+$	$^{36}Cl^-$	
Low Salt	29	0.51 ± 0.05	0.87 ± 0.08	1.71
Normal Salt	59	0.55 ± 0.04	0.80 ± 0.04	1.45
High Salt	77	0.62 ± 0.03	0.89 ± 0.04	1.44

mean sem   n = number of permeability measurements

Rats were adrenalectomised and 10 days later the diffusional permeability to $^{22}Na^+$ and $^{36}Cl^-$ was measured. No difference was found compared to the control rats and no effect of administration of aldosterone for 10 days prior to the experiment was found (table 2).

TABLE 2

EFFECT OF ADRENAL STEROIDS ON DIFFUSIONAL PERMEABILITY TO $^{22}Na^+$ and $^{36}Cl^-$

| | n | Diffusional Permeability µm sec^{-1} | | Ratio |
		$^{22}Na^+$	$^{36}Cl^-$	
Control animals	22	0.49 ± 0.04	0.75 ± 0.05	1.53
Adrenalectomised Animals	24	0.44 ± 0.06	0.75 ± 0.08	1.70
Aldosterone Administered	20	0.52 ± 0.04	0.77 ± 0.06	1.48

mean sem

The diffusional permeability to $^{22}Na^+$ and $^{36}Cl^-$ was determined in papillae from normal rats which were incubated in plasma from rats that had been on a low, normal or high salt diet. The diffusional permeability to $^{22}Na^+$ increased as the salt content of the diet increased and there was a fall in the diffusional permeability to $^{36}Cl^-$ which was not significant. There was a marked change in the ratio of $^{36}Cl^-$: $^{22}Na^+$ diffusional permeability, the net effect of these changes would allow NaCl to more readily enter the lumen of the collecting duct from outside (table 3).

TABLE 3

EFFECT OF PLASMA FROM ANIMALS ON A HIGH, NORMAL OR LOW SALT DIET ON
DIFFUSIONAL PERMEABILITY TO $^{22}Na^+$ and $^{36}Cl^-$

| | n | Diffusional Permeability $\mu m\ sec^{-1}$ | | Ratio |
		$^{22}Na^+$	$^{36}Cl^-$	
Low	14	0.47 ± 0.05	0.79 ± 0.06	1.68
Normal	11	0.47 ± 0.05	0.69 ± 0.08	1.47
High	18	0.59 ± 0.03*	0.65 ± 0.06	1.10

mean sem   *$p < 0.01$

A partially purified extract of "natriuretic factor" provided by Professor
de Wardener was tested in this system. Into a bath containing 15 ml of medium
an amount of extract that was known to cause a natriuresis in rats in water
diuresis was added.(x) This would give a concentration equivalent to or
greater than that which would result in rats assuming an extracellular distribution of the injected substance. In separate experiments the extract was
added to the perfusion fluid to give a concentration equal to ten times that
which would have been achieved in plasma. The extract which has been reported[11]
to have a natriuretic effect in the whole rat had no effect on the diffusional
permeability to $^{22}Na^+$ and $^{36}Cl^-$. The experiments have been performed on two
separate extracts and are presented in table 4. On one occasion there appeared
to be a minor change in permeability but this has not been confirmed in the
other experiments. (table 4)

TABLE 4

EFFECT OF "NATRIURETIC" EXTRACT FROM URINE OF HUMANS ON DIFFUSIONAL
PERMEABILITY TO $^{22}Na^+$ and $^{36}Cl^-$

| | n | Diffusional Permeability $\mu m\ sec^{-1}$ | | | |
| | | Control Values | | Extract | |
		$^{22}Na^+$	$^{36}Cl^-$	$^{22}Na^+$	$^{36}Cl^-$
Extract 1	20	0.42 ± 0.03	0.75 ± 0.05	0.51 ± 0.05*	0.72 ± 0.04
2 x	18	0.57 ± 0.07	0.79 ± 0.09	0.57 ± 0.03	0.87 ± 0.07
2x	4	0.53 ± 0.16	0.71 ± 0.17	0.44 ± 0.09	0.71 ± 0.10
Extract 2					
Perfusate 10x	30	0.59 ± 0.04	0.80 ± 0.07	0.51 ± 0.04	0.71 ± 0.05

mean   sem   * $p < 0.05$ paired "t" test
                $p > 0.01$

Antidiuretic hormone and aldosterone added to the medium had no significant effect on $^{22}Na^+$ or $^{36}Cl^-$ permeability (table 5).

Indomethacin $10^{-5}M$ or Prostaglandin E_2 added to the medium did not alter the diffusional permeability to $^{22}Na^+$ or $^{36}Cl^-$.

TABLE 5

EFFECT OF DIFFERENT SUBSTANCES ON DIFFUSIONAL PERMEABILITY TO $^{22}Na^+$ and $^{36}Cl^-$

		n	Diffusional Permeability $\mu m\ sec^{-1}$ Control	Experimental
ADH 500 µunit/ml	Na^+	6	0.52 ± 0.05	0.50 ± 0.05
	Cl^-	6	0.78 ± 0.09	0.80 ± 0.05
Aldosterone	Na^+	6	0.48 ± 0.05	0.46 ± 0.05
	Cl^-	6	0.75 ± 0.06	0.70 ± 0.04
Indomethacin	Na^+	6	0.57 ± 0.08	0.53 ± 0.08
	Cl^-	6	0.82 ± 0.13	0.84 ± 0.13
Prostaglandin E_2	Na^+	6	0.53 ± 0.09	0.42 ± 0.09
	Cl^-	6	0.74 ± 0.06	0.70 ± 0.17

mean sem

DISCUSSION

In a previous study[12] performed *in vitro* using the same preparation we found no negative potential difference across the collecting duct of the papilla. A slight positive potential difference was found. The resistance of the epithelium was similar to that measured by Rau and Fromter[13] in the hamster and thus we do not believe that that result was an error of measurement. The finding that chloride, a negatively charged ion, has a higher permeability across this epithelium than sodium allows a partial explanation of our results and the negative potential difference during life may result from the diffusion of chloride more rapidly than sodium into the lumen. However, other studies[14,15] indicate that during life that there is net reabsorption of NaCl in the collecting duct system and thus this cannot be the whole explanation.

In the present study only one procedure altered $^{22}Na^+$ diffusional permeability and may also have had an effect on $^{36}Cl^-$ permeability. Plasma from volume expanded rats increased the diffusional permeability of the collecting duct to $^{22}Na^+$ and may have caused a small decrease in $^{36}Cl^-$ permeability. The net result would be that in life after salt loading ions would enter the collecting duct more readily from the interstitium and that there could be addition of NaCl to the urine at the collecting duct level. Sonnenberg[16] has observed that in volume expansion and salt loading that there is entry of salt at this site into the collecting duct system. An additional result of the changes that we have found is that the potential difference in the collecting duct would become less negative without any necessary change in active transport.

We have used an extract of urine supplied by Professor de Wardener to determine if a similar effect was present in that substance. No clearcut effect was obtained and our conclusions are that in that extract this effect has not been observed. We consider this difficult to explain as *in vivo* this extract does cause a natriuresis the nature of which could be readily explained by the present results.

In this preparation no effect on Na^+ or Cl^- permeability was found for a variety of substances. In recent experiments in our laboratory[17] we have shown that salt loading in people with mild hypertension alters the net efflux of $^{22}Na^+$ from red cells that have been preloaded with the isotope. Whether this is an effect on oubain sensitive transport or on the permeability of the red cell to sodium we have not yet determined. It would be intriguing if the change in permeability of the red cell membrane and of the collecting duct epithelium was due to the same factor as de Wardener has suggested.

If we apply these results to the intact animal, salt handling down the nephron would proceed in the following way. In the proximal tubule reabsorption of salt and water is suppressed by volume and salt expansion. More salt and fluid is delivered to the loop of Henle in which net reabsorption of salt and water is increased under these conditions and the net reabsorption of salt and water in the distal tubule is also increased as a consequence of the increased volume flow[6]. If the expansion is due only to increase in plasma volume then the increased reabsorption by the loop of Henle and the distal tubule modulates the proximal tubule effect so that the increase in sodium excretion is small and in proportion to the percentage decrease in Na^+ reabsorption in the proximal tubule. However, if the animal is infused with salt or is previously salt loaded the situation in the collecting duct differs. In this situation active transport of sodium may be inhibited or more likely the entry of Na^+ and Cl^- from the papillary and medullary interstitium into the collecting duct is increased and therefore a massive natriuresis may result. This effect of salt loading would also operate in the absence of any major degree of volume expansion and could be a precise modulator of sodium excretion.

There is evidence that a natriuretic factor is present in plasma and urine of volume expanded animals. Whether there is one or more factors is unclear. This study demonstrates that plasma from volume expanded animals alters the permeability of the epithelium of the collecting duct to sodium in a way which would allow a logical explanation of the nature of natriuresis following a salt or volume load.

ACKNOWLEDGEMENTS

This work was supported by the National Health and Medical Research Council of Australia and by the Australian Kidney Foundation. The stimulation of Professor de Wardener to work in this field is acknowledged. The secretarial help of M. Hayes in dealing with difficult manuscripts is acknowledged.

REFERENCES
1. De Wardener, H.E. *et al* (1961) Clinical Science 21, 249-258.
2. Levinsky, N.S. and Lalone, R.C. (1963) J.Clin. Invest. 42, 1261.
3. Dirks, J.H. *et al* (1965) J. Clin. Invest. 44, 1160.
4. Brenner, B.M. *et al* (1969) Amer. J. of Physiol. 220, 2058.
5. Howards, S.S. *et al* (1968) J. Clin. Invest. 47, 1561-1572.
6. Morgan, T.O. and Berliner, R.W. (1969) Nephron 388-405.
7. Sealey, J.E. *et al* (1969) J. Clin. Invest. 48, 2210-2224.
8. Brown, P.R. *et al* (1972) Kidney International 2, 1-5.
9. Morgan, T.O. *et al* (1968) Amer. J. of Physiol. 214, 574-581.
10. Morgan, T.O. (1974) Clin. and Exp. Pharmacology and Physiology 1, 23-30.
11. Clarkson *et al* (1976) Kidney International 10, 381-394.
12. Morgan *et al* (1978) Abstracts of VII International Congress of Nephrology C12.
13. Rau, W.S. and Fromter, E. (1974) Pflugers Archiv. 351, 113-131.
14. Ullrich, K.J. and Paparassiliou, F. (1979) Pflugers Arch. 379, 49-52.
15. Ozgood, R.W. *et al* (1978) J. Clin. Invest. 62, 311-320.
16. Sonnenberg, H. (1975) Amer. J. of Physiology 228, 565-568.
17. Fitzgibbon, W. *et al* (1980) Abstracts of VII Meeting of International Society of Hypertension. 33.

Hormonal Regulation of Sodium Excretion,
B. Lichardus, R.W. Schrier and J. Ponec, eds.
© 1980 Elsevier/North-Holland Biomedical Press

INHIBITION OF LEUCOCYTE SODIUM TRANSPORT BY THE NATRIURETIC FACTOR OF HUMAN
URINE: DEMONSTRATION OF A LACK OF THE FACTOR IN CIRRHOTIC PATIENTS RETAINING
SODIUM

L. POSTON, S.P. WILKINSON[*], ROGER WILLIAMS

The Liver Unit, King's College Hospital and Medical School, Denmark Hill,
London SE5, England.
[*]Present address: Royal Infirmary, Gloucester, England.

INTRODUCTION

The isotonic expansion of the extracellular fluid volume leads to a natriuresis at least partially independent of changes in the glomerular filtration
rate or to levels of circulating mineralocorticoids. Following the early
experiments of de Wardener et al.[1], in which it was shown that volume expansion
in one dog could lead to a natriuretic response in a second, cross - circulated
animal, it was suggested that a humoral substance other than aldosterone might
be involved in the day-to-day regulation of sodium excretion. The techniques
of ultrafiltration and gel chromatography employed in the search for this
substance have since led to the identification of natriuretic fractions in both
plasma and urine of volume-expanded subjects or animals[2]. Two active fractions
have been isolated from urine. The first, larger molecular weight material[3-6]
when injected into assay rats produces a natriuresis which is slow in onset and
of prolonged duration. The second, smaller molecular weight fraction[6,7] which
appears after the salts when urine is fractionated on Sephadex G-25 invokes a
prompt natriuresis in the assay rat. Both of these fractions also have demonstrable natriuretic activity when isolated from the urine of salt-depleted
subjects, although to a lesser degree[6].

The assays used in the detection of the natriuretic material[2] have included
sodium excretion in the rat, sodium transport in anuran membranes, the uptake
of PAH in renal tubule fragments, the effect of the material on renal Na/K
ATPase and several others. The rat assay, which is the most commonly used, is
hampered by the inherent variability of sodium excretion in the rat and by a
general lack of conformity amongst the various groups which use it. Moreover,
all the techniques of assay have necessarily involved the use of animal tissue
and the extrapolation of results to include human physiology must therefore be
tentative.

In this study we attempted to assay the natriuretic material of human urine

using a sodium transport system of human tissue, that of peripheral blood
leucocytes. The natriuretic material appears to affect sodium transport in a
variety of tissues and it was not unreasonable, therefore, to assume that it would
similarly inhibit sodium transport in leucocytes. However, several studies
have indicated that leucocyte sodium transport mimics that in the nephron during
a state of volume expansion and leucocytes may therefore be 'sensitive' to the
effect of a circulating natriuretic substance. These include the observation
of depressed leucocyte sodium transport during volume expansion by saline
infusion[8], during mineralocorticoid 'escape' in normal subjects[9] and from
patients with severe chronic uraemia[10], all three conditions being associated
with the appearance of highly active natriuretic fractions in the urine.

DEVELOPMENT OF THE ASSAY

As described above, the small molecular weight natriuretic fraction of urine
brings about an almost immediate natriuresis in the assay rat and, because of
this rapid mode of action, was chosen for assay in this study. The fraction
was isolated from the urine of normal subjects both before and after volume
expansion by saline infusion according to the method of Clarkson et al. (1976)[6].
Concentrated urine equivalent to 2 hours of a 24-hour urine collection was
applied to a column of Sephadex G-25 and eluted with the volatile buffer, 0.01M
ammonium acetate. The fraction which appeared immediately after the salts
(Fraction Four, F.IV) was then collected and freeze-dried twice. Leucocytes
were isolated from peripheral venous blood by a method described by Baron and
Ahmed[11]. Leucocyte sodium efflux rates were estimated according to the method
of Hilton and Patrick (1973)[12], which involves the initial loading of leucocytes with ^{22}NaCl and subsequent sampling of the cells at timed intervals. The
rate of efflux of sodium was then calculated from the line of regression of
residual radioactivity within the leucocytes.

Fraction IV equivalent to 0.5ml of an initial 24-hour urine collection
obtained from 8 normal subjects before saline infusion and incubated with
normal leucocytes for 1½ hours had no significant effect on the leucocyte
sodium efflux rate constant. However, incubation of the equivalent amount of
F.IV from the same subjects after volume expansion by saline infusion (20ml
0.9% saline/kg body weight, over 1 hour) resulted in a significant depression
of the leucocyte sodium efflux rate constant (p < 0.001) (Fig. 1).

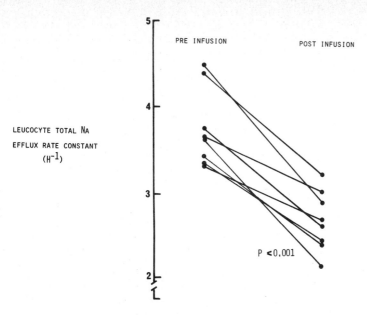

Fig. 1. Sodium efflux in normal leucocytes after preincubation with urine fraction F.IV (0.5 hr) from normal subjects before and after acute saline infusion.

When the quantitiy of F.IV isolated from the urine of subjects before volume expansion was increased to an amount equivalent to 1 hour of the original 24-hour urine collection, a significant depression of the rate of leucocyte sodium efflux was achieved (p < 0.001).

Sodium transport inhibitory activity was thus demonstrated in the small molecular weight fraction (F.IV) isolated from the urine of normal subjects in a state of acute volume expansion and also, to a lesser degree, in the same fraction from subjects on a normal intake of sodium. Sodium transport in the human peripheral blood leucocyte would therefore appear to be a sensitive bioassay for the small molecular weight natriuretic material of urine.

CIRRHOSIS

Renal sodium retention leading to the accumulation of fluid is common in cirrhosis. Aldosterone is likely to be a major factor, the renal sodium excretion being closely related to the plasma aldosterone concentration[13,14]. However, the aldosterone/sodium excretion relationship is abnormal in that for a given sodium excretion the plasma aldosterone concentration has been found to be much lower than in healthy control subjects[13]. This could be explained if the cirrhotic patient had either an increased renal tubular sensitivity to aldosterone or a deficiency of a natriuretic hormone. Since there is some evidence that the liver may be an important source of the natriuretic hormone [5,15], an investigation of the smaller molecular weight urinary natriuretic material was carried out in 23 patients with cirrhosis representing a spectrum with regard to sodium balance. The leucocyte assay described above was used to determine the natriuretic activity of F.IV isolated from the urine of these patients on the fifth day of a 50mM daily sodium diet. Significantly less leucocyte sodium transport inhibitory activity was demonstrated in F.IV from the urine of patients who were in positive sodium balance and accumulating ascites than in the same fraction from those in sodium equilibrium ($p < 0.01$).

Thus, within the limitations of this bioassay, these data suggest that a deficiency of a natriuretic hormone may contribute towards the sodium retention of cirrhosis.

REFERENCES

1. de Wardener, H.E., Mills, I.H., Clapham, W.F. and Hayter, C.J. (1961) Studies on the efferent mechanism of the sodium diuresis which follows the administration of intravenous saline in the dog. Clin. Sci. 21, 249-258.

2. de Wardener, H.E. (1977) Natriuretic hormone. Ed. Rev. Clin. Sci. Molec. Med. 53, 1-8.

3. Krück, F. (1967) Biologischer Nachweis eines humoralen natriuretischen Prinzips im Urin gesunder Menschen. Klin. Wochenschr. 45, 30-34.

4. Viskoper, J.R., Czaczkes, J.W., Schwartz, N. and Ullman, T.D. (1971) Natriuretic activity of a substance isolated from human urine during the excretion of a salt load. Nephron, 8, 540-548.

5. Sealey, J.E. and Laragh, J.H. (1971) Further studies of a natriuretic substance occurring in human urine and plasma. Circ. Res. 28/29, (Suppl. 2), 32-43.

6. Clarkson, E.M., Raw, S.M. and de Wardener, H.E. (1976) Two natriuretic substances in extracts of urine from normal man when salt-depleted and salt-loaded. Kidney Int. 10, 381-394.

7. Favre, H., Hwang, K.H., Schmidt, R.W., Bricker, N.S. and Bourgoignie, J.J. (1975) An inhibitor of sodium transport in the urine of dogs with normal renal function. J. Clin. Invest. 56, 1302-1311.

8. Thomas, R.D., Hilton, P.J., Jones, N.F., Edmondson, R.P.S. and Garcia, B. (1975) Effects of saline infusion and salt depletion on sodium transport by leucocytes in normal man. Clin. Sci. 49, 16P.

9. Poston, L., Wilkinson, S.P., Sewell R. and Williams, R. (1979) Inhibition of leucocyte sodium transport during mineralocorticoid 'escape'. Clin. Sci. 58, 9P.

10. Edmondson, R.P.S., Hilton, P.J., Jones, N.F., Patrick, J. and Thomas, R.D. (1975) Leucocyte sodium transport in uraemia. Clin. Sci. Molec. Med. 49, 213-216.

11. Baron, D.N. and Ahmed, S.A. (1969) Intracellular concentrations of water and of the principal electrolytes determined by analysis of isolated human leucocytes. Clin. Sci. 37, 205-219.

12. Hilton, P.J. and Patrick, J. (1973) Sodium amd potassium flux rates in normal leucocytes in an artificial extracellular fluid. Clin. Sci. Molec. Med. 55, 255-263.

13. Wilkinson, S.P., Jowett, T.P., Slater, J.D.H., Arroyo, V., Moodie, H. and Williams, R. (1979) Renal sodium retention in cirrhosis: relation to aldosterone and nephron site. Clin. Sci. 56, 169-177.

14. Arroyo, V., Bosch, J., Mauri, M., Viver, J., Mas, A., Rivera, F. and Rodes, J. (1979) Renin, aldosterone and renal haemodynamics in cirrhosis with ascites. Eur. J. Clin. Invest. 9, 69-73.

15. Milies, E. (1960) A new diuretic factor of hepatic origin. Acta Physiol. Lat. America, 10, 178-193.

Hormonal Regulation of Sodium Excretion,
B. Lichardus, R.W. Schrier and J. Ponec, eds.
© 1980 Elsevier/North-Holland Biomedical Press

ROLE OF A HUMORAL FACTOR IN LOW RENIN HYPERTENSION

FRANCIS J. HADDY, MOTILAL B. PAMNANI, DAVID L. CLOUGH

Department of Physiology, Uniformed Services University, 4301 Jones Bridge
Road, Bethesda, MD 20014 (USA)

INTRODUCTION

The mechanism of low renin, salt dependent, presumably volume expanded
hypertension is particularly difficult to understand. The renin-angiotensin-
aldosterone and sympathico-adrenal systems are suppressed and hypervolemia,
acting either directly or indirectly via autoregulation, does not seem to be
an adequate explanation for the hypertension. Over the last five years, we
have generated evidence in animals suggesting that it is related to the release of a ouabain-like humoral agent which acts by suppressing the sodium-
potassium pump in vascular and cardiac muscle. It is the purpose of this
paper to review this evidence.

EVIDENCE THAT THE NA^+-K^+ PUMP IS SUPPRESSED

We have used two measures of Na^+-K^+ pump activity in experimental animals,
ouabain-sensitive ^{86}rubidium uptake by blood vessels and Na^+,K^+-ATPase activity
of cardiac microsomes. Rubidium is an ion which substitutes for potassium in
active transport by the pump across cell membranes. It is used in the study
of pump activity because its radioactive form has a longer half life and a
lower energy emission than the radioactive form of potassium. The ouabain-
sensitive rubidium uptake is that uptake related to active transport because
ouabain inhibits the sodium-potassium pump which is responsible for active
transport. Pamnani adapted the rubidium uptake technique to blood vessels and
we first applied the technique to mesenteric arteries and veins of dogs with
one-kidney, one wrapped hypertension[1]. After at least four weeks of sustained
significant hypertension in the experimental animal and at the same time interval in the sham operated control animal, blood vessels were obtained simultaneously from the pair for measurements of ouabain-sensitive and insensitive
^{86}rubidium uptakes. First, the vessels were incubated at 0° C in potassium-
free Krebs-Henseleit solution to depress the sodium-potassium pump and load
the cells with sodium. Next, to stimulate the pump, the vessels were incubated
at 37° C in potassium-free Krebs-Henseleit solution containing 2 mM non-radio-
active rubidium. The solution also contained ^{86}rubidium and its uptake was

measured 18 minutes later. Each vessel was divided in half, one half placed
in media without ouabain and the other in media with ouabain.

Ouabain-sensitive [86]rubidium uptake, which reflects membrane sodium-potassium pump activity, was calculated as the difference between [86]rubidium uptake
without and with ouabain. The [86]rubidium uptake in the presence of ouabain
(ouabain-insensitive uptake) reflects distribution in extracellular space and
passive penetration into cells (determined by cell wall permeability and surface area).

We found that ouabain-sensitive uptake by both arteries and veins from
hypertensive animals was less than that by vessels from the sham operated
normotensive animals. The ouabain-insensitive uptake was not different in the
two groups of animals. Thus the defect was only in the ouabain-sensitive
sodium-potassium pump. Since the defect was also present in veins, it did not
appear to be secondary to increased pressure.

We next examined Na^+,K^+-ATPase activity in a similar model of low renin
hypertension. Like sodium-potassium pump activity in intact cells, the ability
of isolated membranes to split ATP, i.e., the total ATPase activity, is inhibited by addition of ouabain to and removal of potassium from the incubating
medium. Any residual activity is due to Mg^{++}-ATPase. Na^+,K^+-ATPase activity
is then the difference between total ATPase and Mg^{++}-ATPase activities. It
is difficult to isolate membranes from the smooth muscle in blood vessels.
However, this is not the case for heart muscle. Clough, therefore, measured
Na^+,K^+-ATPase activity in microsomes isolated from the left[2, 3] and right[3]
ventricles of rats with one-kidney, one clip hypertension and found it suppressed in both the high and low pressure chambers.

Since then, we have examined ouabain-sensitive rubidium uptake and
Na^+,K^+-ATPase activity in a variety of models of experimental hypertension,
some investigator induced and some genetic in origin. The findings are summarized in Table 1. It is apparent that ouabain-sensitive [86]rubidium uptake
and Na^+,K^+-ATPase activity are reduced only in the investigator induced, low
renin, presumably volume expanded forms of hypertension. These include one-
kidney, one wrapped hypertension in the dog and 1) one-kidney, one clip,
2) one-kidney, DOCA, salt, and 3) reduced renal mass hypertension in the rat.
Pump activity seems to decrease following maneuvers which interfere with water
and salt excretion by the kidney, either mechanical (reduced renal mass, renal
artery constriction) or functional (DOCA). On the other hand, ouabain-sensitive [86]rubidium uptake is increased in two genetic forms of hypertension,
spontaneous and Dahl salt sensitive (ouabain-insensitive ^{86}Rb uptake is also

increased, suggesting that the increased pump activity in these two models is secondary to increased intracellular sodium concentration subsequent to increased permeability).

TABLE 1

[86]RB UPTAKE AND ATPASE ACTIVITY IN BLOOD VESSELS AND HEART OF ANIMALS WITH VARIOUS TYPES OF HYPERTENSION

Type[a]	Blood vessel[b] rubidium uptake		Ref	Ventricular ATPase activity		Ref
	Ouabain sensitive	Ouabain insensitive		Na^+,K^+-	$Mg^{++}-$	
One-kidney, one wrapped	↓	↔	1			
One-kidney, one clip	↓[d]	↔[d]		↓	↑	2, 3
One-kidney, DOCA, salt	↓	↑	4	↓	↑	5
Reduced renal mass	↓	↔	6	↓	↑	7
SHR (relative to WKY)	↑	↑	8	↔	↔	7
Dahl S (high salt)[c]	↑	↑	9	↓[e]	↔[e]	

[a] All rat except one-kidney, one wrapped which was dog.

[b] Tail artery in rat, mesenteric vessels in dog.

[c] Relative to Dahl S on normal salt.

[d] Pamnani, Clough, Haddy - unpublished observation

[e] Clough, Pamnani, Haddy - unpublished observation

EVIDENCE THAT THE PUMP SUPPRESSION RESULTS FROM A HUMORAL AGENT

Since decreased pump activity was seen only in the investigator induced low renin forms of hypertension, we questioned the role of volume expansion. We therefore next measured [86]rubidium uptake in blood vessels of acutely volume expanded rats[10]. We reasoned that if the decreased pump activity is in fact a consequence of expansion of the extracellular fluid volume, acute volume expansion should reproduce the changes in [86]rubidium uptake.

Under pentobarbital anesthesia, normal rats were infused intravenously with enough normal saline to expand extracellular fluid volume by 30%. Paired control rats were sham infused. In the experimental animal, the expansion was maintained for two hrs. At the end of this time, tail arteries were harvested for measurement of ^{86}rubidium uptake and blood was collected and plasma supernates prepared by boiling the plasma.

Ouabain-sensitive ^{86}rubidium uptake was significantly suppressed in the tail arteries from the volume expanded rats and the degree of suppression was similar to that seen in the low renin models of hypertension. Ouabain-insensitive uptake was unaffected, as is the case in most models of low renin hypertension (Table 1).

In another study[11], extracellular volume was expanded with an isoosmotic solution of mannitol rather than normal saline and the changes in rubidium uptake by the tail artery were similar to those seen with saline. Thus the pump suppression appears to result from the excess volume rather than the excess salt.

Volume appears to reduce pump activity by releasing a heat stable humoral agent because when tail arteries from normal rats were incubated in the supernates of boiled plasma prepared from the acutely saline expanded rats, total ^{86}rubidium uptake was suppressed (relative to ^{86}rubidium uptake by tail arteries incubated in supernates of boiled plasma prepared from sham expanded rats)[10, 11]. The sodium and potassium concentrations and the osmolality of the two supernates were not significantly different. Similar changes in rat tail arteries were produced by supernates of plasma prepared from acutely saline expanded dogs, i.e., supernates of boiled plasma from acutely volume expanded dogs reduced total ^{86}rubidium uptake when applied to tail arteries taken from normal rats[11].

These findings encouraged us to examine the plasma in animals with low renin hypertension[11, 12]. We therefore prepared a new series of dogs with one-kidney, one wrapped hypertension. Supernates of boiled plasma from these animals and their sham operated control animals were then applied to tail arteries from normal rats. Ouabain-sensitive ^{86}rubidium uptake by the rat tail arteries was suppressed by the supernates from the hypertensive dogs and ouabain-insensitive ^{86}rubidium uptake was unaffected, just as is the case in the hypertensive animals own vessels (Table 1).

These findings, in total, indicate that sodium-potassium pump activity in animals with low renin hypertension is suppressed by a heat stable humoral agent released by the volume expansion per se.

NATURE OF THE HUMORAL AGENT

In our previous reviews[13-15], we suggested that the pump suppression in blood vessels and heart might result from natriuretic factor because its plasma level rises with volume and because it suppresses sodium pump activity in the renal tubule. Natriuretic factor appears to be a low molecular weight peptide, formed from a larger precursor molecule[16]. Like the humoral pump suppressor observed in our studies, it is heat stable. It probably comes from brain[17] and may be released in response to distention of the pulmonary vascular bed[18]. Recent attempts at purification have met with some success[16, 19, 20]. An approximately 25-fold purification of natriuretic factor from the kidney of the volume expanded rat, achieved by Sephadax gel chromatography and acrylamide gel electrophoresis, has recently been reported[20]. It would be of interest to apply such a partially purified preparation to the rat tail artery to see whether it reduces ouabain-sensitive [86]rubidium uptake. It would also be of interest to inject it intravenously to see whether it raises blood pressure. The old and recent literature in fact suggests the presence of an unknown, slowly acting pressor and sensitizing agent in the blood of animals with low renin hypertension[13-15]. The agent has a molecular weight of about 1000 and, like natriuretic factor and the humoral pump suppressor observed in our studies, it is heat stable[15].

Other agents should also be considered. For example, methylguanidine[21] and vanadate[22, 23] accumulate in the blood during renal insufficiency. Both agents inhibit Na^+, K^+-ATPase activity, constrict blood vessels, and raise blood pressure[21, 23].

HOW PUMP SUPPRESSION MIGHT RAISE BLOOD PRESSURE

Suppression of the sodium-potassium pump in cardiovascular muscle with the cardiac glycosides, for example, has long been known to increase cardiac contractility and produce vasoconstriction[14, 15]. It has more recently been shown that pump suppression also increases the responses of blood vessels to vasoactive agents and raises the blood pressure (particularly if diuresis cannot occur)[14, 15]. These changes are not unlike those seen in experimental low renin hypertension[14, 15]. Increased cardiac contractility, vasoconstriction, and increased vascular responses to vasoactive agents all occur in experimental low renin hypertension[14, 15].

While it is clear that pump suppression stimulates the heart and blood vessels, the cellular mechanism is not so clear[14, 15]. Both electrogenic depolarization and the Na-Ca exchange mechanism may be involved[14, 15].

SUMMARY

Recent studies suggest that the sodium-potassium pump is suppressed in

384

vascular and cardiac muscle of animals with low renin hypertension. This is of interest because induced pump suppression in normal animals, with cardiac glycosides, for example, reproduces many of the hemodynamic changes seen in low renin hypertension. The pump suppression in animals with low renin hypertension appears to result from a heat stable humoral agent. An effort should be made to determine whether this agent is natriuretic factor.

REFERENCES

1. Overbeck, H.W., Pamnani, M.B., Akera, T., Brody, T.M., and Haddy, F.J. (1976) Circ. Res. (Suppl 2), 48-52.

2. Clough, D.L., Pamnani, M.B., Overbeck, H.W., and Haddy, F.J. (1977) Fed. Proc. 36, 491.

3. Clough, D.L., Pamnani, M.B., Overbeck, H.W., and Haddy, F.J. (1977) Physiologist 20, 18.

4. Pamnani, M.B., Clough, D.L., and Haddy, F.J. (1978) Clin. Sci. Mol. Med. 55, 41s-43s.

5. Clough, D.L., Pamnani, M.B., and Haddy, F.J. (1978) Clin. Res. 26, 361.

6. Huot, S., Pamnani, M., Clough, D., and Haddy, F. (1980) Fed. Proc. 39, 1188.

7. Clough, D., Pamnani, M., Huot, S., and Haddy, F. (1980) Physiologist, in press.

8. Pamnani, M.B., Clough, D.L., and Haddy, F.J. (1979) Jap. Heart J. 20 (Suppl 1), 228-230.

9. Pamnani, M., Clough, D., Huot, S., and Haddy, F. (1980) Fed. Proc. 39, 812.

10. Pamnani, M.B., Clough, D.L., Steffen, R.P., and Haddy, F.J. (1978) Physiologist 21, 88.

11. Pamnani, M.B., Clough, D.L., Huot, S.J., and Haddy, F.J. (1980) Mechanisms of Vasodilatation, ed by Vanhoutte, P., Raven Press, New York, in press.

12. Pamnani, M., Huot, S., Steffen, R., and Haddy, F. (1980) Physiologist, in press.

13. Haddy, F.J. and Overbeck, H.W. (1976) Life Sciences 19, 935-948.

14. Haddy, F., Pamnani, M., and Clough, D. (1978) Clin. Exp. Hypertension 1, 295-336.

15. Haddy, F.J., Pamnani, M.B., and Clough, D.L. (1979) Life Sciences 24, 2105-2118.

16. Gruber, K.A. and Buckalew, V.M., Jr. (1978) Proc. Soc. Exptl. Biol. Med. 159, 463-467.

17. Bealer, S., Haywood, J.R., Johnson, A.K., Buckalew, V.M., and Brody, M.J. (1979) Fed. Proc. 38, 1232.

18. Epstein, M. (1976) Circ. Res. 39, 619-628.

19. Licht, A., Stein, S., Udenfriend, S., and Bricher, N.S. (1978) Proc. Amer. Soc. Neph. 11, 133.

20. Raghavan, S.R.V. and Gonick, H.C. (1980) Proc. Soc. Exptl. Biol. Med. 164, 101-104.

21. Haddy, F.J. (1974) Arch. Int. Med. 133, 916-931.

22. Bello-Reuss, E.N., Grady, T.P., Mazumdar, D.C. (1979) Ann. Int. Med. 91, 743.

23. Inciarte, D.J., Steffen, R.P., Dobbins, D.E., Swindall, B.T., Johnston, J., and Haddy, F.J. (1980) Am. J. Physiol., in press.

Hormonal Regulation of Sodium Excretion,
B. Lichardus, R.W. Schrier and J. Ponec, eds.
© 1980 Elsevier/North-Holland Biomedical Press

THE NATRIURETIC HORMONE AND ESSENTIAL HYPERTENSION

HUGH de WARDENER and GRAHAM MacGREGOR
Department of Medicine, Charing Cross Hospital Medical School, Fulham Palace
Road, London W6 8RF, England

In a stock colony of rats the incidence of hypertension increases with
age[1,2]. With inbreeding between rats which develop hypertension, and those
that do not it is possible to obtain two strains of rats[3,4]. One develops
hypertension within 50 days (the spontaneously hypertensive strain S.H.S.) and
in the other the blood pressure does not rise at any time throughout it's life
(the normotensive rat). It has also been demonstrated that the prevalence of
hypertension in a stock colony is directly related to the intake of sodium[5].
And that by in-breeding between those rats which develop hypertension on a high
sodium intake and those that do not it is possible to obtain two strains of
rats[6-8]. One develops hypertension on a high sodium intake early in life
(the sodium sensitive strain) and the other does not develop hypertension on a
high sodium intake (the sodium resistant strain). It appears therefore that
hypertension in the rat is genetically determined.

The genetic fault appears to reside in the kidney for renal cross-transplan-
tation experiments in both hypertensive strains of rat (S.H.S. and S.S.) have
demonstrated that the hypertension 'follows' the kidney[9-15]. A kidney from a
normotensive donor placed into a potentially hypertensive rat before or after
the age at which hypertension usually becomes manifest will either prevent the
hypertension or lower the pressure to normal. Alternatively transplantation
of a kidney from a young normotensive donor from one of the two hypertensive
strains into a normotensive strain of rat causes the recipient to develop hypertension. There is considerable, though mainly circumstantial, evidence that
the genetic fault in the kidney is related to a difficulty in sodium excretion,
which tends to increase the extracellular fluid volume. There is the finding
of a persistently low plasma renin activity in the sodium sensitive hypertensive strain[16]; a transient period of sodium retention and low plasma renin
activity in the spontaneous hypertensive rat[17-19]; and in both strains an
accelerated natriuresis after an acute intravenous saline load[18-20]. Though
all these observations are compatible with a rise in extracellular fluid it is
usually not possible to detect a statistically significant and persistent rise
in extracellular fluid in the adult hypertensive rat of either of these two
strains prone to develop hypertension.

In both hypertensive strains of rats there are a number of observations which support directly and indirectly that the hypertension is related to a circulating substance which inhibits sodium transport. (1) Small intravenous injections of plasma from a spontaneously hypertensive rat increase the vascular reactivity of a recipient specially prepared rat[21]; (2) cross circulation of the hindquarters between hypertensive and normotensive rats increases the arterial resistance of the vascular bed of the normotensive rat[22], and (3) impairment of Na^+ - K^+ membrane transport has been observed in the arteries[23-26], and the red cells[27-30] of both hypertensive strains.

The way in which an increase in the concentration of a circulating sodium transport inhibitor might cause hypertension has been reviewed by Blaustein[31]. He has pointed out that the intracellular calcium concentration which determines the tension of the smooth muscle in arteries is in turn dependent on the intracellular sodium concentration. And that the intracellular sodium concentration is in turn dependent on the activity of the main Na^+ - K^+ pump. Therefore an interference with net sodium transport which causes a rise in intracellular sodium will in turn cause a rise in intracellular calcium concentration and an increase in arteriolar tone.

Overall these observations suggest that hypertension in the rat is due to an interlocking set of mechanisms which begins with a genetically abnormal kidney. This tends to cause sodium retention which stimulates a compensatory rise in the concentration of a circulating natriuretic substance, the activity of which is dependent on it's being a sodium transport inhibitor. The presence of such substances in the blood and urine have been demonstrated in acute and chronic volume expansion experiments in both man and animals. The evidence suggests that such a substance may be responsible for the demonstrable impairment in Na^+ - K^+ transport in the arterial smooth muscle and red cells of the hypertensive strains of rats. And that the hypertension is a consequence of the impairment of Na^+ - K^+ transport in the arteries.

In man, as in the rat, essential hypertension is genetically determined[32], it's prevalence increases with age[33], and it is related to sodium ingestion[34], (Fig.). Hypertension is rare in peoples which ingest less than 60 mEq of sodium per day[34-36]. It is very common when the sodium intake is more than 400 mEq/day[37-39]. There is no comparable direct evidence to that obtained with cross transplantation in the rat, that the kidneys are responsible for the hypertension. But the large proportion of hypertensive patients with low plasma renin activity[40], the observation that normotensive children of hypertensive parents have an accelerated natriuresis with an acute intravenous

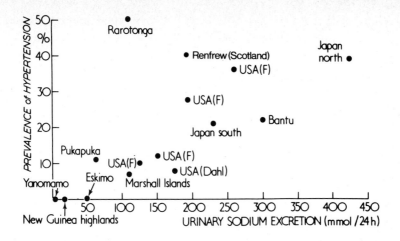

Fig. Geographical distribution of the relationship between the prevalence of hypertension and urinary sodium excretion (Hypertension defined as diastolic pressure > 90mmHg and/or systolic pressure > 140mmHg). Data obtained from following references: Yanomamo[35], New Guinea Highlands[36], Eskimo[34], Marshall Islands[34], U.S.A.(F) (Table 6)[41], Pukapuka and Rarotonga[42], Japan South[39], Japan North[37], Bantu[43].

saline load[44]; and that such children also have an increased renal plasma flow[45], is compatible with their having, as in the rat, a tendency for an increased extracellular fluid volume. As in the rat there is some direct evidence that the hypertension is associated with a circulating substance[46,47]. And, as in the rat, there is also indirect evidence which is compatible with the presence of a circulating sodium transport inhibitor. This consists of the many observations which demonstrate that there is a generalised disturbance of $Na^+ - K^+$ transport. These have been observed in the arteries[48], red cells[49-55], leucocytes[56,57] and lymphocytes[58] of patients with essential hypertension. And some workers have also found these disturbances to be present in the normotensive children of hypertensive parents[49,55]. In contrast, the abnormalities of $Na^+ - K^+$ transport demonstrated in the red blood cells[53] and leucocytes[59] of patients with hypertension are not present in those who have been treated with diuretics.

The accumulation of similarities between hypertension of unknown cause in rats and man suggests that the mechanism responsible for the hypertension in both may be the same. Accordingly it is proposed that essential hypertension in man is due to an inherited abnormality of the kidney, which, when sodium intake is greater than about 50mEq/day, causes a tendency to retain sodium.

390

This leads to an increase in the circulating concentration of a sodium transport inhibitor, the effect of which on the arteries is to increase the intracellular calcium concentration and thus the arterial pressure.

In support of this hypothesis Poston et al[60] find that incubation of leucocytes from a normal subject in the plasma of a hypertensive patient induces the same inhibition of Na^+ - K^+ transport in the normal white cells as is present in the patient's own white cells.

REFERENCES

1. Medoff, H.S. and Bongiovanni, A.M. (1945) Am. J. Physiol. 143, 297-299.
2. Okamoto, K. and Aoki, K. (1963) Jpn. Circ. J, 27, 282-293.
3. Bianchi, G., Fox, U. and Imbasciati, E. (1974) Life Sci, 14, 339-347.
4. Smirk, F.H. and Hall, W.H. (1958) Nature, 182, 727-728.
5. Meneely, G.R., Tucker, R.G., Darby, W.J. and Auerbach, S.H. (1953) Ann. intern. Med, 39, 991-998.
6. Dahl, L.K. (1962) Brookhaven Lecture Ser. 12.
7. Dahl, L.K., Heine, M. and Tassinar, L. (1962) J. Exp. Med. 115, 1173-1190.
8. Dahl, L.K. and Schackow, E. (1964) Can. Med. Assoc. J, 90, 155-160.
9. Bianchi, G., Fox, U., Di Francesco, G.F., Bardi, U. and Radice, M. (1973) Clin. Sci. Mol. Med, 45, 135-139.
10. Bianchi, G., Fox, U., Di Francesco, G.F., Giovannetti, A.M. and Pagetti,D. (1974) Clin. Sci. Mol. Med, 47, 435-448.
11. Dahl, L.K. and Heine, M. (1975) Circ. Res, 36, 692-696.
12. Dahl, L.K., Heine, M. and Thompson, K. (1972) Proc. Soc. Exp. Biol, 140, 852-856.
13. Dahl, L.K., Heine, M. and Thompson, K. (1974) Circ. Res, 34, 94-101.
14. Fox, U. and Bianchi, G. (1976) Clin. Exp. Pharmacol. Physiol. (Suppl) 3, 71-74.
15. Tobian, L., Coffee, K., McCrea, P. and Dahl, L. (1966) J. Clin. Invest, 45, 1080.
16. Iwai, J., Dahl, L.K. and Knudsen, K.D. (1973) Circ. Res. 32, 678-684.
17. Bianchi, G., Baer, P.G., Fox, U., Duzzi, L., Pagetti, D. and Giovannetti, A.M. (1975) Circ. Res. (Suppl) 36 & 37, I-153 - I-161.
18. Bianchi, G., Baer, P.G., Fox, U. and Guidi, E. (1977) Postgrad. Med. J. (Suppl 2) 53, 123-135.
19. Bianchi, G., Fox, U., Pagetti, D., Caravaggi, A.M., Baer, P.G. and Baldoli, E. (1975) Kidney Int (Suppl) 8, 165-173.
20. Ben-Ishay, D., Knudsen, K.D. and Dahl, L.K. (1973) J. Lab. Clin. Med, 82, 597-604.
21. Self, L.E., Battarbee, H.D., Gaar, K.A. Jr. and Meneely, G.R. (1976) Proc. Soc. Exp. Biol. Med, 153, 7-12.

22. Tobian, L., Pumper, M., Johnson, S. and Iwai, J. (1979) Clin. Sci, 57, 345s-347s.

23. Altman, J., Garay, R., Papadimitriou, A. and Worcel, M. (1977) Br. J. Pharmacol. 59, 496.

24. Jones, A.W. (1973) Circ. Res, 33, 563-572.

25. Madden, J.A., Smith, G.A. and Llaurado, J.G. (1979) Clin. Sci, 56, 471-478.

26. Wei, J-W, Janis, R.A. and Daniel, E.E. (1976) Circ. Res, 39, 133-140.

27. Ben-Ishay, D., Aviram, A. and Viskoper, R. (1975) Experientia, 31, 660-662.

28. Friedman, S.M., Nakashima, M., McIndoe, R.A. and Freidman, C.L. (1976) Experientia, 32, 476-478.

29. Postnov, YU.V., Orlov, S., Gulak, P. and Schevchenko, A. (1976) Pfleugers Arch, 365, 257-263.

30. Postnov, YU.V., Orlov, S.N. and Pokudin, N.I. (1979) Pfleugers Arch, 379, 191-195.

31. Blaustein, M.P. (1977) Am. J. Physiol. 232(3), C165-C173.

32. Pickering, G. (1968) High Blood Pressure, Churchill, London, pp.236-290.

33. Miall, W.E. (1959) Br. Med. J, 11, 1204-1210.

34. Dahl, L.K. (1961) Am. J. Cardiol, 8, 571-575.

35. Oliver, W.J., Cohen, E.L. and Neel, J.V. (1975) Circulation, 52, 146-151.

36. Sinnett, P.F. and White, H.M. (1973) J. Chronic Dis, 26, 265-290.

37. Fukuda, T. (1954) Chiba, Igakki, Zasshi (J. Chiba Med. Soc), 29, 490-502.

38. Sasaki, N. (1964) Geriatrics, 19, 735-744.

39. Takamatsu, M. (1955) J. Sci. Lab. (Rodo Kagaku), 31, 349-370.

40. Dunn, M.J. and Tannen, R.L. (1974) Kidney Int. 5, 317-325.

41. Dawber, T.R., Kannel, W.B., Kagan, A., Donabedian, R.K. and McNamara, P.M. (1967) Epidemiology of Hypertension, Grune and Stratton, New York, pp.255-288.

42. Prior, I.A.M., Grimley Evans, J., Harvey, H.P.B., Davidson, F. and Lindsey, M. (1968) New Eng. J. Medicine, 279, 515-520.

43. Isaacson, L.C., Modlin, M. and Jackson, W.P.U. (1963) Lancet, 1, 946.

44. Wiggins, R.C., Basar, I. and Slater, J.D.H. (1978) Clin. Sci. Mol. Med, 54, 639-647.

45. Bianchi, G., Picotti, G.B., Bracchi, G., Cusi, D., Gatti, M., Lupi, G.P., Ferrari, P., Barlassina, C., Colombo, G. and Gori, D. (1978) Clin. Sci. Mol. Med, 55, 367s-371s.

46. Michelakis, A.M., Mizukoshi, H., Huang, C., Murakami, K. and Inagami, T. (1975) J. Clin. Endocrinol. Metab, 41, 90-96.

47. Mizukoshi, H. and Michelakis, A.M. (1972) J. Clin. Endocrinol. Metab. 34, 1016-1024.

48. Tobian, L.Jr. and Binion, J.T. (1952) Circulation, 5, 754-758.

49. Garay, R.P. and Meyer, P. (1979) Lancet, 1, 349-353.

50. Gessler Von U. (1962) Z. Kreislaufforsch, 51, 177-183.

51. Henningsen, N.C., Mattsson, S., Nosslin, B., Nelson, D. and Ohlsson, O. (1979) Clin. Sci, 57, 321s-324s.

52. Losse, H., Wehmeyer, H. and Wessels, F. (1960) Klin. Wochenschr, 38, 393-395.

53. Postnov, YU.V., Orlov, S.N., Shevchenko, A. and Adler, A.M. (1977) Pfleugers Arch, 371, 263-269.

54. Wessels, V.F., Junoe-Hulsing, G. and Losse,H. (1967) Z. Kreislaufforsch, 56, 374-380.

55. Wessels, V.F., Zumkley, H. and Losse, H. (1970) Z. Kreislaufforsch, 59, 415-416.

56. Canessa, M., Adragna, N., Connolly, T., Solomon, H. and Tosteson, D.O. (1979) Abstract VIth Int. Soc. Hypertension, Goteborg.

57. Edmondson, R.P.S., Thomas, R.D., Hilton, P.J., Patrick, J. and Jones, N.F. (1975) Lancet, 1, 1003-1005.

58. Ambrosioni, E., Tartagni, F., Montebugnoli, L. and Magnani, B. (1979) Clin. Sci, 57, 325s-327s.

59. Thomas, R.D., Edmondson, R.P.S., Hilton, P.J. and Jones, N.F. (1975) Clin. Sci. Mol. Med, 48, 169s-170s.

60. Poston, L., Sewell, R., Williams, R., Richardson, P. and de Wardener, H.E. (1980) Int. Symposium on Intracellular Electrolytes and Arterial Hypertension, G. Thieme, (in press).

Hormonal Regulation of Sodium Excretion,
B. Lichardus, R.W. Schrier and J. Ponec, eds.
© 1980 Elsevier/North-Holland Biomedical Press

OUABAIN RADIORECEPTOR ASSAY FOR NATRIURETIC FACTOR

TIMOTHY BOHAN, LINCOLN POTTER AND JACQUES J. BOURGOIGNIE
with the technical assistance of MELANIE ASHBY
Laboratory of the Howard Hughes Medical Institute, the Departments of Medicine and Pharmacology, University of Miami School of Medicine, Miami, Florida 33101.

INTRODUCTION

Any attempt at isolating and purifying a compound requires an assay preparation in which the activity of the biologic substance under scrutiny can be quantitated precisely. This requirement is dictated not only by the need to compare activities of different samples but to support studies on purification. A standard unit of reference therefore must be available. Although we have described a dose dependent inhibition of short circuit current in the isolated toad bladder with natriuretic factor extracted from urine of chronically uremic patients and the possibility of developing in this preparation a semiquantitative assay using ammonium chloride as a standard of reference[1], the toad bladder lacks specificity, sensitivity and reproducibility.

Inhibition of $(Na^+ + K^+)$-ATPase activity by a low molecular weight natriuretic factor extracted from plasma and kidney of volume expanded rats has been described[2]. We therefore explored the possibility that the low molecular weight natriuretic factor described by us in serum and urine of patients and dogs with chronic renal insufficiency also possessed $(Na^+ + K^+)$-ATPase inhibitory activity. For this purpose, we have used a ouabain binding receptor assay. Indeed, in canine whole tissue homogenate of left ventricle, the initial velocity of ATP plus Mg^{2+} plus Na^+ supported (^3H)-ouabain binding bears a direct relationship to $(Na^+ + K^+)$-ATPase activity of partially purified microsomal fraction from the same tissue[3].

Using an ATP plus Mg^{2+} plus Na^+ supported (^3H)-ouabain binding receptor assay, we report the inhibition of ouabain binding in renal cortical membranes by natriuretic factor from urine of chronically uremic dog.

METHODS

Natriuretic factor preparation

Urine was collected from a dog with a remnant kidney and chronic renal

insufficiency of 6 months duration (exogenous creatinine clearance 10 ml/
min). The animal received a diet containing about 120 meq Na^+. Twenty-
four urine samples, obtained under metabolic conditions, were lyophilized,
applied to a 95 x 2.5 cm column of Sephadex G-25 and eluted with 10 mM ammonium acetate at pH 6.8 as previously described[4,5]. The Na^+-and K^+-free
fraction (10 tubes of 12 ml/each), which elutes immediately after the salt
peak and has been shown to contain natriuretic activity, was collected,
lyophilized to dryness and reconstituted in a volume of distilled water so
that one ml of fraction was equivalent to 2 hours of original urine. The
sample was frozen until tested in our standard preparation of isolated toad
bladder[5] and in the ouabain radiobinding assay.

Tissue homogenate

Kidneys were removed from a normal dog under pentobarbital anesthesia.
The cortical tissue was immediately dissected, rinsed in chilled saline,
homogenized (10% w/v) with a Polytron in 50 mM Tris-HCl buffer (pH 7.5)
and filtered. After centrifugation at 5000 rpm for 20 minutes, the supernatant was decanted, the pellet resuspended in Tris-HCl buffer, homogenized,
centrifuged again, filtered through a tea filter and suspended in 9 volumes
of 50 mM Tris-HCl (pH 7.5). This homogenate was separated in multiple one
ml aliquots and frozen at -20 C.

Ouabain receptor assay

The receptor assay was performed, as described with heart membranes by
Gelbart and Goldman[3], in a solution having the following composition (final
volume 1 ml): Tris-HCl 50 mM (pH 7.4), $MgCl_2$ 3 mM, NaCl 100 mM, EGTA 1 mM,
ATP (Na salt-vanadium free) 5 mM, in the presence of 100 µl of homogenate,
1×10^{-8} M (^{3}H)-ouabain (specific activity 14.4 Ci/mmol) and varying concentrations of cold ouabain (from 1×10^{-9} to 1×10^{-6} M) or natriuretic
factor*.

RESULTS

In agreement with previous observations from this laboratory, the fraction of urine from the uremic dog inhibited short-circuit current across
the standard preparation of isolated toad bladder. After one hour of expo-

---

*The concentration of (3H)-ouabain (10^{-8}M) was in excess so that its free
concentration in the absence of cold ouabain or inhibitor changed by less
than 10 percent during the course of incubation. Under these conditions
the kinetics of the binding reaction become pseudo-first-order (at least
in heart membranes), and the rate of formation of the ouabain-receptor complex is proportional to the concentration of free binding sites[3].

sure to an amount of fraction equivalent to 1 hour of urine, short circuit current decreased from 48 to 33 μAmp, a 31 percent inhibition, while it did not change in a time control preparation from the same bladder observed concurrently but not exposed to the fraction.

Fig. 1 depicts the (^3H)-ouabain displacement in renal cortical membranes by unlabeled ouabain and urine fraction from the uremic dog. Increasing concentrations of ouabain displaced the (^3H)-ouabain bound to the renal membranes in a dose related fashion. In the presence of 3×10^{-9} M ouabain, 95 percent of the (^3H)-ouabain remained bound to the receptors. Fifty percent inhibition of binding occurred in the presence of 4×10^{-8} M ouabain and 100 percent in the presence of 3×10^{-7} M ouabain, the 3 percent (^3H)-ouabain still bound at that concentration representing non-specific non-ATP dependent binding.

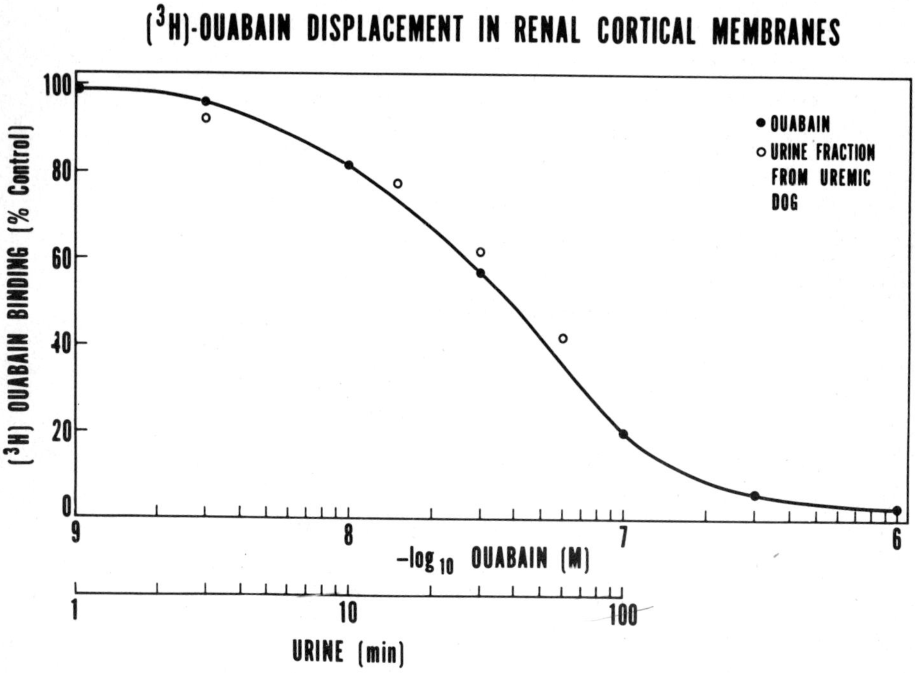

(^3H)-OUABAIN DISPLACEMENT IN RENAL CORTICAL MEMBRANES

Fig. 1. (^3H)-ouabain displacement in renal cortical membranes by unlabeled ouabain and urine fraction from uremic dog. Each value is the mean of triplicate determinations.

A similar displacement of (^3H)-ouabain was evident when the receptor assay was performed in the presence of the urine fraction instead of unlabeled ouabain. The equivalent of 3 minutes of original urine had little effect on binding of (^3H)-ouabain. In contrast, the equivalents of 15, 30, and 60 minutes of original urine inhibited binding by 22, 38, and 58 percent, respectively. This inhibition corresponds to that achieved by 1.25×10^{-8} M, 2.5×10^{-8} M and 4.8×10^{-8} M cold ouabain, respectively, for a mean ouabain-like activity of 4.9×10^{-8} M in one hour of urine. When the same urine sample was retested one week later it yielded values equivalent to 7.4×10^{-9} M, 1.6×10^{-8} M, and 6.4×10^{-8} M ouabain with the 15, 30 and 60 min. samples, respectively, for an average ouabain-like activity of 4.2×10^{-8} M in one hour of urine.

DISCUSSION

Binding of (^3H)-ouabain to whole tissue homogenate is a convenient method for estimating $(Na^+ + K^+)$-ATPase activity. An excellent and direct correlation (p<0.01) was found between the two activities in canine cardiac tissue[3]. The assay offers the advantage of methodological simplicity and reproducibility; multiple samples can be processed in a single assay.

The present results demonstrate displacement of (^3H)-ouabain from membrane receptors of renal cortical tissue by a low molecular weight fraction of urine from a chronically uremic dog. This fraction contains natriuretic factor and showed biological activity in inhibiting the short circuit current of a toad bladder preparation. The radiobinding assay shows dose-response relationship, reproducibility and sensitivity with an equivalent of 15 min of original urine readily demonstrating inhibitory activity. The displacement of (^3H)-ouabain from its receptors by the low molecular weight fraction of our uremic dog superimposes on the displacement curve produced by unlabeled ouabain demonstrating specificity of competition.

These results suggest that natriuretic factor may have a glycosidic nature, although other factors like potassium[6], calcium[7], and vanadium ions also inhibit ouabain-binding onto membrane receptors. Rigorous selection of a potassium-free fraction and the presence of EGTA in the incubation medium make it unlikely that potassium or calcium ions were responsible for the observed displacement. Although increased vanadium concentrations have been found in patients with chronic renal disease[8], vanadium elutes with the salt peak on Sephadex G-25 (I.H. Mills, personal communication).

Endogenous digitalis-like activity has been previously described in biological specimens. While not found in serum of frog Rana pipiens or human serum, digitalis-like activity has been detected in the serum of toad Bufo marinus in apparent concentrations of 2.5×10^{-5} M by radioreceptor competition assay and 10^{-7} M by immunologic assay[9,10]. Because of suggestive evidence that the central nervous system may be the source of natriuretic factor[11], the brain has been explored as a source of a factor with ouabain-like properties. A low molecular weight, basic, nonpeptidic factor that inhibits active sodium transport across anuran membranes, ouabain binding to frog urinary bladder and $(Na^{+}+K^{+})$-ATPase, has been prepared from bovine hypothalami[12]. Endogenous digitalis-like activity has also been found in guinea pig brain[13]. In the latter study, however, although the extract prevented binding of (^{3}H)-ouabain to brain microsomes in a dose-dependent manner, the extract and the unlabeled ouabain did not displace the (^{3}H)-ouabain in a superimposable fashion. Finally, Gruber et al[14] also demonstrated by radioimmunoassay an endogenous digoxin-like substance in plasma of dog, sheep and man.

All the experiments reported so far, however, do not demonstrate a direct relationship between this endogenous cardiac glycoside-like material and sodium regulation. Nevertheless, such a substance might represent an endogenous regulator of membrane $(Na^{+}+K^{+})$-ATPase and thereby be an integral component of the control system regulating sodium excretion by the kidneys.

ACKNOWLEDGEMENTS

This work was supported by NIH Research Grant AM19822 and with funds from the American Heart Association and its Florida affiliate.

REFERENCES

1. Licht, A., Fine, L. and Bourgoignie, J.J. (1978) Contributions to Nephrology 13,3-11.

2. Gonick, H.C. (1978) Natriuretic Hormone, Springer-Verlag, Berlin pp. 108-122.

3. Gelbart, A. and Golldman, R.H. (1977) Biochim. Biophys. Acta, 481, 689-694.

4. Bourgoignie, J.J., Hwang, K., Ipakchi, E. and Bricker, N.S. (1974) J. Clin. Invest., 53,1559-1567.

5. Bourgoignie, J.J., Klahr, S. and Bricker, N.S. (1971) J. Clin. Invest., 50,303-312.

6. Sweadner, K.J. and Goldin, S.M. (1980) New England J. Med., 302, 777-783.

7. Godfraind, T., De Pover, A., and Verbeke, N. (1977) Biochim. Biophys. Acta, 481, 202-211.

8. Bello-Reuss, E.N., Grady, T.P. and Mazumbar, D.C. (1979) Ann. Int. Med., 91, 743.

9. Flier, J.S. (1978) Nature, 274, 285-286.

10. Flier, J.S., Maratos-Flier, E., Pallotta, J.A. and McIsaac, D. (1979) Nature, 279, 341-343.

11. Kaloyanides, G.J., Balabanian, M.B. and Bowman, R.L. (1978) J. Clin. Invest., 62, 1288-1295.

12. Haupert, G.T., Jr. and Sancho, J.M. (1979) Proc. Natl. Acad. Sci., 76, 4658-4660.

13. Fishman, M.C. (1979) Proc. Natl. Acad. Sci., 76, 4661-4663.

14. Gruber, K.A., Whitaker, J.M., Plunkett, W.C. and Buckalew, V.M., Jr. (1979) Kidney Intern., 16, 817.

Hormonal Regulation of Sodium Excretion,
B. Lichardus, R.W. Schrier and J. Ponec, eds.
© 1980 Elsevier/North-Holland Biomedical Press

NATRIURETIC HORMONE: BIOLOGIC EFFECTS AND PROGRESS IN IDENTIFICATION AND
ISOLATION

NEAL S. BRICKER and AMNON LICHT
University of California, Los Angeles, School of Medicine, Los Angeles, CA.,
90024, U.S.A.

INTRODUCTION

The regulation of the constancy of extracellular fluid (ECF) volume in
mammalian species is directed by and under the aegis of a complex, highly
sophisticated and, under most circumstances, remarkably effective biologic
control system. The principal determinant of the ECF volume is the total amount
of extracellular sodium with the water content being determined by the sodium.
The maintenance of a constant ECF volume thus depends upon the continuing
ability to prevent either the net loss or the net gain of sodium from the body
and this in turn demands that external balance be preserved for sodium by maintaining excretion rates from the body equal to acquisition rates. The principal
and generally the only source of acquisition of new sodium on a continuing basis
is the sodium chloride in the diet; the principal organ of excretion of sodium
is the kidney. Hence, the rate of renal excretion of sodium must remain closely attuned to the contemporaneous rate of sodium ingestion if the maintenance
of sodium homeostasis is to be accomplished. Moreover, this most important of
all renal functions must be accomplished with precision in the face of potentially wide and random variations, whether from meal to meal, day to day, or
one period of life to another, in sodium intake.

If there is an error in the regulation of sodium excretion which results
either in the net loss or net gain of this cation from the ECF, the typical
consequence will be a parallel loss or gain of ECF volume. The maintenance of
external sodium balance, therefore, is critical to the maintenance of ECF
volume, and hence to the integrity of the cardiovascular system. One biologic
expression of this coupling between ECF sodium content and ECF water content
is the fact that the entrance or loss of sodium into the ECF appears to be
monitored by a biologic control system which detects translocations of some
function of volume from the steady state, rather than by a detector element
sensitive to changes in the concentration of sodium per se. The design of this
"volume control system" is understood only in outline form and the specific
elements and events involved in its operation largely remain to be delineated.

However, it seems likely that in addition to the "detector element," there may
be an "integrator element," probably located in the central nervous system which
receives, collates and interprets messages from all the detector elements in
the body, assuming that there are multiple such elements. Thus, if there is an
internal translocation of ECF volume from the lower extremities into the more
cephalad portions of the body (such as occurs in water immersion, bedrest,
application of lower extremity pressure suits, and exposure to the weightless
environment of space), it presumably is the integrator element that gives prior-
ity to the expansion of intrathoracic volume rather than to the contraction of
lower extremity volume and initiates a natriuresis. The opposite situation
obtains with translocation of ECF into the lower extremities during quiet standing, application of tourniquets to the thighs, etc. The final element in the
control system is the "effector element." It is the charge of this component
of the system to transmit the information to the end organ, the nephron, and
to effect the modulation of the rate of sodium transport so as to change the
rate of sodium excretion in the appropriate quantity and direction required for
the restoration of the initial steady state.

Much emphasis has been directed in recent years to defining the nature of
the effector element of the control system. A number of factors are known to be
capable of influencing sodium excretion. These include: 1) aldosterone activity; 2) intrarenal "physical forces" (i.e., changes in arterial blood pressure,
filtration fraction, peritubular capillary hydrostatic and oncotic pressures,
hematocrit, medullary blood flow, etc.); 3) changes in single nephron GFR
(SNGFR); 4) redistribution of glomerular plasma flow and SNGFR between superficial and juxtamedullary nephrons; 5) prostaglandin activity; 6) activity of
the kallekrein-kinin system; and 7) the putative natriuretic hormone (NH). Because of the extreme importance of the volume control system to survival, as
well as to continued well-being, it seems quite likely that at least several of
the foregoing events or substances can exercise a physiologic effect on the
rates of sodium excretion. It also seems likely that each of these could, under
certain adverse circumstances, become the major modulator of sodium excretion.
However, if this control system is like many other biologic control systems,
only one substance will serve as the final modulator of sodium excretion, though
it may be assisted and/or supported by the effects of one or more of the other
factors. It is our view that the most likely candidate for the "definitive
modulator" is the natriuretic hormone, despite its putative nature. The present
paper is directed to the status of current research on the effects and chemical
nature of this substance.

THE EVIDENCE FOR THE EXISTENCE OF NH

Although the search for natriuretic hormone began almost two decades ago, it has continued to elude definitive characterization and synthesis. Yet, there is a compelling body of data which supports its existence and a growing body of data about its nature and biologic properties. In the discussion we will summarize data from several laboratories engaged in the pursuit of NH; however, a principal purpose of the presentation will be to review the data, including very recent observations, that have been obtained in our laboratories.

Because the site of production of NH is unknown, most attempts to isolate the hormone have been made using either blood or urine under conditions where NH concentrations should be maximized (i.e., during high rates of sodium excretion per nephron). A number of states exist in nature wherein values for fractional excretion of sodium (FE_{Na}) are elevated, either acutely or chronically; but in the extreme renal salt wasting states (i.e., post-obstructive diuresis and the diuretic phase of acute tubular necrosis), the high FE_{Na} values are due to a functional defect in the nephron. To obtain values for FE_{Na} of 20% or greater in normal animals or human beings by oral or intravenous administration of sodium is extremely difficult, and with the intravenous route the natriuresis is accompanied by profound alterations in cardiovascular function which can interfere seriously with interpretation of the data. One situation in which values for FE_{Na} increase progressively and appropriately with time to values as high as 40 to 50% on a *normal salt intake* is in advanced chronic renal disease (CRD). In a normal person ingesting 7 grams of salt per day (120 mEq of Na), at a GFR of 120 ml/min, external sodium balance requires a fractional excretion rate (averaged over a 24 hour period) of 0.5%. However, with each 50% reduction of GFR, FE_{Na} doubles with the same salt intake and it is not unusual for a non-dialyzed patient with a GFR as low as 2 ml per minute to be able to continue to maintain external sodium balance on the same 7 g salt diet. To accomplish this requires a fractional excretion rate of over 30%. Thus, in the transition from the GFR of 120 to 2, over a sixty-fold increase occurs in the fraction of filtered sodium excreted by each surviving nephron. It should be emphasized again, that this remarkable natriuresis per nephron evolves with *no increase* in the amount of sodium entering the ECF daily and thus no apparent change in what the detector element of the volume control system "sees."

Because of the foregoing observation, we initiated our search for NH in uremic patients. In both the serum and the urine of patients and dogs with advanced CRD, a low molecular weight fraction of a Sephadex G-25 gel filtration eluate was found to inhibit sodium transport across the isolated frog skin and toad

402

bladder and to increase sodium excretion by the unanesthetized rat. The same
Sephadex fraction obtained from serum and urine of normal subjects did not produce inhibition unless the dose was markedly increased. There thus was an elevation both in the circulating level of the factor and in its rate of renal
excretion, a combination which indicates that it is not retained in the blood
by virtue of failure of excretion but rather is produced in increased quantity
(with or without a prolongation of biologic half life).

In most of the subsequent studies from this and other laboratories, serum
and urine have been used as the source of NH and initial purification has begun
with gel filtration (either Sephadex G-25 or Biogel P-2). However, studies have
also been described in which kidney and brain homogenates have been employed as
a source and there also have been reports of a high molecular weight fraction
obtained with Sephadex G-50 or G-75 which inhibits sodium transport. The latter
may well be a precursor of the low molecular weight (approximately 500 Daltons)
natriuretic factor (NF), rather than a separate natriuretic hormone. In any
event, the majority of data in the literature represent studies with the low
molecular weight material.

In addition to uremia, NF has been demonstrated in the following circumstances: 1) normal individuals on a high salt diet[1]; 2) normal dogs on a high
salt diet and mineralocorticoid hormone following "escape"[2]; 3) normal subjects
exposed to immersion in water to the level of neck[3]; 4) normal subjects wearing
a lower extremity and abdominal "pressure suit"[4]; 5) normal subjects during
bedrest natriuresis; 6) patients with aldosterone secreting tumors[5]; 7) patients with head trauma and associated natriuretic state[6]; 8) patients with
Bartter's Syndrome[7].

The clinical and experimental states wherin natriuretic activity has not been
demonstrated using the same dosage and the same bioassay techniques, include:
1) uremic patients with high rates of protein excretion, hypoalbuminemia, renal
sodium retention and edema[8]; 2) uremic dogs in which the adaptive natriuresis
per nephron has been prevented by reducing dietary salt intake in exact proportion
to the reduction in GFR[9]; 3) the patients cited above with aldosterone secreting tumors following removal of the tumors[5]; 4) patients with head trauma in
whom a natriuretic state has not developed[6].

THE BIOLOGIC EFFECTS OF NF

The biologic systems in which natriuretic factor inhibits sodium transport
include: 1) the kidneys of normal male rats[1], 2) the kidneys of salt loaded
uremic rats[8], 3) the isolated frog skin[10], 4) the isolated urinary bladder

of the toad^2, 5) the isolated perfused cortical collecting tubule of the rabbit[11], 6) isolated epithelial cells obtained from the urinary bladder of the toad[12], 7) the "MDCK" tissure culture line of epithelial cells originally obtained from canine kidneys[12], 8) red blood cells[12], 9) rabbit and rat kidney slice uptake of PAH (a sodium dependent transport mechanism)[13]. Some inhibition of sodium reabsorption also has been demonstrated in the proximal convoluted tubules of rats using the recollection micropuncture technique[14]; however studies cited above on the isolated tubule suggest that the primary site of action in the nephron is "down stream."

In addition, NF also has been found by some investigators to inhibit Na-K-ATPase activity[15], to increase intracellular sodium content of isolated toad bladder epithelia and to decrease pyruvate oxidation by the same cells[16].

The bioassay systems used for evaluating the presence of biologically active natriuretic factor have been developed from the biologic effects of the factor cited above. The two systems used most extensively have been the isolated toad bladder (or frog skin) in which the effect of the addition of the factor to the serosal (i.e., blood) side of the membrane on transcellular sodium transport is measured using the short-circuit current; the natriuretic effect of NF when given intravenously to either normal Sprague Dawley rats[1] or to uremic rats with a single "remnant" kidney which have been maintained on a 2% saline solution in lieu of drinking water for 24 to 36 hours before performance of the assay[8]. In addition, some investigators have used inhibition of Na-K-ATPase activity as the index of biologic activity[17]. Finally, the effects of the fraction on sodium efflux by MDCK and other isolated tissue cells have been used in preliminary studies in order to obtain a bioassay that utilizes smaller quantities of NF, thereby leaving larger quantities for purification studies.

Further biologic and physiologic affects of NF are: 1) In the isolated perfused tubule[11], the isolated toad bladder[2] and the isolated frog skin[10], inhibition of transepithelial sodium transport occurs only when NF is added from the blood side of the membrane (i.e., peritubular capillary surface of the tubule, serosal surface of the bladder and the inside of the frog skin). 2) In the isolated perfused tubule, there is a reduction in the transepithelial potential difference (i.e., the intraluminal negativity becomes less)[11]. 3) In the isolated tubule, the natriuretic factor decreases sodium efflux from lumen to basolateral surface but it does not affect the unidirectional flux in the opposite direction[11]. 4) The natriuresis produced by NF is not associated with a change in GFR, PAH clearance or filtration fraction[8]. 5) The natriuresis is not associated with a change in systemic blood pressure[8]. 6) The onset

of action of NF takes place in all systems within ten minutes. 7) The natriuresis produced by NF is not associated with a kaliuretic or calciuric response
but the phosphate excretion rate increases[18]. 8) In the MDCK cell system, the
inhibition of sodium efflux is not associated with a measurable inhibition of
rubidium influx[12].

PHYSICAL AND CHEMICAL CHARACTERISTICS OF NF

The physical and chemical characteristics of NF include: 1) The biologic
activity of the active fraction persists at -80°C for at least a year. It also
is resistant to boiling. 2) The active fraction is retarded on Sephadex G-25,
appearing in the eluate (using ammonium acetate pH 6.8 as the buffer) after the
salt peak[10]. 3) The active fraction is contained in a portion of the eluate
that has minimal conductivity[10]. 4) The molecular weight of the fraction obtained from uremic patients and dogs, normal human beings and normal mineralocorticoid "escaped" dogs is approximately 500-1000 Daltons[10]. 5) The active
fraction is acidic and non-volatile[19]. 6) The active fraction is water soluble[19]. 7) The active fraction is insoluble in some organic solvents (ether
and chloroform) but it appears to be soluble in certain other organic solvents
with high dielectric constants suggesting that the hormone is polar in nature[19].
8) NF has been found to be soluble in isobutanol at pH of 1.5 by one group[20],
but insoluble by a different group[19]. 9) NF is inactivated or the activity
markedly decreased by acid hydrolysis[21]. 10) With reverse phase high performance liquid chromatography (see below) the biologic activity present in the
G-25 active fraction persists in a peak which contains an active amine group[22].
11) The G-25 fraction with biologic activity has been found to be inactivated
by leucine aminopeptodase (using 4 bioassay systems) by one group[21] but to be
unaffected by a second group[20]. Similar contradictory data have been observed
with pepsin hydrolysis[20]. Both groups have found that trypsin and chymotrypsin
do not inactivate the factor and pronase and subtilysin also have been found to
have no effect on natriuretic activity of the active fraction obtained from the
urine of normal man[20]. However, prolidase, a proteolytic enzyme, was found to
destroy the natriuretic activity of NF dissolved in 95% acetone[20]. 12) The
activity of the Sephadex G-25 fraction is removed by filtration through charcoal[21].

EVIDENCE FOR A PHYSIOLOGIC ROLE OF NF IN THE REGULATION OF SODIUM EXCRETION

The evidence supporting a correlation between NF activity and the contemporaneous patterns of sodium excretion has been included in the section on biologic
effects of the factor. Noteworthy among these are: 1) When the adaptive

natriuresis per nephron is either prevented in the uremic dog by proportional reduction of sodium or is absent in uremic man by virtue of the coexistence of the nephrotic syndrome, NF activity is not demonstrable. 2) The incidence of positive bioassays in mineralocorticoid hormone "escaped" dogs using both the isolated toad bladder and the unanesthetized uremic rat correlates closely with the degree of sodium retention prior to the onset of "escape"[2]. 3) The same patients in whom assays were positive with functioning aldosterone secreting tumors became negative after surgical removal of the tumors[5]. 4) Occasional patients with CRD and uremia have negative bioassays for reasons which remain unknown at this time. Two such patients have been subjected to water immersion in order to produce acute natriuretic stimuli. In both, the increase in sodium excretion above control levels was attended by a positive bioassay for NF. 5) Not only is NF activity demonstrable in the urine of non-uremic dogs and man with high values for FE_{Na} due to a variety of causes, but if the dose of the NF containing fraction of the gel filtration eluate is increased by tenfold natriuretic activity is found in normal individuals on a normal salt diet. The latter observation suggests that NF exists under conditions of day to day living, but that the bioassay technique employed is not sensitive enough to detect endogenous levels using the same "hourly equivalents" of original urine that produce positive bioassays in natriuretic states.

PROGRESS IN ISOLATION OF NF

The biologically active fraction obtained from gel filtration has been subjected to a series of chromatographic steps using high pressure liquid chromatography and a series of selected ion exchange resins. Using urine from mineralocorticoid escaped dogs and uremic patients, four succesive chromatographic steps have been employed. With each, a technique of "stream-sampling" has been used whereby a small percentage (i.e., less than 5%) of each fraction of eluate collected is diverted through the automated stream-sampling system; fluorescamine, a highly fluorescent compound with a high affinity for active amine groups is added and the fluorescent pattern monitored continuously. The major portion of each eluate fraction is collected using a conventional fraction collector and is available for further study and processing. At each stage of purification, each of the fractions was tested for biologic activity and only the active fraction was used in the subsequent chromatographic separation. With the first HPLC step, a cation exchange resin was employed. Six fluorescent fractions were obtained, only one of which was biologically active. When this fraction designated as F-I was chromatographed on reverse phase resin, five fractions were obtained. Only one of these was positive. This fraction designated as (F-I)$_5$ was next rechromatographed using other cation exchange resin. Two major peaks were obtained. These were designated as N and H. One, N, was naturally fluorescent; the other, H, did not appear in the absence of fluorescamine but was present as a highly fluorescent peak in the presence of fluorescamine. When the two peaks were split and subjected separately to bioassay, only the fluorescamine positive, peak H, was found to be biologically active. Amino acid analysis was performed on the (F-I)$_5$ fraction prior to separating the N and H peaks; only eight amino acids, all of which were neutral or acidic were detected. Thus, if natriuretic hormone is a peptide, it should not contain more than these eight amino acids.

In the process of purification described above, biologic activity was lost at each step. Thus, it took approximately 20 times as much material, using the number of hours of original urine as the frame of reference, to obtain a comparable natriuretic response in the rat with fraction H as with the post-salt peak obtained from the initial Sephadex G-25 chromatographic step. Because of this loss of biologic activity, recent efforts have been made to modify and shorten the separation procedure. The Sephadex G-25 fraction with biologic activity has been processed through a monitoring system using reverse phase liquid chromatography. A number of fluorescent peaks were obtained; however, the area of the eluate containing biologic activity, in studies to date, appears to be substantially more active than the H peak obtained in the multiple step procedure described above. It also appears to be relatively pure.

Future efforts at purification will be performed using both peak H and the biologically active fraction from the reverse phase chromatography. Once sufficient material is collected, the purity of each of the two fractions will be established, the peptidic nature of the inhibitor will be re-examined and if NF is a low molecular weight peptide further determination of its amino acid composition will be undertaken. Thereafter, efforts will be directed at determining the structure of the molecule and finally attempts will be made to sequence and synthesize it. The availability of pure natriuretic hormone should permit the design of experiments aimed at making the small molecule antigenic so as to produce antibodies for a specific radioimmunoassay or radio-receptor assay which would detect physiologic levels in health and in a variety of disease states.

SUMMARY

The regulation of sodium excretion is among the most important and efficient of life processes. There is strong evidence, albeit in part circumstantial, that a biologic control system oriented to the maintenance of a normal ECF

volume serves in the role of a sodium control system maintaining total sodium
excretion rates equal to contemporaneous rates of sodium entry into the ECF
(allowing for any extrarenal losses of this cation). The means by which the
nephrons, which in health reabsorb over 99% of the sodium filtered at the glomeruli in subjects on an average salt diet, are "instructed " to change the net
rate of reabsorption of sodium from the glomerular filtrate are not fully understood; but the modulator must be capable of operating with sufficient precision
and subtlety to change tubular sodium reabsorption by as little as 1 out of 400
filtered sodium ions. The inability to make these changes with accuracy would
lead to major abnormalities of ECF volume and thus cardiovascular integrity
within a relatively short time. But the mechanisms that modulate tubular reabsorption of sodium also must serve to effect continued external balance throughout the course of chronic progressive renal disease,since a modest change in
salt intake in a patient with a very low GFR may require changes in sodium excretion per nephron many orders of magnitude greater than those required in
health.

   The list of potential modulators of sodium excretion has been presented in
the body of the chapter. From the multiple potential effector elements, we have
attempted to collate those data that favor the existence of a natriuretic hormone as a physiologic entity and the evidence and information, some phenomeno-
logic in nature, that supports the view that this putative hormone could be a
definitive modulator of sodium excretion. The biologic effect of the inhibitor
of sodium transport present in serum, urine and possibly kidney and brain homogenates has been reviewed and what is known of its physical character has been
described.

   If the putative hormone is shown to be a real hormone and if its role in
biology is, as our bias leads us to believe, the "fine dial" of the sodium control system, its isolation, synthesis, and the development of techniques for
measuring circulating levels in health and disease could provide a major break-
through in the understanding of a large number of pathologic disorders of salt
and water regulation. Moreover, the availability of the pure hormone could add
a potent therapeutic tool to the armamentarium presently available for treating
certain disorders of volume regulation. Finally, if the high levels of natriuretic hormone, presumed to exist in advancing uremia act to inhibit the extrusion of sodium from cell types other than tubular epithelial cells, NH could be
a potent uremic toxin[23], and new insight into major abnormalities of the uremic
state plus new approaches to conservative therapy of uremia would inevitably
emerge.

408

REFERENCES

1. Brown, P.R., et al. (1972) Kidney Int., 2, 1-5.
2. Favre, H., et al. (1975) J. Clin. Invest., 56, 1302-1311.
3. Epstein, M., et al. (1978) Kidney Int., 13, 152-158.
4. Danovitch, G.M., et al. Unpublished observation.
5. Vanlanthem, M., et al. (1979) J. d'Urolog. Nephrol.,85, 569-573.
6. Klahr, S. and Rodriguez, H.J. (1975) Nephron, 15, 387-408.
7. Bricker, N.S., et al. Unpublished observation.
8. Bourgoignie, J.J., et al. (1974) J. Clin. Invest., 53, 1559-1567.
9. Schmidt, R.W., et al. (1974) J. Clin. Invest., 53, 1736-1741.
10. Bourgoignie, J.J., et al. (1971) J. Clin. Invest., 50, 303-311.
11. Fine, L.G., et al. (1976) J. Clin. Invest., 58, 590-597.
12. Licht, A., et al. Unpublished observation.
13. Bricker, N.S., et al. (1968) Nature, 219, 1058-1059.
14. Weber, H., et al. (1974) Amer. J. Physiol. 226, 419-425.
15. Gonick, H.C., and Salldanha, L.F., (1975) J.Clin. Invest. 56, 247-255.
16. Kaplan, M.A., et al. (1974) J. Clin. Invest. 53, 1568-1577.
17. Raghavan, S.R.V. and Gonick, H.C. (1980) Proc. Soc. Exp. Biol. Med. 164, 101-104.
18. Licht, A., et al. Unpublished observation.
19. Bourgoignie, J.J., et al. (1972) J. Clin. Invest. 51, 1519-1527.
20. Clarkson, E.M. (1979) Kidney Int., 16, 710-721.
21. Bourgoignie, J.J., et al. (1978) International Symposium. G. Thieme Verlag/Bonn, pp. 122-130.
22. Licht, A., et al. (1978) Biochem. Soc. Trans. 6, 837-839.
23. Bricker, N.S., et al. (1970) Arch. Inter. Med., 126, 860-869.

AUTHOR INDEX